Age of Onset of Mental Disorders

Giovanni de Girolamo
Patrick D. McGorry • Norman Sartorius
Editors

Age of Onset of Mental Disorders

Etiopathogenetic and Treatment Implications

Springer

Editors
Giovanni de Girolamo
Unit of Psychiatric Epidemiology and Evaluation
IRCCS St John of God Clinical Research Center
Brescia
Italy

Patrick D. McGorry
Orygen The National Centre of Excellence
University of Melbourne
Victoria
Australia

Norman Sartorius
Association for the Improvement of Mental Health Programmes
Geneva
Switzerland

ISBN 978-3-319-72618-2 ISBN 978-3-319-72619-9 (eBook)
https://doi.org/10.1007/978-3-319-72619-9

Library of Congress Control Number: 2018957691

This Springer imprint is published by the registered company Springer Nature Switzerland AG
The registered company address is: Gewerbestrasse 11, 6330 Cham, Switzerland

Foreword

This is an important book. It presents the first in-depth investigation of the age of onset (AOO) distributions of common mental disorders, a critical and, until recently, neglected aspect of mental disorder population dynamics. As the editors of this fascinating compilation point out in their introduction, AOO distributions have profound implications, not the least of which are the far greater importance of mental disorders than physical disorders in influencing the life trajectories of children, adolescents, and young adults due to the typically earlier AOOs of mental than physical disorders and the fact that early-onset disorders seldom are treated until after they have persisted for a number of years.
The editors note in their introductory chapter that research over the past two decades has shown that timely interventions with prodromal or incident cases of early-onset mental disorders can be effective in delaying, and sometimes even preventing, onset as well as in reducing lifetime persistence and severity once onset occurs. The editors expand on this theme in the concluding chapter, where they describe innovative early-intervention programmes that have been proven effective in reducing the burden of mental disorders. The monograph would have been enhanced if these innovative early intervention studies had been a more central focus on the disorder-specific chapters (e.g. Correll et al. 2018; Donaldson et al. 2015; Hawkins et al. 2008; van der Gaag et al. 2013).

The chapters in this volume focused much more on three broad areas of more basic research that have expanded in response to the successes of early intervention research: improving estimation of AOO distributions; discovering reliable prodromal patterns that provide targets for preventive intervention; and investigating potentially modifiable pathways that link early-onset to persistence-severity.

With regard to estimating AOO, the material reviewed in the chapters makes it clear that even though broad consistencies exist in basic epidemiological data on AOO distributions for the mental disorders considered here, considerable uncertainty exists beyond these basics. This is true in large part because mental disorders are accretion disorders, that is, disorders in which early signs and symptoms are often present for many years before the disorders declare themselves. This makes it difficult to know exactly what we mean by an "onset." In addition, and possibly as a result of the fact that so many early-onset mental disorders have an insidious onset, it is uncommon for people with mental disorders to seek treatment for incident episodes unless these episodes are either very severe or persist for a number of years (Wang et al. 2007). As a result of this fact, information about AOO distributions comes largely, although not entirely (e.g. Fogel et al. 2006), from retrospective reports based on epidemiological samples. Recall bias in these reports can distort estimates. Although innovative methods exist to reduce this bias to some extent by splicing together synthetic AOO curves in ways that reduce length of recall (Eaton et al. 2012), these methods were not used in any of the chapters in the volume.

So much uncertainty exists about AOO due to these limitations that several of the chapters in this volume were devoted almost entirely to reviewing and evaluating the descriptive evidence on AOO distributions (e.g. the Dagani et al. chapter on bipolar disorder and the Legerstee et al. chapter on anxiety disorders). In one case, the Chanen et al. chapter on personality disorders, the authors went so far as to abandon hope of determining AOO in any serious way, noting that clinically significant paediatric manifestations of personality pathology are the norm among people with personality disorders and that these early manifestations are typically so non-specific and intertwined with Axis I disorders that it is possible to define clear disorder onsets only as end points that typically occur in the transition to adulthood.

Interestingly, most of the chapters that focused on describing AOO distributions were concerned more with central tendency (i.e. mean or median AOO) than dispersion (i.e. the breadth of the age range in which onsets occur), although the few chapters that considered dispersion found it to be as striking as central tendency in differentiating among mental disorders. This is made clear in the Chanen et al. chapter on personality disorders, which, as noted in the last paragraph, distinguished between a prodromal paediatric phase and a syndromal phase that typically begins in the transition to adulthood; the Legerstee et al. chapter on anxiety disorders, which emphasised the importance of an early childhood risk window for the fear disorders as compared to a later and broader risk window for other anxiety disorders; the Kelly et al. and Connor et al. chapters, which noted that a relatively narrow risk window in adolescence and young adulthood exists for onset of substance use disorders; and the Coghill et al. chapter on attention deficit hyperactivity disorder (ADHD), where the authors noted new evidence suggesting that there might be a wider risk window than was previously thought to be the case.

The second of the three areas of research noted above, on the discovery of reliable prodromal signs and symptoms that could provide targets for preventive intervention, is hampered by the fact that it is often unclear which of these signs and symptoms are causal risk factors. This, in turn, leads to uncertainties about how to intervene to prevent progression even after reliable predictors of onset are found. A number of chapters in this volume note these uncertainties. Yet, surprisingly little emphasis was placed in these chapters on the investigations of researchers in developmental psychopathology (Lewis 2014), youth mental health (Rice et al. 2018), and early high-risk (Hartmann et al. 2018) who address these uncertainties by carrying out fine-grained longitudinal studies and interventions during the years prior to typical AOO to document reliable markers of incipient psychopathology and to evaluate causal hypotheses. In recent years, this type of research has become increasingly interdisciplinary and focused on biomarkers. Although as-yet of uncertain clinical value, epigenetics has been a focus of much of the latter work, given that mental disorders are known to cluster in families and environmental risk factors are thought to interact with genetic predispositions (Hyde 2015).

It is sometimes possible to make inferences about causal pathways by inspecting subgroup AOO distributions, as in the hypothesis described by Häfner in his chapter on schizophrenia about the role of oestrogen in explaining sex differences in schizophrenia, a hypothesis that was originally proposed based on observed sex differences in AOO distributions of schizophrenia related to ages of menarche and menopause. A similar kind of work has been carried out to investigate the extent to which sex hormones explain the well-known higher prevalence of major depression among women than men (Angold and Costello 2006). Implications of this work for preventive intervention have also been considered (Adam et al. 2008).

An important exception to the lack of focus on pre-onset interventions was found in the chapters on substance use disorders (SUDs), where a good deal of attention was focused on pre-disorder precursors and preventive interventions. This is, in some ways, not surprising, though, as there are clear behavioural characteristics of precursors to SUDs, such as early first use, rapid progression from first use to regular use, and binge use (in the case of alcohol), all of which have long been known to predict SUD onset. As reviewed in the SUD chapters, interventions designed to influence these earlier stages have been carried out and have been found to predict the subsequent onset and progression of SUDs. These studies are also unique among those considered in this volume to consider restricted access to means as a focus of preventive intervention, although this is also a focus, and the subject of considerable controversy in the USA with regard to firearms, in research on risk factors for suicide (Yip et al. 2012).

The third of the three areas of investigation I noted earlier involves pathways that link early-onset with later disorder persistence-severity. A number of chapters comment on studies of this sort. A major interest of researchers working in this area is in sorting out the relative importance of several different pathways that could all plausibly be involved as causes of these predictive associations. Speaking broadly, these include the possibility that early-onset disorders themselves have biological effects, possibly related to critical periods in brain development, that account for the associations of early AOO with persistence-severity (see the discussion of "susceptibility windows" in the chapter by Fiorito et al.); that comorbid condition either cause and/or are caused by early-onset disorders and account for the associations of early onset of these disorders with subsequent persistence-severity; and that the more extreme negative effects of early-onset than later-onset disorders cases on developmental trajectories account for the associations of early-onset with persistence-severity (see the discussion of the earlier AOO of schizophrenia among men than women leading to great disruption in developmental trajectories described in the chapter by Häfner).

The possibility of early-onset disorders having unique biological effects was discussed by Miettunen et al. in their chapter on schizophrenia spectrum disorder, where they suggested that early AOO is associated with increased cognitive deficits and brain alterations that lead to subsequent persistence-severity. Yet the evidence reviewed in that chapter focused more on documenting predictive mediation than evaluating the extent to which these biomarkers might be causal mediators. This is a challenging area of investigation, but one that needs to be tackled to make progress in understanding the translational implications of information about biological determinants of the effects of early onset.

One of the most interesting programmes of research on this topic was initiated by Post (2015), who suggested that major depressive episode recurrence creates increased reactivity via epigenetic mechanisms that, in turn, promote further severity-persistence. This work highlights the importance of distinguishing between the effects of AOO and the effects of duration of untreated disorder. The two are related, of course, due to the fact that the treatment rate is lower for early-onset than later-onset disorders, leading to early-onset cases having a longer duration of untreated prevalence. The clinical importance of the distinction can be seen by noting that efforts to reduce episode duration would imply that the kinds of treatments developed to promote rapid episode remission, which currently are used mostly for severe cases, might also make sense to consider as first-line treatments for incident episodes (e.g. Canuso et al. 2018). If episode recurrence is more important, in comparison, then maintenance medications, which currently are recommended primarily for patients with recurrent or chronic disorders (e.g. Gelenberg et al. 2010), might be considered as preventive interventions against recurrence among incident cases. Or, given concerns about negative effects of long-term medication administered after incident episodes, non-pharmacologic treatments focused on preventing recurrence might be investigated as treatments-of-choice for early-onset incident cases (e.g. Huijbers and Speckens 2015).

Another potentially important set of pathways involves the mediating effects of secondary comorbid mental disorders of the associations of early-onset primary mental disorders with persistence-severity of those disorders and with other negative life course outcomes associated with these early-onset primary disorders. Although most of the chapters in this volume commented on the fact that early-onset disorders are associated with high comorbidity, few of them discussed the possibility that this comorbidity could account for the associations of early-onset with subsequent persistence-severity of the primary disorders or with negative life course outcomes associated with these disorders. Furthermore, none of the chapters discussed the value of developing preventive interventions for patients with refractory early-onset disorders to prevent the onset of secondary disorders in the hopes that such preventive interventions, if successful, might influence the persistence-severity of the primary disorders. For example, we know that youngsters with ADHD are at increased risk of numerous negative life course outcomes because of secondary comorbid disorders that intervene between temporally primary ADHD and these outcomes and that often persist even after the ADHD remits (Kessler et al. 2014). The investigation of these mediating associations and the implementation-evaluation of interventions designed to prevent onset of the secondary disorders that mediate the effects of early-onset primary disorders on these outcomes could have great clinical significance. This is especially true given that very high proportions of mental disorders, and especially severe-persistent mental disorders, are secondary comorbid disorders associated with early-onset primary disorders (Kessler and Price 1993).

A related possibility is that early-onset disorders are more persistent-severe than later-onset disorders because they have more negative life course consequences that lead to subsequent disorder persistence-severity. This could occur either because early-onset disorders occur during critical periods of life course development or because their longer durations, partially influenced by their low rates of treatment, put people with early onsets at risk for longer periods of time than if their disorders had later AOOs. In either of these cases, interventions aimed at preventing these negative life course consequences might be effective in reducing persistence-severity of early-onset disorders even if these disorders were refractory. Given that research exists on secondary preventive interventions designed to avert these effects, this focus needs much more serious attention in a monograph on AOO. A good example is clinical research on paediatric-onset anxiety disorders, which are known to be associated with a wide range of later-life impairments due to the fact that anxious youth are at increased risk of using alcohol and illicit drugs for self-medication (Menary et al. 2011). This maladaptive coping style, in turn, leads to other negative outcomes that can exacerbate anxiety. So strong is this pattern that some psychological interventions for adolescent anxiety disorder include a component to prevent self-medication by promoting the use of more productive coping strategies (Kendall et al. 2004).

One gets the impression from the reviews in this volume that the natural history of research in a number of disorder-specific areas is poised to begin launch initiatives aimed at tracing out mediating processes of the sort sketched out in the last three paragraphs. The closing chapter by the editors is especially exciting in pointing to translational implications of doing this. The next generation of AOO research will likely use AOO as a point of departure for investigating other key characteristics of mental disorder population dynamics by developing, implementing, and refining coordinated interventions that begin much earlier in the life course than current treatments and lead to a dramatic reduction in the global burden of mental disorders. Although the next part of the script is yet to be clearly specified, the current volume at least provides a solid foundation for this next generation of research.

Ronald C. Kessler
Department of Health Care Policy,
Harvard Medical School,
Boston, MA, USA

References

Adam EK, Sutton JM, Doane LD, Mineka S. Incorporating hypothalamic-pituitary-adrenal axis measures into preventive interventions for adolescent depression: are we there yet? Dev Psychopathol. 2008;20(3):975–1001.

Angold A, Costello EJ. Puberty and depression. Child Adolesc Psychiatr Clin N Am. 2006;15(4):919–37.

Canuso CM, Singh JB, Fedgchin M, Alphs L, Lane R, Lim P, et al. Efficacy and safety of intranasal esketamine for the rapid reduction of symptoms of depression and suicidality in patients at imminent risk for suicide: results of a double-blind, randomized, placebo-controlled study. Am J Psychiatry. 2018;175(7):620–30.

Correll CU, Galling B, Pawar A, Krivko A, Bonetto C, Ruggeri M, et al. Comparison of early intervention services vs treatment as usual for early-phase psychosis: a systematic review, meta-analysis, and meta-regression. JAMA Psychiatry. 2018;75(6):555–65.

Donaldson JM, Wiskow KM, Soto PL. Immediate and distal effects of the good behavior game. J Appl Behav Anal. 2015;48(3):685–9.

Eaton WW, Alexandre P, Kessler RC, Martins SS, Mortensen PB, Rebok GW, et al. The population dynamics of mental disorders. In: Public mental health. Oxford, United Kingdom: Oxford University Press; 2012.

Fogel J, Eaton WW, Ford DE. Minor depression as a predictor of the first onset of major depressive disorder over a 15-year follow-up. Acta Psychiatr Scand. 2006;113(1):36–43.

Gelenberg AJ, Freeman MP, Markowitz JF, Thase ME, Trivedi MH, Van Rhoads RS. Practice guideline for the treatment of patients with major depressive disorder. 3rd ed. American Psychiatric Association; 2010.

Hartmann JA, Nelson B, Ratheesh A, Treen D, McGorry PD. At-risk studies and clinical antecedents of psychosis, bipolar disorder and depression: a scoping review in the context of clinical staging. Psychol Med. 2018;1–13.

Hawkins JD, Kosterman R, Catalano RF, Hill KG, Abbott RD. Effects of social development intervention in childhood 15 years later. Arch Pediatr Adolesc Med. 2008;162(12):1133–41.

Huijbers M, Speckens A. Mindfulness-based cognitive therapy as an alternative to maintenance antidepressant medication to prevent relapse and recurrence in depression. Evid Based Ment Health. 2015;18(4):126.

Hyde LW. Developmental psychopathology in an era of molecular genetics and neuroimaging: a developmental neurogenetics approach. Dev Psychopathol. 2015;27(2):587–613.

Kendall PC, Safford S, Flannery-Schroeder E, Webb A. Child anxiety treatment: outcomes in adolescence and impact on substance use and depression at 7.4-year follow-up. J Consult Clin Psychol. 2004;72(2):276–87.

Kessler RC, Price RH. Primary prevention of secondary disorders: a proposal and agenda. Am J Community Psychol. 1993;21(5):607–33.

Kessler RC, Adler LA, Berglund P, Green JG, McLaughlin KA, Fayyad J, et al. The effects of temporally secondary co-morbid mental disorders on the associations of DSM-IV ADHD with adverse outcomes in the US National Comorbidity Survey Replication Adolescent Supplement (NCS-A). Psychol Med. 2014;44(8):1779–92.

Lewis M. Toward the development of the science of developmental psychopathology. In: Lewis M, Rudolph KD, editors. Handbook of developmental psychopathology. 3rd ed. New York: Springer; 2014.

Menary KR, Kushner MG, Maurer E, Thuras P. The prevalence and clinical implications of self-medication among individuals with anxiety disorders. J Anxiety Disord. 2011;25(3):335–9.

Post RM. Heading off depressive illness evolution and progression to treatment resistance. Dialogues Clin Neurosci. 2015;17(2):105–9.

Rice SM, Purcell R, McGorry PD. Adolescent and young adult male mental health: transforming system failures into proactive models of engagement. J Adolesc Health. 2018;62(3S):S9–17.

van der Gaag M, Smit F, Bechdolf A, French P, Linszen DH, Yung AR, et al. Preventing a first episode of psychosis: meta-analysis of randomized controlled prevention trials of 12 month and longer-term follow-ups. Schizophr Res. 2013;149(1–3):56–62.

Wang PS, Angermeyer M, Borges G, Bruffaerts R, Tat Chiu W, DE Girolamo G, et al. Delay and failure in treatment seeking after first onset of mental disorders in the World Health Organization's World Mental Health Survey Initiative. World Psychiatry. 2007;6(3):177–85.

Yip PS, Caine E, Yousuf S, Chang SS, Wu KC, Chen YY. Means restriction for suicide prevention. Lancet. 2012;379(9834):2393–9.

Contents

Contributors

Phillip Asherson MRC Social Genetic and Developmental Psychiatry (SGDP), Institute of Psychiatry, London, UK

Ross J. Baldessarini Harvard Medical School, Boston, MA, USA

International Consortium for Bipolar and Psychotic Disorder Research, Mailman Research Center, McLean Hospital, Belmont, MA, USA

Ralph Brinks Hiller Research Unit for Rheumatology, Medical Faculty of the University Hospital Düsseldorf, Düsseldorf, Germany

Institute for Biometry and Epidemiology, German Diabetes Center, Düsseldorf, Germany

Paolo Busetto Department of Neuroscience, Psychiatric Clinic, University of Padova, Padova, Italy

Andrew M. Chanen Orygen, The National Centre of Excellence in Youth Mental Health, Melbourne, VIC, Australia

Centre for Youth Mental Health, The University of Melbourne, Melbourne, VIC, Australia

Orygen Youth Health, Melbourne, VIC, Australia

David Coghill Departments of Paediatrics and Psychiatry, University of Melbourne, Parkville, VIC, Australia

Murdoch Children's Research Institute, Melbourne, VIC, Australia

Royal Children's Hospital, Melbourne, VIC, Australia

Enrico Collantoni Department of Neuroscience, Psychiatric Clinic, University of Padova, Padova, Italy

Jason P. Connor Faculty of Medicine, The University of Queensland, Royal Brisbane and Women's Hospital, Herston, QLD, Australia

Centre for Youth Substance Abuse Research, Faculty of Health and Behavioural Sciences, The University of Queensland, St Lucia, QLD, Australia

Jessica Dagani Unit of Psychiatric Epidemiology and Evaluation, IRCCS St John of God Clinical Research Center, Brescia, Italy

Giovanni de Girolamo Unit of Psychiatric Epidemiology and Evaluation, IRCCS St John of God Clinical Research Center, Brescia, Italy

Jasmijn M. de Lijster Department of Child and Adolescent Psychiatry/Psychology, Erasmus MC—Sophia Children's Hospital, Rotterdam, The Netherlands

Gwen C. Dieleman Department of Child and Adolescent Psychiatry/Psychology, Erasmus MC—Sophia Children's Hospital, Rotterdam, The Netherlands

Bram Dierckx Department of Child and Adolescent Psychiatry/Psychology, Erasmus MC—Sophia Children's Hospital, Rotterdam, The Netherlands

Stephen V. Faraone Departments of Psychiatry and of Neuroscience and Physiology, SUNY Upstate Medical University, Syracuse, NY, USA

Angela Favaro Department of Neuroscience, Psychiatric Clinic, University of Padova, Padova, Italy

Giovanni Fiorito Italian Institute for Genomic Medicine, (IIGM, ex HuGeF), Turin, Italy

Heinz Häfner Schizophrenia Research Group, Central Institute of Mental Health, Medical Faculty Mannheim, Heidelberg University, Mannheim, Germany

Wayne D. Hall Centre for Youth Substance Abuse Research, Faculty of Health and Behavioural Sciences, The University of Queensland, St Lucia, QLD, Australia

Queensland Centre for Mental Health Research, School of Public Health, The University of Queensland, The Park Centre for Mental Health Treatment, Research and Education, Wacol, QLD, Australia

National Addiction Centre, Institute of Psychiatry, Psychology and Neuroscience, King's College London, London, UK

Annika Hoyer Institute for Biometry and Epidemiology, German Diabetes Center, Düsseldorf, Germany

Johanna Immonen Center for Life Course Health Research, University of Oulu, Oulu, Finland

Medical Research Center Oulu, Oulu University Hospital and University of Oulu, Oulu, Finland

Matti Isohanni Center for Life Course Health Research, University of Oulu, Oulu, Finland

Erika Jääskeläinen Center for Life Course Health Research, University of Oulu, Oulu, Finland

Medical Research Center Oulu, Oulu University Hospital and University of Oulu, Oulu, Finland

Department of Psychiatry, Research Unit of Clinical Neuroscience, University of Oulu, Oulu, Finland

Department of Psychiatry, Oulu University Hospital, Oulu, Finland

Adrian B. Kelly School of Psychology and Counselling, Queensland University of Technology, Brisbane, QLD, Australia

Sandra Landwehr Kassenärztliche Vereinigung Nordrhein, Düsseldorf, Germany

Matthew Large School of Psychiatry, University of New South Wales, Sydney, NSW, Australia

Prince of Wales Hospital Sydney, Sydney, NSW, Australia

Jeroen S. Legerstee Department of Child and Adolescent Psychiatry/Psychology, Erasmus MC—Sophia Children's Hospital, Rotterdam, The Netherlands

Patrick D. McGorry Orygen The National Centre of Excellence in Youth Mental Health and Centre for Youth Mental Health, University of Melbourne, Parkville, VIC, Australia

John J. McGrath Queensland Centre for Mental Health Research, The Park Centre for Mental Health, Wacol, QLD, Australia

Queensland Brain Institute, University of Queensland, St Lucia, QLD, Australia

National Centre for Register-Based Research, Aarhus BSS, Aarhus University, Aarhus, Denmark

Jouko Miettunen Center for Life Course Health Research, University of Oulu, Oulu, Finland

Medical Research Center Oulu, Oulu University Hospital and University of Oulu, Oulu, Finland

Olav Nielssen Macquarie University, Sydney, NSW, Australia

School of Psychiatry, University of New South Wales, Sydney, NSW, Australia

St Vincents Hospital, Sydney, NSW, Australia

Luis A. Rohde Department of Psychiatry, Federal University of Rio Grande do Sul, Porto Alegre, Brazil

Hospital de Clínicas de Porto Alegre, Porto Alegre, Brazil

Carlotta Sacerdote Città della Salute e della Scienza University-Hospital and CPO-Piemonte, Turin, Italy

Paolo Santonastaso Psychiatric Clinic, University of Padova, Padova, Italy

Department of Neuroscience, Psychiatric Clinic, University of Padova, Padova, Italy

Norman Sartorius Association for the Improvement of Mental Health Programmes (AMH), Geneva, Switzerland

Giulia Signorini Unit of Psychiatric Epidemiology and Evaluation, IRCCS St John of God Clinical Research Center, Brescia, Italy

Katherine N. Thompson Orygen, The National Centre of Excellence in Youth Mental Health, Melbourne, VIC, Australia

Centre for Youth Mental Health, The University of Melbourne, Melbourne, VIC, Australia

Elisabeth M. W. J. Utens Department of Child and Adolescent Psychiatry/Psychology, Erasmus MC—Sophia Children's Hospital, Rotterdam, The Netherlands

Research Institute of Child Development and Education, University of Amsterdam, Amsterdam, The Netherlands

Academic Centre for Child Psychiatry the Bascule/Department Child and Adolescent Psychiatry, Academic Medical Centre, Amsterdam, The Netherlands

Frank C. Verhulst Department of Child and Adolescent Psychiatry/Psychology, Erasmus MC—Sophia Children's Hospital, Rotterdam, The Netherlands

Child and Adolescent Mental Health Center, Mental Health Services, Capital Region of Denmark/Department of Clinical Medicine, Faculty of Health and Medical Sciences, Copenhagen University Hospital/University of Copenhagen, Copenhagen, Denmark

Paolo Vineis Italian Institute for Genomic Medicine, Turin, Italy

MRC-PHE Centre for Environment and Health, School of Public Health, Imperial College, London, UK

Megan Weier Centre for Youth Substance Abuse Research, Faculty of Health and Behavioural Sciences, The University of Queensland, St Lucia, QLD, Australia

National Drug and Alcohol Research Centre, The University of New South Wales, Sydney, NSW, Australia

Nefize Yalin Centre for Affective Disorders, Department of Psychological Medicine, Institute of Psychiatry, Psychology and Neuroscience, King's College of London, London, UK

Allan H. Young Centre for Affective Disorders, Department of Psychological Medicine, Institute of Psychiatry, Psychology and Neuroscience, King's College of London, London, UK

Carola Zieldorff Department of Child and Adolescent Psychiatry/Psychology, Erasmus MC—Sophia Children's Hospital, Rotterdam, The Netherlands

Introduction: Relevance of the Age of Onset of Mental Disorders to Research in Psychiatry and to the Organization of Services for People with Mental Illness

1

Giovanni de Girolamo, Patrick D. McGorry, and Norman Sartorius

1.1 Introduction

Early intervention for potentially serious illnesses is a fundamental principle accepted in all the major areas of health care and especially among the non-communicable diseases that cause the majority of disease burden in developed countries. However, it is only in recent years that it has become part of the landscape in mental health care. Beginning with psychotic illnesses and the apparently unpromising domain of schizophrenia, an inexorable accumulation of evidence, which has now satisfied the Cochrane level 1 criterion, has demonstrated that early intervention can:

- Improve the early course and outcome of mental disorders.
- Reduce suffering of those affected by such disorders.
- Help to maintain social links and developmental trajectory of people affected and their place in the community.

From the public health point of view, it is therefore important to know at what age an illness begins because this will allow the effective organization and targeting of mental health and other social services to reduce its impact. In addition to guiding

G. de Girolamo (✉)
Unit of Psychiatric Epidemiology and Evaluation, IRCCS St John of God Clinical Research Center, Brescia, Italy
e-mail: gdegirolamo@fatebenefratelli.eu

P. D. McGorry
Orygen The National Centre of Excellence, University of Melbourne, Parkville, VIC, Australia
e-mail: Pat.mcgorry@orygen.org.au

N. Sartorius
Association for the Improvement of Mental Health Programmes (AMH), Geneva, Switzerland
e-mail: sartorius@normansartorius.com

G. de Girolamo et al. (eds.), *Age of Onset of Mental Disorders*,
https://doi.org/10.1007/978-3-319-72619-9_1

the location, style and culture in designing services and targeting people early in the course of their illness, knowledge about the age of onset (AOO) may provide important clues and a window into the pathogenesis of mental illness and the links that may exist between mental disorders and a variety of biological and psychosocial maturation processes. For all these reasons, the study of AOO has great theoretical and clinical relevance and could have a tremendous impact both on service configuration as well as for the content and deployment of interventions.

A key initial step is clearly to delineate and define the AOO of various types of mental disorders: yet it is surprising to discover that there are no systematic reviews of knowledge about the AOO or mode of onset of most mental disorders. There are publications which present the findings about the AOO of specific mental disorders, but no overall review of the issues related to onset of mental illness across the diagnostic spectrum, nor a synthesis of our knowledge from a transdiagnostic perspective. For this reason, this book seeks to explore, map and capture the present state of knowledge of AOO for a spectrum of key mental disorders.

In this introductory piece, we will offer some general thoughts about AOO in mental disorders and will highlight some problems faced by research in this area.

1.2 Age, Development and Diseases

Disease develops at all stages throughout our lifetime. As Kessler et al. (2007) observed, the study of AOO enables us to calculate projected lifetime risk of disorders and contributes to understand the topography of onset and to clarify the etiopathogenesis of disorders. Such information allows primary prevention, prevention of secondary disorders and early intervention strategies, to all be conceptualized and deployed in an efficient, timely and cost-effective manner.

AOO can profoundly affect the clinical presentation, course and outcome of all human disorders, as it is intertwined with an internal, inherited biological 'clock', which shapes and modulates the action of genes and the environment. Thus, AOO is a disease *modifier*, which differentially shapes the clinical presentation and severity of a disorder in relation to the age of an affected individual. One example of this pathoplasticity is the propensity for psychotic symptoms to characterize a range of mental disorders in young people which are less prone to feature in the same disorders later in life.

Age is a unifying factor in which monogenic and multifactorial conditions can be brought together conceptually: 'It is a part of the lore of human genetics that the younger cases of a disease with a broad span of ages at onset may be more severely affected and more likely to have similarly afflicted relatives. Accordingly, age at onset, defined as the age when symptoms become overt, is also a useful criterion for establishing heterogeneity of cause. The question is, Why does a particular person contract diabetes or gout at age 8 rather than at 35 or at 80 years?' (Childs and Scriver 1986). A possible answer is that there are different causes simultaneously in action.

1.3 Options for the Definition of the Age of Onset: Their Advantages and Disadvantages

There are several different operational criteria that we could adopt to define the 'age of onset' of a disease/disorder. These are not necessarily mutually exclusive and have been used to a varying degree in epidemiological and clinical research. They involve different dating in the longitudinal trajectory of an individual's life and have different implications for public health, for conducting research on the etiopathogenesis of disorders and for intervention planning. It can even be argued that for many conditions it is possible to identify multiple and different AOOs, in relation to the objectives of the inquiry.

1.3.1 Criterion 1: The Age When the First Morpho-functional Pathological Processes, Which Lead to a Disorder (e.g. Cellular, Receptor or Genetic Alterations or Changes), Appear

From a heuristic point of view, the initial change in a human genome may be considered as the 'onset' of a cascade of molecular events which lead to a dysfunction in complex brain neuro-circuitry. This then passes in ascending order to specific functions and ultimately to complex behavioural and cognitive patterns that are finally revealed in the clinical presentation of a specific disorder. It must be said that it is very difficult, both conceptually and operationally, to establish this precise timing.

To give an example from oncology, cancer initiates with a single mutation in a cell. This mutation causes irreversible damage to the DNA and is called the initiator. An initiator, however, does not immediately cause cancer. The mutated cell needs the continuous action of a promoter to turn into cancer. A promoter is a noncarcinogenic substance that, when applied repeatedly, amplifies cancer-inducing effects of the initiator. They induce the proliferation (reproduction) of the cell, giving rise to many daughter cells containing the mutation created by the initiator. At this point, the mass of mutated cells is usually a benign tumour. Cancer starts when cells begin to grow out of control. These biological processes can occur months or years before a cancer becomes clinically evident and a patient requires diagnosis and treatment. A further simple example from general medicine is that of prediabetes which can be recognized in asymptomatic individuals as a precursor of the clinical diabetic state: thus, the AOO of prediabetes differs from the AOO of frank diabetes. A similar picture can be applied to the neurobiological changes predating the appearance of signs and symptoms of certain mental disorders. As with cancer, these subtle biological processes of change reflecting brain abnormalities in childhood and adolescence can substantially predate the onset of a disorder.

This conceptual framework is at the forefront of the well-known neurodevelopmental model of schizophrenia, which 'In its simplest form this model posits that schizophrenia is the behavioral outcome of an aberration in neurodevelopmental processes that begins long before the onset of clinical symptoms and is caused by a combination of environmental and genetic factors' (Rapoport et al. 2005). Subjects who later develop schizophrenia are more likely than healthy subjects to have experienced pre- or perinatal adverse events or to have been exposed to potentially harmful stressors. They also exhibit increased rates of minor physical anomalies, which are soft indicators of disturbed prenatal development, as well as minor deviations in motor, cognitive and social development. These observations strongly suggest that abnormalities in brain function are present very early in life in individuals who later develop schizophrenia.

Recent research has challenged this simple perspective, and it is now less clear when these disturbances actually emerge, that is, early in development or, increasingly likely, also during the latent or early symptomatic prodromal periods. This has led to a revision of the neurodevelopmental model suggesting that 'quantitative pathogenic biological events are present in early life that undergo various developmental stages predisposed by complex genetic influences and environmental "hits" that continue through all phases of the illness.... Alternatively, the available evidence may be explained as reflecting an interaction between the timing of a hit (i.e., maturational stages) with the age of onset of the disorder' (Gogtay et al. 2011).

The theoretical implication of this model is that the 'true' onset of the pathway which, with the interplay of a variety of risk and protective factors, can ultimately lead to the emergence of a psychotic disorder can be dated well before the appearance of the specific signs or symptoms of illness, particularly for late macro-phenotypes like schizophrenia. Although this is heuristically true, nobody (as also shown in the chapter on the AOO of schizophrenia) has ever fixed the AOO of the schizophrenia spectrum disorder at birth. The start of neurobiological changes, which after many years can lead to an overt disorder, may be considered as a precursor pathway for preventive purposes, to identify high-risk subjects and to decrease these risk factors, improve protective factors and strengthen individual resilience. Although the neurodevelopmental model has been mainly developed for schizophrenia, it can also be applied to a variety of other severe mental disorders, such as bipolar disorder, anorexia nervosa and other major syndromes.

In summary, the first criterion to establish AOO proves to be theoretically and heuristically appropriate and can be of great value in the biological investigation of pathways leading to the development of a full-blown disorder. However, it is of limited clinical utility in dating the start of necessary clinical interventions.

1.3.2 Criterion 2: The Age When the First Signs of a Disorder Appear (e.g. Cognitive Dysfunctions)

The second criterion for establishing the AOO of mental disorders entails the appearance of pathological signs, which are not necessarily recognized by the patient and his relatives but may be detectable when investigated with appropriate tools. These signs coincide with the so-called endophenotypes and are defined 'as biological or psychological phenomena of a disorder believed to be in the causal chain between genetic contributions to a disorder and diagnosable symptoms of psychopathology' (Miller and Rockstroh 2016). Another definition of an endophenotype posits that it 'is a quantitative biological trait that is reliable in reflecting the function of a discrete biological system and is reasonably heritable, and as such is more closely related to the root cause of the disease than the broad clinical phenotype' (Wong et al. 2011). Endophenotypes are biological or psychological, to the extent that there is a foreseeable causal path from the gene through endophenotype(s) to phenotype (clinical expression). Therefore, the causal pathway to illness begins with genes and proceeds with the development of endophenotypes, and these should meet specific criteria, as lucidly suggested by Lenzenweger (2013): (1) they should be associated with disorders; (2) they should be heritable (at odds with a biomarker, which need not be heritable); (3) they should be largely independent (traceable in the individual whether or not the disorder is active); (4) within families, endophenotype and illness co-segregate and are more frequent among the ill relatives of ill subjects; and (5) the endophenotype is 'a trait that can be measured reliably, and it is ideally more strongly associated with the disease of interest than with other psychiatric conditions'.

A large body of research has investigated the endophenotypes (DiLalla et al. 2017; Miskowiak et al. 2017) of specific disorders, in particular schizophrenia, with the hope that identifying these variables would reliably allow us to recognize high-risk individuals. This in turn would allow early interventions, ultimately aimed at averting the full-blown disorder. Some trials targeting very-high-risk groups are based on the identification of non-manifest signs of dysfunction in people already at high risk for familiarity (Ising et al. 2017; Pfennig et al. 2014). Research on mental disorder AOO has rarely used this criterion to date the onset of a disorder, although identification of this crucial time point in the pathway to an overt clinical syndrome should be considered clinically and is theoretically very important.

1.3.3 Criterion 3: The Age When the First Symptoms of a Disorder Appear (e.g. Depressed Mood)

The third criterion for defining mental disorder AOO is perhaps the most widely used in clinical settings, that is, the appearance of a symptom specific for a single disorder, pointing to a change from a condition, self-rated and/or perceived by others, of normality or well-being to an ill state. The emergence of a clearly depressed mood, with biological correlates such as alterations in sleep pattern, lack of energy, loss of pleasure, etc., indicates that something has changed and that a 'disturbance' has arisen. The same might be said in the context of a psychotic condition, with the appearance of positive symptoms (e.g. delusions and hallucinations), while the dating of negative symptoms has traditionally been difficult to establish, because of their usual slow onset, which are often misrecognized and misunderstood. A key advance in recent years is that subthreshold stages of illness which in retrospect can be termed 'prodromes' (provided a more specific disorder does in fact develop) have been recognized and characterized (Addington et al. 2015; Goulding et al. 2013; Van Meter et al. 2016). This has in turn led to the formulation of clinical staging models which have moved forward the timing for AOO to the earliest treatable stage (Agius et al. 2010; Duffy 2014; Kapczinski et al. 2014).

The appearance of a symptom (or of a symptom constellation) does sometimes lead to referral to a professional or to a service, although in the absence of novel and accessible mental health cultures and structures this contact often is missed or delayed. Indeed, many epidemiological studies have shown that there is often a long period of time between symptom(s) onset, albeit severe (e.g. hallucinations and delusions in the case of schizophrenia spectrum disorders), and the first contact with a service and the start of treatment. This has led to the development of the well-known concept of 'duration of untreated illness' (DUI) (Altamura et al. 2013; Dell'Osso and Altamura 2010; Ghio et al. 2014; Murru and Carpiniello 2018). Therefore, the third criterion used to establish the onset for a disorder and define AOO should be taken with caution and cannot be interpreted as the 'true' onset of a disorder, often being preceded by a subthreshold stage, which acts as leverage for the development of the full-blown syndrome. It is important to note that such a full-blown syndrome becomes typically a late macro-phenotype, such as schizophrenia or bipolar disorder, only diagnosable months or years after a need for care linked to an earlier stage of syndromal development or micro-phenotype has clearly manifested.

1.3.4 Criterion 4: The Age When the First Overt Episode of a Disorder Appears (e.g. First Psychotic Episode)

Many mental disorders either remain silent for months, in some cases for years, or build up gradually accumulating symptoms and functional impairments too, until an acute episode of illness supervenes or manifests itself as a behavioural precipitant, such as a suicide attempt, and often requires immediate care and treatment. This is a relatively common situation for psychotic disorders, generally preceded by a DUI that generally spans over months and can exceed several years. Unlike the first three types of onset, an acute illness episode is always easily recognizable and so can be dated precisely, though a not common onset in psychosis. Nevertheless, for many years, the emergence of an acute psychotic episode has been conventionally acknowledged as a critical time point in the individual lifespan and in the longitudinal trajectory of the disorder, although, as explained before, morpho-functional alterations of specific biological, neuropsychological and behavioural pathways have been in place for years. In the case of stress-related disorders (e.g. PTSD, acute stress disorder), however, it can be argued that the onset of the disorder should be dated to the time of exposure to the stressful event, although vulnerability factors (and, conversely, resilience) predated the clinical presentation. Even here, however, the emergence of PTSD is often delayed to sometime after the traumatic stressor.

1.3.5 Criterion 5: The Age of the First Contact with Any Health Service

For many years, epidemiological and health service research has assigned a key role to when the person, spontaneously or stimulated by family members, friends, etc., makes an initial contact with any health service. This 'pathway' to care has been recognized as crucial from a longitudinal perspective. Though this first contact cannot be considered the 'true' onset of a disorder, the first contact with a service is a 'strong' dating event that allows us, considering the DUI, to trace back to the 'true' AOO of the disorder. This 'hard' criterion, as well as the date of first hospitalization, is usually used by national and local psychiatric case registers to analyse pathways to care and treatment and allows us to build models to analyse the 'attraction' capacity or accessibility of the services themselves. The implicit assumption in this approach, that the majority of psychotic patients eventually come to clinical attention, is possibly true, making this approach useful for studying psychotic AOO. This assumption is highly debatable, however, and is certainly much less useful for less common mental disorders which cause less impairment, as the majority of people with such disorders often do not come to clinical attention.

There have been cross-national studies which have carefully investigated the delay in pathways to care present in different settings. In the World Mental Health Survey Initiative, it was found that while in some countries most patients with lifetime disorders eventually make treatment contact with a (health or non-health) care agency, there is tremendous between-country variation, less for mood disorders (88.1–94.2%) than for anxiety (27.3–95.3%), impulse control (33.9–51.8%) or substance disorders (52.7–76.9%) (Wang et al. 2007). However, in this large epidemiological survey, delay among those who eventually made treatment contact was significant, ranging from 6 to 8 years for mood disorders and 9–23 years for anxiety disorders. Poor access to treatment and delay among those who eventually made treatment contact were both associated with early AOO in an older cohort and with selected socio-demographic characteristics such as being male, married and poorly educated.

Another strong demonstration of DUI comes from a meta-analysis on the length of the interval between onset and the initial management of bipolar disorder. In this study, Dagani et al. (2017) analysed 27 studies, reporting 51 samples and a total of 9415 patients. The pooled estimate for the interval between the onset of bipolar disorder and its management was 5.8 years (95% confidence interval [CI], 4.8–6.8), pointing to a long time of untreated disorder and great possibilities for earlier intervention that could modify course and outcome of the disorder.

1.3.6 Criterion 6: The Age of the First Pharmacological Treatment

In many mental disorders, the first presentation of the disorder is difficult to disentangle, and even severe disorders may exhibit initial mild, non-specific signs and symptoms. In these cases, the clinician often adopts a 'waiting' stance and tries to watch the disorder course closely, in the hope that the natural course will allow a definite diagnostic conclusion. This period of latency can also be substantial. Thus, in many epidemiological studies, the establishment of the AOO has overlapped with the start of initial pharmacological treatment, which should logically flow from a definite diagnostic formulation.

1.3.7 Criterion 7: The Age of the First Hospitalization

In-patient care remains the mainstream of intensive treatment for many severe patients, particularly patients with psychotic disorders, and is an essential component of any well-integrated system of psychiatric care. Several studies have shown that up to 90% of patients suffering from a psychotic disorder do have a hospital admission during their life, which however can take place long after the 'true' onset of the disorder. In addition to symptom severity, sometimes hospital care is also affected by the nature and extent of social support, the burden of which lies principally on patients' families (Magliano et al. 2002). Family members mediate a large proportion of admission requests and frequently accompany patients to services (Preti et al. 2009).

For this reason, the establishment of AOO of severe disorders based on first hospitalization rarely coincides with the 'true' start of the pathological processes that lead to a full-blown disorder. However, as for the first contact with a service, it is a 'hard' variable and does allow for precise dating, which can provide valuable information for epidemiological research and for the planning of optimal service configurations. And indeed, as shown in Haefner's chapter, the first hospitalization for a psychotic episode has been widely used in studies focusing on the AOO of schizophrenia, and a substantial difference in the age at first hospitalization between patients of male and female gender has been demonstrated. Nevertheless, the validity of this strategy must be questioned for the reasons already given.

1.4 Methods for Assessing the Age of Onset, Their Advantages and Shortcomings

There are two basic strategies to obtain information about AOO. The most common strategy is based on retrospective investigation, which may involve the patient as well as relatives, friends, etc. A second strategy involves the conduct of prospective cohort studies that can enrol and follow up sizeable numbers of healthy individuals for years, picking up those who become ill over time.

Retrospective reports from community-based surveys, typically of an incomplete range of disorders, are often hampered by recall bias, making the timing of the disorder onset uncertain. Retrospective measures of treated incidence samples even for psychotic disorders are known to be incomplete. Certainly, for the mood, anxiety, substance use and personality disorders, where treated incidence and prevalence are low as a proportion of the total, AOO data found in this way may be of uncertain accuracy. Moffitt et al. (2010) provided a clear example of these problems. The authors followed up the representative 1972–1973 Dunedin New Zealand birth cohort ($N = 1037$) to age 32 years (achieving a 96% retention) and compared it with the National New Zealand Mental Health Survey (NZMHS), as well as with two US samples. The prevalence of lifetime disorder at the age of 32 years approximately doubled in prospective as compared with retrospective data for all disorder types assessed. In the case of children and adolescents, Angold et al. (1996) showed that when symptoms persisted longer than 3 months, the month of onset usually cannot be accurately reported, while with symptoms lasting a year or more, even the year of onset is usually uncertain.

A recall bias exists whenever the information, in this case for AOO, is retrospectively provided by the interviewed subject or by a key informant. The greater the temporal distance between the assessment and presumed AOO, the greater the risk of a recall bias. The recall bias can act in all directions, anticipating or postponing the 'true' AOO, often in an unintentional attempt to explain the disorder onset and 'anchor' its start to an event or to a series of events of emotional or personal significance.

It should also be emphasized that the recall bias does not necessarily coincide with a mnemonic gap (Raphael 1987). Indeed, having two groups of patients with different disorders who are compared about their AOOs, if the mnemonic gap occurs equally in the two groups, there will be no recall bias! However, memory failure will lead to a measurement error, which in turn leads to a loss of statistical power.

On the other hand, a study aimed at investigating the reliability of self-reported AOO of common mental disorders and their association with patient and disorder characteristics found that self-reports may be more accurate than generally thought (Barkow et al. 2002). In this study, a total of 1031 primary care patients with at least one lifetime psychiatric diagnosis were asked to report AOO of their disorders at baseline and after 1 year. Intra-class correlation coefficients (ICC) for AOO information were calculated for individual disorders: ICC were high and lay between 0.67 (generalized anxiety disorder) and 0.79 (dysthymia). Factors associated with reliability were different for different disorders: gender for depressive episodes; gross national product per year per inhabitant for dysthymia; age for pain disorder; years of formal education for dysthymia, generalized anxiety disorder and agoraphobia; and number of lifetime diagnoses for depression and agoraphobia. The authors' conclusion was that self-reported AOO is more reliable than is generally considered. However, reliability is not the same thing as validity, which must still be somewhat questionable.

The second theoretical alternative to relying on retrospective AOO reports is to carry out large long-term prospective surveys to estimate incidence directly. Numerous studies of this sort exist in the well-funded fields of cancer epidemiology and cardiovascular epidemiology. Comparable studies of mental disorders do not exist, although valuable information was obtained in cohort studies aimed at tracking main developmental paths and timely identify the onset of many disorders. These include, among others, the British 1946 birth cohort study (Kuh et al. 2011), the

1972–1973 Dunedin New Zealand birth cohort (Moffitt et al. 2007), the Avon Longitudinal Study of Parents and Children (Niarchou et al. 2015), the Dutch TRAILS study (Ormel et al. 2015) and the Generation R study (Tiemeier et al. 2012).

All these investigations have provided, and will provide for many years to come, substantive materials to precisely date the onset of many mental disorders, to identify their precursors and to link different AOO to variable courses and outcomes.

1.5 Clinical Consequences of Different AOO

Several studies have emphasized a relationship between the AOO of certain disorders and the course of illness. For instance, in schizophrenia earlier onset (before 18 years of age) has been associated with a more chronic form of the disorder (for reviews, see Kyriakopoulos and Frangou 2007; Vyas et al. 2011), and more severe cognitive deficits (Rajji et al. 2009), with impairments in general intellectual ability (IQ), attention, executive function and memory consistently found in early-onset cases of schizophrenia (Frangou 2010).

These findings support the view that the severity of the disease process may be associated with different AOO. Indeed, late adolescence is probably a critical period in brain development, making it particularly vulnerable for the onset of psychopathology. It is likely that the appearance of disturbed and dysfunctional behaviours is more frequent and occurs in more severe forms when the biological maturation of the central nervous system and personal maturation is nearly completed. This is the time when interpersonal relationships, schooling, occupation as well as areas which require a subtle affective tuning (affective relationships, sexual intercourse, etc.) set the stage, as is the case during the second decade of life. In other words, this developmental period is not only the most vulnerable one for the onset of major mental disorders, but if such disorders do emerge then, they are more disruptive to the trajectories of social and vocational functioning and of personal development.

Therefore, under certain conditions, allocation to specific diagnostic categories is influenced by knowledge of AOO. Moreover, the culture of the service and treatment decisions vary with the AOO and the duration of disorder. Also, the decision on establishing a primary and a secondary disorder (comorbidity and sequencing issues) depends on exact AOO, and this decision has direct implications for the treatment of mental disorders.

1.6 Public Health Consequences of Different AOO

Knowledge of the distribution of AOO across the lifespan is critical for designing service models and prevention programmes that target at risk populations. Models of care that are directed towards high onset periods ensure that service structures and treatment approaches align with the developmental, cultural and psychosocial needs of patients. The majority of mental disorders have been shown to emerge during early life, particularly during the transition from adolescence to adulthood

(Kessler et al. 2005). Yet traditional and current service models for mental disorders, with a paediatric-adult split, create discontinuity in care that can lead to service disengagement or inaccessible services during a critical window for intervention. This can exacerbate the individual and societal impacts of mental disorders, which include reduced educational attainment, employment prospects and life expectancy and increased risk of drug and alcohol misuse, suicide, violent behaviour and physical illness. Consequently, mental disorders are a leading cause of disability for young people (Gore et al. 2011) and are projected to have the greatest impact on global economic growth of all non-communicable diseases (Bloom et al. 2011). Prevention and early intervention of mental disorders are imperative to reduce the burden of mental disorders; however, this has been undermined by the trend of focusing on acute or chronic mental health care. Understanding AOO provides opportunities to rebuild our mental health system with services that improve access, timing of treatment and outcomes at critical time points, which would provide a substantial economic return on investment (Campion and Knapp 2018).

1.7 Plan of the Book

This book begins with an examination of AOO in physical illness and how this knowledge can be translated to mental health (Chap. 2). This is followed by a report of the results from a long-term study on the association between AOO and the epidemiology of schizophrenia (Chap. 3). The book then examines the age of onset for a range of mental disorders that includes schizophrenia spectrum disorders (Chap. 4), bipolar disorder (Chap. 5), unipolar depression (Chap. 6), anxiety (Chap. 7), substance (Chap. 8) and alcohol use disorders (Chap. 9), personality disorder (Chap. 10), eating disorders (Chap. 11), ADHD (Chap. 12) and the dementias (Chap. 13). We conclude the book with a discussion on the implications of AOO on age-specific mental health interventions (Chap. 14).

Conclusion

DeLisi (1992), in a way channelling Emil Kraepelin, has stated that for schizophrenia 'Age of onset is the single most important clue to the etiology of illness'. Indeed, the study of AOO is a critical element to understand the clinical presentation, projected course and potential risk factors for a range of mental disorders and to inform the development of prevention and early intervention strategies. There are, however, methodological challenges to researching AOO, which include defining AOO and the reliance on retrospective data as opposed to well-powered long-term prospective data. From a treatment perspective, AOO is a key factor for determining the most appropriate and effective organization of mental health services. Early intervention models that are guided by the timing and emergence of mental disorders offer critical opportunities to reduce the individual, societal and economic burden of these disorders. This book is intended as an aid to promote research initiatives and clinical innovations which may ultimately improve the course and outcome of mental disorders.

References

Addington J, Liu L, Buchy L, et al. North American Prodrome Longitudinal Study (NAPLS 2): the prodromal symptoms. J Nerv Ment Dis. 2015;203:328–35.

Agius M, Goh C, Ulhaq S, et al. The staging model in schizophrenia, and its clinical implications. Psychiatr Danub. 2010;22:211–20.

Altamura AC, Camuri G, Dell'Osso B. Duration of untreated illness and duration of illness in anxiety disorders: assessment and influence on outcome. Mod Trends Pharmacopsychiatry. 2013;29:111–8.

Angold A, Erkanli A, Costello EJ, Rutter M. Precision, reliability and accuracy in the dating of symptom onsets in child and adolescent psychopathology. J Child Psychol Psychiatry. 1996;37(6):657–64.

Barkow K, Heun R, Ustün TB, et al. Test-retest reliability of self-reported age at onset of selected psychiatric diagnoses in general health care. Acta Psychiatr Scand. 2002;106:117–25.

Bloom DE, Cafiero ET, Jané-Llopis E, et al. The global economic burden of non-communicable diseases. Geneva: World Economic Forum; 2011.

Campion J, Knapp M. The economic case for improved coverage of public 182 mental health interventions. Lancet Psychiatry. 2018;5:103–5.

Childs B, Scriver CR. Age at onset and causes of disease. Perspect Biol Med. 1986;29:437–60.

Dagani J, Signorini G, Nielssen O, et al. Meta-analysis of the interval between the onset and management of bipolar disorder. Can J Psychiatry. 2017;62:247–58.

Dell'Osso B, Altamura AC. Duration of untreated psychosis and duration of untreated illness: new vistas. CNS Spectr. 2010;15:238–46.

DeLisi LE. The significance of age of onset for schizophrenia. Schizophr Bull. 1992;18(2):209–15.

DiLalla LF, McCrary M, Diaz E. A review of endophenotypes in schizophrenia and autism: the next phase for understanding genetic etiologies. Am J Med Genet C Semin Med Genet. 2017;175:354–61.

Duffy A. Toward a comprehensive clinical staging model for bipolar disorder: integrating the evidence. Can J Psychiatry. 2014;59:659–66.

Frangou S. Cognitive function in early onset schizophrenia: a selective review. Front Hum Neurosci. 2010;29(3):79. https://doi.org/10.3389/neuro.09.079.2009.

Ghio L, Gotelli S, Marcenaro M, et al. Duration of untreated illness and outcomes in unipolar depression: a systematic review and meta-analysis. J Affect Disord. 2014;152–154:45–51.

Gogtay N, Vyas NS, Testa R, et al. Age of onset of schizophrenia: perspectives from structural neuroimaging studies. Schizophr Bull. 2011;37:504–13.

Gore FM, Bloem PJ, Patton GC, et al. Global burden of disease in young people aged 10-24 years: a systematic analysis. Lancet. 2011;377:2093–102.

Goulding SM, Holtzman CW, Trotman HD, et al. The prodrome and clinical risk for psychotic disorders. Child Adolesc Psychiatr Clin N Am. 2013;22:557–67.

Ising HK, Lokkerbol J, Rietdijk J, et al. Four-year cost-effectiveness of cognitive behavior therapy for preventing first-episode psychosis: the Dutch Early Detection Intervention Evaluation (EDIE-NL) Trial. Schizophr Bull. 2017;43:365–74.

Kapczinski F, Magalhães PV, Balanzá-Martinez V, et al. Staging systems in bipolar disorder: an International Society for Bipolar Disorders Task Force Report. Acta Psychiatr Scand. 2014;130:354–63.

Kessler RC, Berglund P, Demler O, et al. Lifetime prevalence and age-of-onset distributions of DSM-IV disorders in the National Comorbidity Survey Replication. Arch Gen Psychiatry. 2005;62:593–602.

Kessler RC, Amminger GP, Aguilar-Gaxiola S, et al. Age of onset of mental disorders: a review of recent literature. Curr Opin Psychiatry. 2007;20:359–64.

Kuh D, Pierce M, Adams J, et al. Cohort profile: updating the cohort profile for the MRC National Survey of Health and Development: a new clinic-based data collection for ageing research. Int J Epidemiol. 2011;40:e1–9.

Kyriakopoulos M, Frangou S. Pathophysiology of early onset schizophrenia. Int Rev Psychiatry. 2007;19:315–24.

Lenzenweger MF. Thinking clearly about the endophenotype-intermediate phenotype-biomarker distinctions in developmental psychopathology research. Dev Psychopathol. 2013;25:1347–57.

Magliano L, Marasco C, Fiorillo A, et al. The impact of professional and social network support on the burden of families of patients with schizophrenia in Italy. Acta Psychiatr Scand. 2002;106:291–8.

Miller GA, Rockstroh BS. Progress and prospects for endophenotypes for schizophrenia in the time of genomics, epigenetics, oscillatory brain dynamics, and the Research Domain Criteria. In: Abel T, Nickl-Jockschat T, editors. The neurobiology of schizophrenia. 2016. p. 17–38.

Miskowiak KW, Kjærstad HL, Meluken I, et al. The search for neuroimaging and cognitive endophenotypes: a critical systematic review of studies involving unaffected first-degree relatives of individuals with bipolar disorder. Neurosci Biobehav Rev. 2017;73:1–22.

Moffitt TE, Harrington H, Caspi A, et al. Depression and generalized anxiety disorder: cumulative and sequential comorbidity in a birth cohort followed prospectively to age 32 years. Arch Gen Psychiatry. 2007;64:651–60.

Moffitt TE, Caspi A, Taylor A, et al. How common are common mental disorders? Evidence that lifetime prevalence rates are doubled by prospective versus retrospective ascertainment. Psychol Med. 2010;40:899–909.

Murru A, Carpiniello B. Duration of untreated illness as a key to early intervention in schizophrenia: a review. Neurosci Lett. 2018;16:59–67.

Niarchou M, Zammit S, Lewis G. The Avon Longitudinal Study of Parents and Children (ALSPAC) birth cohort as a resource for studying psychopathology in childhood and adolescence: a summary of findings for depression and psychosis. Soc Psychiatry Psychiatr Epidemiol. 2015;50:1017–27.

Ormel J, Raven D, van Oort F, et al. Mental health in Dutch adolescents: a TRAILS report on prevalence, severity, age of onset, continuity and co-morbidity of DSM disorders. Psychol Med. 2015;45:345–60.

Pfennig A, Leopold K, Bechdolf A, et al. Early specific cognitive-behavioural psychotherapy in subjects at high risk for bipolar disorders: study protocol for a randomised controlled trial. Trials. 2014;15:161.

Preti A, Rucci P, Santone G, et al. Patterns of admission to acute psychiatric inpatient facilities: a national survey in Italy. Psychol Med. 2009;39:485–96.

Rajji TK, Ismail Z, Mulsant BH. Age at onset and cognition in schizophrenia: meta-analysis. Br J Psychiatry. 2009;195:286–93.

Raphael K. Recall bias: a proposal for assessment and control. Int J Epidemiol. 1987;16:167–70.

Rapoport JL, Addington AM, Frangou S, et al. The neurodevelopmental model of schizophrenia: update 2005. Mol Psychiatry. 2005;10:434–49.

Tiemeier H, Velders FP, Szekely E, et al. The Generation R Study: a review of design, findings to date, and a study of the 5-HTTLPR by environmental interaction from fetal life onward. J Am Acad Child Adolesc Psychiatry. 2012;51:1119–35.

Van Meter AR, Burke C, Youngstrom EA, et al. The bipolar prodrome: meta-analysis of symptom prevalence prior to initial or recurrent mood episodes. J Am Acad Child Adolesc Psychiatry. 2016;55:543–55.

Vyas NS, Patel NH, Puri BK. Neurobiology and phenotypic expression in early onset schizophrenia. Early Interv Psychiatry. 2011;5:3–14.

Wang PS, Aguilar-Gaxiola S, Alonso J, et al. Use of mental health services for anxiety, mood, and substance disorders in 17 countries in the WHO world mental health surveys. Lancet. 2007;370:841–50.

Wong EH, Fox JC, Ng MY, et al. Toward personalized medicine in the neuropsychiatric field. Int Rev Neurobiol. 2011;101:329–49.

Lessons from Knowledge on the Correlates of the Age of Onset of Physical Illness

2

Giovanni Fiorito, Carlotta Sacerdote, and Paolo Vineis

Epidemiologists in the last century observed that, in general, the risk of non-communicable diseases increases with age, sometimes exponentially (Fisher and Hollomon 1951). The recognition that ageing is a major risk factor for cancer, neurodegenerative disorders, diabetes, cardiovascular diseases and other diseases has stimulated research on the molecular basis of this association. In many types of cancer, incidence rates tend to increase approximately logarithmically with age (Armitage and Doll 1954). In fact, population cancer data rarely perfectly fit the log scale model, the deviation from the hypothetical log linearity model providing interesting clues on disease aetiology. The plot of the number of cancer cases per year in a particular age group divided by the number of people in that age group on a log–log scale is used in descriptive epidemiology to show the positive acceleration of chronic diseases with age.

Monogenic diseases or inherited genetic defects (i.e. bilateral retinoblastoma) are individually rare and affect approximately 1% of the human population overall (Nagy et al. 2004). In contrast, the causes of major common diseases often involve both susceptibility genes and their interactions with the environment.

In a first simplified model, assuming that the main non-communicable diseases are caused by gene–environment interactions, ageing can be considered a marker of the accumulation of exposure to modifiable risk factors. According to this

G. Fiorito
Italian Institute for Genomic Medicine, (IIGM, ex HuGeF), Turin, Italy

C. Sacerdote
Città della Salute e della Scienza University-Hospital and CPO-Piemonte, Turin, Italy
e-mail: carlotta.sacerdote@cpo.it

P. Vineis (✉)
Italian Institute for Genomic Medicine, Turin, Italy

MRC-PHE Centre for Environment and Health, School of Public Health, Imperial College, London, UK
e-mail: p.vineis@imperial.ac.uk

G. de Girolamo et al. (eds.), *Age of Onset of Mental Disorders*,
https://doi.org/10.1007/978-3-319-72619-9_2

hypothesis, diseases with a late onset could mainly be attributed to cumulative environmental exposures, while diseases in early life could be attributable to genetic defects. It is a common observation that genetically predisposed individuals develop chronic diseases with an earlier age of onset than patients with sporadic diseases (Brandt et al. 2008; Garber and Offit 2005).

The apportionment of the weight of genetic and environmental agents in disease aetiology is complicated by the role of epigenetic changes. Epigenetic mechanisms do not alter the genetic code of an individual but affect the transcriptional programme of cells in response to environmental challenges. The aetiological models become more complex considering that (1) not only life-course exposures but also in utero exposures may affect organ-specific gene programming; (2) some of the epigenetic changes are heritable; and (3) part of epigenetic modulation is reversible throughout life.

In gene–environment interactions, the extent to which incidence patterns change depends on the dosage and the duration of exposure (Peto et al. 1991). For several common exposures, age is a proxy for duration of exposure.

2.1 Models of Environmental Influences

2.1.1 Cumulative Exposure Model: The Example of Lung Cancer and Smoking

Induction of lung cancer by tobacco smoking is a clear example of the powerful effect of duration of exposure, with cancer arising at a younger age when exposure started early or very early in life (Doll and Peto 1978). Conversely, cessation of smoking is followed by a "freezing" of cancer incidence. Since in never smokers lung cancer continues to rise with age, after many years (>25) the incidence rate of ex-smokers almost meets the rate of never smokers. The cumulative risk of lung cancer drops from >16% (cumulative risk to the age of 75 years) to 5% when comparing individuals who smoked without interruption from the age of 20 years with individuals who stopped at the age of 50 years (with a cumulative risk of 1% for never smokers) (Vineis et al. 2004) (Fig. 2.1). Thus, tobacco-induced lung cancer is a clear example of a cumulative effect throughout ageing, which can be interpreted as the extent of smoking duration.

Long-term exposure to carcinogens such as those contained in tobacco smoke is able to induce molecular changes that involve DNA damage and epigenetic changes. Freezing of cancer risk after cessation of exposure suggests that the mechanisms involved are likely to include epigenetic events because mutations or chromosome damage are fixed after cell replication (note: risk "freezes" in absolute terms if we use rates or cumulative risks and it decreases if we use relative measures such as relative risks compared to never smokers). Notably, it seems that ex-smokers never really reach the risk of never smokers, which means that some mutations have been fixed in early stages and have become permanent. What happens in ex-smokers has been described in an effective way by John Cairns:

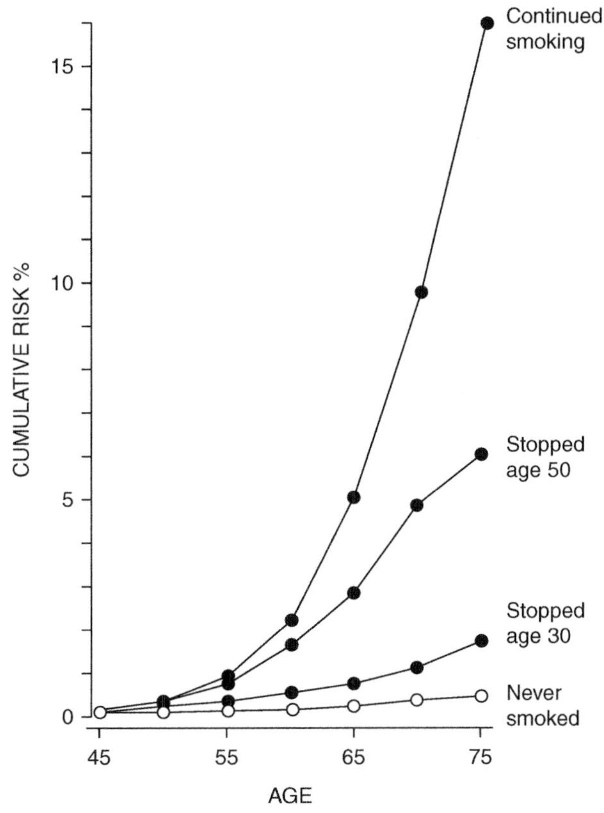

Fig. 2.1 Cumulative risk of lung cancer mortality among men in the UK who smoke, according to the age when they stopped smoking. Figure adapted from the original by permission of the (Peto et al. 2000)

"At any moment, the frequency of any class of cancer presumably reflects the number of cells that have undergone all but the final step in carcinogenesis, multiplied by the rate of whatever happens to be the final step. If this final step required DNA damage, the death rate from lung cancer would quickly drop when the mutagenic stimulus (smoking) was removed. In fact … at that point the death rate shows no decline and for the next 10–20 years actually stays roughly at the level it had reached in the year before the smoker stopped smoking …. This suggests that the final step … is an event of a different kind from the steps that lead to the accumulation of mutant cells because, unlike the earlier steps, it does not have to be stimulated by the toxicity and mutagenicity of tobacco …. It must, however, be a rare event because the incidence of lung cancer in ex-smokers, even in those who smoked for >40 years, is <1% a year" (Cairns 2006).

Cairns continues by suggesting that what happens is an epigenetic event at the stem cell level:

"Normally, each time a stem cell divides, its two daughters have different fates: one has to replace its parent and stay within the confines of the stem cell niche, while the other is programmed to differentiate and multiply and eventually all its descendants die and are discarded. The final step could be the rare failure of this dichotomy, when a fully mutant cancerous stem cell produces a daughter cell that is freed from some non-genetic imperative to differentiate and die (an event analogous to Prehn's 'symmetrical division')" (Cairns 2006).

Studying the timing of carcinogenic events has provided important hints on the putative mechanisms of cancer onset, i.e. of the processes that lead to the first malignant cell (M-cell). With a mathematical approach, we compared two models for lung carcinogenesis: an evolutionary model based on the Wright–Fisher (WF) process and the MVK model of Moolgavkar, Venzon and Knudson, also known as the two-stage clonal expansion model. The main result of our study on lung cancer was that with both models (WF and MVK) we obtained similar values for the median waiting time to the first M-cell and that there was a dominating effect of clonal cell selection in carcinogenesis. Both the WF and MVK models predicted waiting times that are consistent across several previously reported datasets. Thus, while both mutation and selection seem necessary for carcinogenesis, the model comparison suggests that the formation of the first M-cell is driven mainly by clonal expansion of selectively advantageous cells, whereas the effect of the mutation rate appears smaller (Schöllnberger et al. 2010). We hypothesised that carcinogenesis is a Darwinian process involving stem cells that acquire selective advantage due to epigenetic (i.e. reversible) changes (Vineis et al. 2010; Vineis 2015). This is compatible with the observation that risk in ex-smokers freezes but never reaches exactly the risk of never smokers. A full description of how stem cell methylation can serve as a kind of memory—similar to immunological memory—has been reported elsewhere (Vineis et al. 2017).

2.1.2 Susceptibility Windows: Breast Cancer and Relevance of Exposure at Puberty

The model proposed by Peto et al. for carcinogenesis, according to which the risk of disease is strictly related to dosage and duration of exposure, assuming age as a proxy of the duration of exposure, is not always appropriate. An example of a disease with a "susceptibility window" for exposure is breast cancer. In fact, breast cancer aetiology has been described with several pathways, most of which have their origins in early life (Trichopoulos et al. 2005). There is evidence that a larger number of undifferentiated cells in the breast might increase breast cancer risk, because undifferentiated cells seem to have a higher probability of being transformed into M-cells than differentiated cells (Bodicoat et al. 2014). Furthermore, hormones, such as oestrogens, increase cell proliferation, raising the chance of detrimental mutations occurring during DNA replication. These pathways suggest that there is a "susceptibility window" to endogenous exposure at the time of puberty, which could potentially affect breast cancer risk since the number of undifferentiated breast cells increases rapidly during puberty. It has been hypothesised that earlier thelarche (breast development) and/or menarche are associated with a higher risk of breast cancer because earlier thelarche/menarche involve exposure to oestrogens during a phase in which the breast comprises a high number of undifferentiated cells. In fact, the breast comprises predominantly undifferentiated, proliferating cells until the first full-term pregnancy and lactation, at which point a large proportion of breast cells differentiate fully (Apter and Vihko 1983).

Another "susceptibility window" when the breast tissue is particularly vulnerable to carcinogenic stimuli is the interval between menarche and first pregnancy. The longer this interval, the greater a woman's breast cancer risk is (Colditz et al. 2014). Full-term pregnancy induces cellular differentiation and molecular changes including a decrease in the number of hormone-sensitive luminal cells, making breast tissue less susceptible to carcinogens (Meier-Abt and Bentires-Alj 2014).

2.1.3 Developmental Origin of Health and Disease Hypothesis (DOHAD): The Case of Early Socioeconomic Status and Diabetes

The simplified model of balance between genetics and environmental agents in disease aetiology, in which age can be considered a proxy of the duration of exposure, is complicated by in utero exposures and the heritability of the epigenetic changes.

The Thrifty Phenotype Hypothesis is the theory that under- or malnutrition during gestation could permanently influence the body's structure and function, contributing to adult disease (Hales and Barker 1992). The Thrifty Phenotype Hypothesis has then been closely linked with biological embedding, the process through which external exposures "get under the skin" to influence human biological processes (Juarez et al. 2014), and with the Developmental Origin of Health and Disease (DOHAD) hypothesis. Biological embedding has been hypothesised to occur through three different processes, which may often co-exist.

The first process involves plasticity. Development is plastic so as to allow an organism to respond to its surrounding environment, especially very early in development, when cells and tissues are differentiating. At these critical windows of development, plasticity is heightened since proper growth and differentiation depends on nutrient availability, chemical signals from surrounding tissues, as well as environmental signals (Gluckman et al. 2008). An example of this process is exposure to diethylstilbestrol (DES) during gestation, which can cause subfertility and cancer in reproductive organs in the offspring. Another example is benzene exposure. There is evidence that maternal exposure to benzene is associated with a higher risk of childhood leukaemia (Carlos-Wallace et al. 2016). Chromosome translocations and epigenetic changes have been shown to be present in blood spots collected at birth (Greaves and Wiemels 2003). The genotoxic action of benzene induces multiple detrimental genetic changes, and it is likely that benzene exposure in mothers can cause abnormalities in foetal haematopoietic stem cells. In utero exposure can be the initiator of childhood leukaemia, even without any further exposure to benzene in children in early life.

Second, studies have shown that exposures can leave their mark on the biology of an organism throughout life (Fig. 2.2). In fact, certain exposures can have a stronger effect during a sensitive period, but they can affect biological processes, weakly, also outside sensitive periods. This is because maladaptive responses (Gluckman et al. 2008) may not lead to adverse phenotypic changes at the time of exposure but may accumulate, persist or even be reinforced for years, increasing the risk of

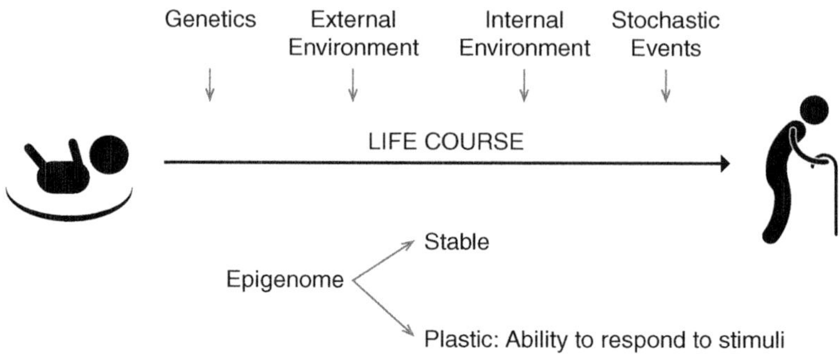

Fig. 2.2 Lifetime epigenomic plasticity decline. Although some components of the epigenome are stable, there is also great plasticity allowing the epigenome to respond to events throughout the life course. This plasticity is heightened during developmentally critical windows. Reproduced with permission from Demetriou et al. (2015)

dysfunction and disease years after the period of exposure. This is a second process through which external exposures can be internalised to influence health—the cumulative effects process.

A third process through which biological embedding can occur is through pathway effects, i.e. certain early life events can direct individuals into different life trajectories leading to different ageing experiences and life expectancies. Examples include early life socioeconomic position (SEP), which can limit an individual's educational opportunities, which can in turn lead to unfavourable circumstances and adverse health behaviours in adulthood with the associated shorter life expectancy.

2.1.3.1 Examples from Recent Research

Study of the impact of early life on subsequent disease is a very active area of research and in this section, we describe recent examples. In their study, Fantin et al. (2016) used data from 4437 girls and 4337 boys born in 2000–2001 in the UK (Millennium Cohort Study). The children's body mass index (BMI) was measured at ages 3, 5, 7 and 11 years. They described the children's environment using social class and behaviours within the family. At the age of 3 years, there was no link between the environment and children's BMI. In contrast, there was a clear link between the environment and BMI slopes between 3 and 11 years of age. At the age of 11 years, they calculated that if all children had the most favourable environment, mean BMI would be reduced by 0.91 kg/m^2 (95% confidence interval [CI] 0.57–1.26) for boys and by 1.65 kg/m^2 (95% CI 1.28–2.02) for girls (Fantin et al. 2016).

A second study comes from the multicentre Lifepath network on the impact of early socioeconomic status (SES) on ageing (McCrory et al. 2017). McCrory et al. aimed to investigate the independent and synergistic effects of childhood and adult SEP, as well as the effect of social mobility, on type 2 diabetes (T2D) risk in later life. Cross-sectional data from The Irish Longitudinal Study of Ageing (TILDA) (n = 4998), a nationally representative probability sample of adults aged 50 years and older, were analysed. Compared to high SEP, low SEP in both childhood (odds ratio [OR]: 1.84, 95% CI 1.00–3.37) and adulthood (OR: 1.78, 95% CI 1.01–3.14) were independently associated with T2D in adult women. Women remaining in low SEP at both timepoints were at greatest risk of T2D (OR: 2.51, 95% CI 1.24–5.06) compared with those classified as "Stable High". This study confirms a strong association between low SEP and T2D in women which persists from childhood through to adulthood, suggesting an early imprinting associated with a poor living environment.

2.1.4 Epigenetic Age Acceleration

A recent interesting development in the biology of ageing and the impact of age on disease is the concept of epigenetic age acceleration (AA). DNA methylation is well-known for being one of the main molecular mechanisms implicated in cell differentiation and cellular response to ageing (Bell et al. 2012; Day et al. 2013). Recent studies on a genome-wide scale indicate a global increase in epigenetic drift with age (Teschendorff et al. 2013; Tan et al. 2016). The concept of epigenetic drift can be described through studies involving monozygotic twins: twins are epigenetically very similar at birth and in the first years of life, when they share the same environment and similar exposures, but become more and more epigenetically different with ageing as their exposures begin to differ (Martin 2005).

Several age-dependent differentially methylated CpG sites for specific biological fluids or particular tissues have been identified through epigenome-wide association studies (EWAS) in the last few years (Zykovich et al. 2014; Teschendorff et al. 2010; Garagnani et al. 2012). Interestingly, more than 95% of the age-associated CpGs (±500 base pairs) are located near the transcriptional start site of the associated gene, suggesting a role in the regulation of gene expression (Rakyan et al. 2010).

The concept of the "epigenetic clock" was introduced in 2013 by Steve Horvath (Horvath 2013). He developed a multi-tissue predictor of chronological age, based on a set of 353 CpGs whose DNA methylation is strongly correlated with chronological age across different tissues and cell types. These were identified using 82 publicly available DNA methylation datasets involving about 8000 samples and 51 different healthy tissues and cell types.

Although epigenetic age and chronological age are highly correlated across study populations, there is significant inter-individual variability (Horvath 2013; Weidner et al. 2014). This means that an individual's DNA methylation age is more similar to their chronological age than for other individuals (Jones et al. 2015). Also, the gap between epigenetic age and chronological age tends to increase with ageing. Such phenomenon could be explained by the "accumulation of exposures" hypothesis (Horvath 2013; Weidner et al. 2014; Jones et al. 2015) (Fig. 2.3). Accordingly, the concept of AA was introduced, with AA defined as the epigenetic age minus chronological age (Horvath 2013). Individuals with positive AA values (biological age greater than their chronological age) are experiencing accelerated ageing and vice versa.

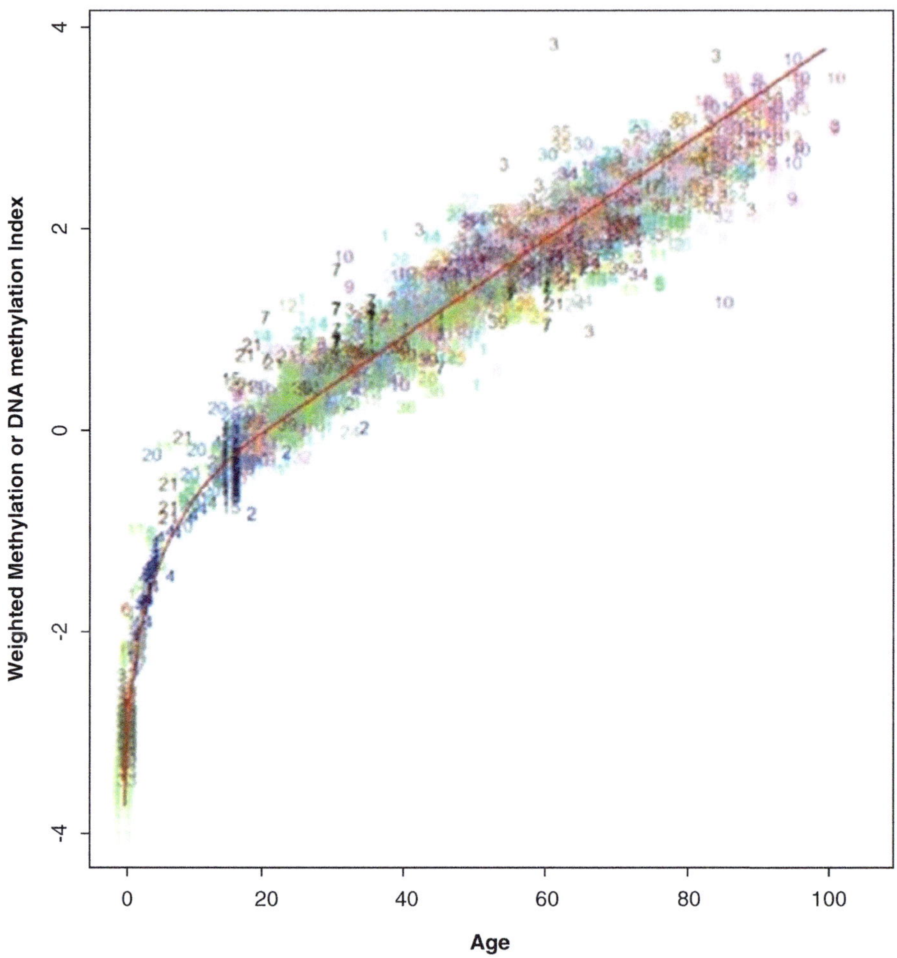

Fig. 2.3 Weighted average of the 353 clock CpGs versus chronological age. The rate of change of the red curve can be interpreted as the tick rate. The deviation of biological age from chronological age increases with age, supporting the hypothesis of the epigenetic drift as a consequence of the accumulation of the exposures. Figure adapted from the original and reproduced by permission from Horvath (2013)

2.1.4.1 Association of Age Acceleration with Unhealthy Lifestyle and Ageing-Related Diseases

In his original publication, Horvath (2013) explained accelerated epigenetic ageing in cancer tissues compared with normal tissues as a consequence of the extremely high rate of cell proliferation in cancer cells, and because several biological functions are enriched in the genes located near the 353 age-dependent CpGs. Gene set enrichment analysis indicated "cell death/survival" and "cellular growth/development" as the most significantly enriched biological functions. Significant overlap has been observed also for disease-related gene sets such as "cancer", "endocrine system disorder", "hereditary disorders" and "reproductive system diseases".

Since then, several studies have described the association of accelerated epigenetic ageing with unhealthy lifestyle habits and complex diseases risk factors such as obesity (Nevalainen et al. 2017; Horvath et al. 2014), smoking (Beach et al. 2015), alcohol intake (Beach et al. 2015; Quach et al. 2017), poor physical activity and unhealthy diet (Quach et al. 2017). Other examples concern the association of epigenetic AA with long-term exposure to air pollution (Ward-Caviness et al. 2016), lifetime stress (Zannas et al. 2015), early occurrence of menopause in women (Quach et al. 2017; Levine et al. 2016) and low education (Quach et al. 2017). Also, AA is associated with several age-related chronic conditions and unhealthy status, providing further evidence that the epigenetic clock is a powerful biomarker of healthy ageing. For instance, the epigenetic age of blood predicts all-cause mortality (Chen et al. 2016; Marioni et al. 2015a, b; Perna et al. 2016), frailty (Breitling et al. 2016), lung cancer (Levine et al. 2015a, b), and cognitive and physical functioning (Marioni et al. 2015a, b). Furthermore, the utility of the epigenetic clock using various tissues and organs has been demonstrated in applications surrounding Alzheimer's disease (Levine et al. 2015a, b), centenarian status (Horvath et al. 2015b), Down syndrome (Horvath et al. 2015a), Huntington's disease (Horvath et al. 2016), osteoarthritis (Vidal-Bralo et al. 2016) and Parkinson's disease (Horvath). The epigenetic clock seems to be not only dependent on endogenous and exogenous exposures. A slow epigenetic ageing has also been described as a heritable trait in a study in which the blood of the offspring of Italian semi-super-centenarians (i.e. participants aged 105 years or older) was shown to have a lower epigenetic age than that of age-matched controls (Horvath et al. 2015b).

2.1.4.2 Epigenetic Clock in Newborns and Children

Recent research shows that effects of in utero and early life exposures may be stored in cells through epigenetic modifications that can be sustained for decades (Joubert et al. 2016a, b; Guida et al. 2015; Demetriou et al. 2015). As a consequence, researchers have started to study the effect of early childhood exposure on epigenetic ageing, providing strong evidence that AA in children is associated with prenatal (in utero) and early life exposure. For this purpose, studies involving mother–offspring pairs are very useful. Associations between AA and sex, weight at birth, caesarean section birth and maternal characteristics during pregnancy, such as smoking habits, weight gain/loss during pregnancy, BMI, and selenium and cholesterol level have been described recently (Simpkin et al. 2016; Javed et al. 2016). Knight and colleagues (2016) recently developed a cord-blood methylation-based predictor of gestational age based on 148 CpGs. Gestational age is often used as a proxy for developmental maturity by clinicians and researchers, and it is usually estimated from the first day of the last menstrual cycle. According to Horvath's definition of AA, the gestational AA is defined as the difference between the DNA methylation measure and the estimated gestational age. Further studies are needed to assess whether the epigenetic gestational AA is a good predictor of child cognitive and physical development, though preliminary results are promising (Knight et al. 2016).

2.1.4.3 Reversibility of the Effect

Due to the relative importance of early life exposure on accelerated ageing, one of the open questions in this research field is whether the effect is reversible or not. No studies to date have investigated whether changes in lifestyle conditions (e.g. a weight-loss diet or quitting smoking) decelerate the ageing process. In a recent study investigating the association of AA with SES in more than 5000 individuals, the biological age of low SES individuals was estimated to be on average 1 year higher than for high SES subjects. Interestingly, AA was more noticeable in individuals whose SES started low and remained low later in life than in those whose status improved during the life course, while intermediate changes were found in subjects whose SES declined from high to low. This pattern of findings is compatible with some degree of reversibility of the effect and further supports the relative importance of the early life childhood social environment.

Conclusions

The age of onset of chronic diseases is a crucial variable to consider both in research settings and clinical practice, since there is increasing evidence of a strict association with aetiology, treatment options and prognosis.

Age can be considered not only a marker of the accumulation of exposure to modifiable risk factors but also an indication of the existence of susceptibility windows in a specific period of life (including intrauterine and early postnatal life), within an epidemiological life course perspective of chronic disease onset.

Several theories have been proposed (and described here) to link age and chronic diseases, none of which appears to be completely satisfactory for all diseases. Their interplay, however, is likely to address the complexity of the problem.

Most of the hypotheses on the role of environmental exposures in disease onset and then, most of the examples here proposed, have been historically developed for cancer models. However, the same pathogenetic models can be applied to several other chronic diseases, such as neurological and psychiatric diseases. Understanding the link between the age of onset and environmental exposures is of utmost importance in aetiological research on all chronic diseases.

References

Apter D, Vihko R. Early menarche, a risk factor for breast cancer, indicates early onset of ovulatory cycles. J Clin Endocrinol Metab. 1983;57:82–6.

Armitage P, Doll R. The age distribution of cancer and a multi-stage theory of carcinogenesis. Br J Cancer. 1954;8:1–12.

Beach SR, Dogan MV, Lei MK, Cutrona CE, Gerrard M, Gibbons FX, Simons RL, Brody GH, Philibert RA. Methylomic ageing as a window onto the influence of lifestyle: tobacco and alcohol use alter the rate of biological ageing. J Am Geriatr Soc. 2015;63:2519–25.
Bell JT, Tsai PC, Yang TP, Pidsley R, Nisbet J, Glass D, Mangino M, Zhai G, Zhang F, Valdes A, Shin SY, Dempster EL, Murray RM, Grundberg E, Hedman AK, Nica A, Small KS, MuTHER Consortium, Dermitzakis ET, McCarthy MI, Mill J, Spector TD, Deloukas P. Epigenome-wide scans identify differentially methylated regions for age and age-related phenotypes in a healthy ageing population. PLoS Genet. 2012;8:e1002629.
Bodicoat DH, Schoemaker MJ, Jones ME, McFadden E, Griffin J, Ashworth A, Swerdlow AJ. Timing of pubertal stages and breast cancer risk: the Breakthrough Generations Study. Breast Cancer Res. 2014;16:R18.
Brandt A, Bermejo JL, Sundquist J, Hemminki K. Age of onset in familial cancer. Ann Oncol. 2008;19:2084–8.
Breitling LP, Saum KU, Perna L, Schöttker B, Holleczek B, Brenner H. Frailty is associated with the epigenetic clock but not with telomere length in a German cohort. Clin Epigenetics. 2016;8:21.
Cairns J. Cancer and the immortal strand hypothesis. Genetics. 2006;174:1069–72.
Carlos-Wallace FM, Zhang L, Smith MT, Rader G, Steinmaus C. Parental, in utero, and early-life exposure to benzene and the risk of childhood leukemia: a meta-analysis. Am J Epidemiol. 2016;183:1–14.
Chen BH, Marioni RE, Colicino E, Peters MJ, Ward-Caviness CK, Tsai PC, Roetker NS, Just AC, Demerath EW, Guan W, Bressler J, Fornage M, Studenski S, Vandiver AR, Moore AZ, Tanaka T, Kiel DP, Liang L, Vokonas P, Schwartz J, Lunetta KL, Murabito JM, Bandinelli S, Hernandez DG, Melzer D, Nalls M, Pilling LC, Price TR, Singleton AB, Gieger C, Holle R, Kretschmer A, Kronenberg F, Kunze S, Linseisen J, Meisinger C, Rathmann W, Waldenberger M, Visscher PM, Shah S, Wray NR, McRae AF, Franco OH, Hofman A, Uitterlinden AG, Absher D, Assimes T, Levine ME, Lu AT, Tsao PS, Hou L, Manson JE, Carty CL, LaCroix AZ, Reiner AP, Spector TD, Feinberg AP, Levy D, Baccarelli A, van Meurs J, Bell JT, Peters A, Deary IJ, Pankow JS, Ferrucci L, Horvath S. DNA methylation-based measures of biological age: meta-analysis predicting time to death. Aging. 2016;8:1844–65.
Colditz GA, Bohlke K, Berkey CS. Breast cancer risk accumulation starts early: prevention must also. Breast Cancer Res Treat. 2014;145:567–79.
Day K, Waite LL, Thalacker-Mercer A, West A, Bamman MM, Brooks JD, Myers RM, Absher D. Differential DNA methylation with age displays both common and dynamic features across human tissues that are influenced by CpG landscape. Genome Biol. 2013;14:R102.
Demetriou CA, van Veldhoven K, Relton C, Stringhini S, Kyriacou K, Vineis P. Biological embedding of early-life exposures and disease risk in humans: a role for DNA methylation. Eur J Clin Investig. 2015;45:303–32.
Doll R, Peto R. Cigarette smoking and bronchial carcinoma: dose and time relationships among regular smokers and lifelong non-smokers. J Epidemiol Community Health. 1978;32:303–13.
Fantin R, Delpierre C, Dimeglio C, Lamy S, Barboza Solís C, Charles MA, Kelly-Irving M. Disentangling the respective roles of the early environment and parental BMI on BMI change across childhood: a counterfactual analysis using the Millennium Cohort Study. Prev Med. 2016;89:146–53.
Fisher JC, Hollomon JH. A hypothesis for the origin of cancer foci. Cancer. 1951;4:916–8.
Frank SA. Dynamics of cancer. Incidence, inheritance, and evolution. Princeton and Oxford: Princeton University Press; 2007.
Garagnani P, Bacalini MG, Pirazzini C, Gori D, Giuliani C, Mari D, Di Blasio AM, Gentilini D, Vitale G, Collino S, Rezzi S, Castellani G, Capri M, Salvioli S, Franceschi C. Methylation of ELOVL2 gene as a new epigenetic marker of age. Aging Cell. 2012;11(6):1132–4.
Garber JE, Offit K. Hereditary cancer predisposition syndromes. J Clin Oncol. 2005;23(2):276–92.
Gluckman PD, Hanson MA, Cooper C, Thornburg KL. Effect of in utero and early-life conditions on adult health and disease. N Engl J Med. 2008;359:61–73.

Greaves MF, Wiemels J. Origins of chromosome translocations in childhood leukaemia. Nat Rev Cancer. 2003;3:639–49.

Guida F, Sandanger TM, Castagné R, Campanella G, Polidoro S, Palli D, Krogh V, Tumino R, Sacerdote C, Panico S, Severi G, Kyrtopoulos SA, Georgiadis P, Vermeulen RC, Lund E, Vineis P, Chadeau-Hyam M. Dynamics of smoking-induced genome-wide methylation changes with time since smoking cessation. Hum Mol Genet. 2015;24:2349–59.

Hales CN, Barker DJ. Type 2 (non-insulin-dependent) diabetes mellitus: the thrifty phenotype hypothesis. Diabetologia. 1992;35:595–601.

Horvath S. DNA methylation age of human tissues and cell types. Genome Biol. 2013;14:R115.

Horvath S, Ritz BR. Increased epigenetic age and granulocyte counts in the blood of Parkinson's disease patients. Aging. 2015;7:1130–42.

Horvath S, Erhart W, Brosch M, Ammerpohl O, von Schönfels W, Ahrens M, Heits N, Bell JT, Tsai PC, Spector TD, Deloukas P, Siebert R, Sipos B, Becker T, Röcken C, Schafmayer C, Hampe J. Obesity accelerates epigenetic ageing of human liver. Proc Natl Acad Sci. 2014;111:15538–43.

Horvath S, Garagnani P, Bacalini MG, Pirazzini C, Salvioli S, Gentilini D, Di Blasio AM, Giuliani C, Tung S, Vinters HV, Franceschi C. Accelerated epigenetic ageing in Down syndrome. Aging Cell. 2015a;14:491–5.

Horvath S, Pirazzini C, Bacalini MG, Gentilini D, Di Blasio AM, Delledonne M, Mari D, Arosio B, Monti D, Passarino G, De Rango F, D'Aquila P, Giuliani C, Marasco E, Collino S, Descombes P, Garagnani P, Franceschi C. Decreased epigenetic age of PBMCs from Italian semi-supercentenarians and their offspring. Aging. 2015b;7:1159–70.

Horvath S, Langfelder P, Kwak S, Aaronson J, Rosinski J, Vogt TF, Eszes M, Faull RL, Curtis MA, Waldvogel HJ, Choi OW, Tung S, Vinters HV, Coppola G, Yang XW. Huntington's disease accelerates epigenetic ageing of human brain and disrupts DNA methylation levels. Aging. 2016;8:1485–512.

Javed R, Chen W, Lin F, Liang H. Infant's DNA methylation age at birth and epigenetic ageing accelerators. Biomed Res Int. 2016;2016:4515928.

Jones MJ, Goodman SJ, Kobor MS. DNA methylation and healthy human ageing. Aging Cell. 2015;14:924–32.

Joubert BR, den Dekker HT, Felix JF, Bohlin J, Ligthart S, Beckett E, Tiemeier H, van Meurs JB, Uitterlinden AG, Hofman A, Håberg SE, Reese SE, Peters MJ, Andreassen BK, Steegers EA, Nilsen RM, Vollset SE, Midttun Ø, Ueland PM, Franco OH, Dehghan A, de Jongste JC, Wu MC, Wang T, Peddada SD, Jaddoe VW, Nystad W, Duijts L, London SJ. Maternal plasma folate impacts differential DNA methylation in an epigenome-wide meta-analysis of newborns. Nat Commun. 2016a;7:10577.

Joubert BR, Felix JF, Yousefi P, Bakulski KM, Just AC, Breton C, Reese SE, Markunas CA, Richmond RC, Xu CJ, Küpers LK, Oh SS, Hoyo C, Gruzieva O, Söderhäll C, Salas LA, Baïz N, Zhang H, Lepeule J, Ruiz C, Ligthart S, Wang T, Taylor JA, Duijts L, Sharp GC, Jankipersadsing SA, Nilsen RM, Vaez A, Fallin MD, Hu D, Litonjua AA, Fuemmeler BF, Huen K, Kere J, Kull I, Munthe-Kaas MC, Gehring U, Bustamante M, Saurel-Coubizolles MJ, Quraishi BM, Ren J, Tost J, Gonzalez JR, Peters MJ, Håberg SE, Xu Z, van Meurs JB, Gaunt TR, Kerkhof M, Corpeleijn E, Feinberg AP, Eng C, Baccarelli AA, Benjamin Neelon SE, Bradman A, Merid SK, Bergström A, Herceg Z, Hernandez-Vargas H, Brunekreef B, Pinart M, Heude B, Ewart S, Yao J, Lemonnier N, Franco OH, Wu MC, Hofman A, McArdle W, Van der Vlies P, Falahi F, Gillman MW, Barcellos LF, Kumar A, Wickman M, Guerra S, Charles MA, Holloway J, Auffray C, Tiemeier HW, Smith GD, Postma D, Hivert MF, Eskenazi B, Vrijheid M, Arshad H, Antó JM, Dehghan A, Karmaus W, Annesi-Maesano I, Sunyer J, Ghantous A, Pershagen G, Holland N, Murphy SK, DeMeo DL, Burchard EG, Ladd-Acosta C, Snieder H, Nystad W, Koppelman GH, Relton CL, Jaddoe VW, Wilcox A, Melén E, London SJ. DNA methylation in newborns and maternal smoking in pregnancy: genome-wide consortium meta-analysis. Am J Hum Genet. 2016b;98(4):680–96.

Juarez PD, Matthews-Juarez P, Hood DB, Im W, Levine RS, Kilbourne BJ, Langston MA, Al-Hamdan MZ, Crosson WL, Estes MG, Estes SM, Agboto VK, Robinson P, Wilson S,

Lichtveld MY. The public health exposome: a population-based, exposure science approach to health disparities research. Int J Environ Res Public Health. 2014;11:12866–95.

Knight AK, Craig JM, Theda C, Bækvad-Hansen M, Bybjerg-Grauholm J, Hansen CS, Hollegaard MV, Hougaard DM, Mortensen PB, Weinsheimer SM, Werge TM, Brennan PA, Cubells JF, Newport DJ, Stowe ZN, Cheong JL, Dalach P, Doyle LW, Loke YJ, Baccarelli AA, Just AC, Wright RO, Téllez-Rojo MM, Svensson K, Trevisi L, Kennedy EM, Binder EB, Iurato S, Czamara D, Räikkönen K, Lahti JM, Pesonen AK, Kajantie E, Villa PM, Laivuori H, Hämäläinen E, Park HJ, Bailey LB, Parets SE, Kilaru V, Menon R, Horvath S, Bush NR, LeWinn KZ, Tylavsky FA, Conneely KN, Smith AK. An epigenetic clock for gestational age at birth based on blood methylation data. Genome Biol. 2016;17:206.

Levine ME, Hosgood HD, Chen B, Absher D, Assimes T, Horvath S. DNA methylation age of blood predicts future onset of lung cancer in the women's health initiative. Aging (Albany NY). 2015a;7(9):690–700.

Levine ME, Lu AT, Bennett DA, Horvath S. Epigenetic age of the pre-frontal cortex is associated with neuritic plaques, amyloid load, and Alzheimer's disease related cognitive functioning. Aging. 2015b;7:1198–211.

Levine ME, Lu AT, Chen BH, Hernandez DG, Singleton AB, Ferrucci L, Bandinelli S, Salfati E, Manson JE, Quach A, Kusters CD, Kuh D, Wong A, Teschendorff AE, Widschwendter M, Ritz BR, Absher D, Assimes TL, Horvath S. Menopause accelerates biological ageing. Proc Natl Acad Sci U S A. 2016;113:9327–32.

Marioni RE, Shah S, McRae AF, Ritchie SJ, Muniz-Terrera G, Harris SE, Gibson J, Redmond P, Cox SR, Pattie A, Corley J, Taylor A, Murphy L, Starr JM, Horvath S, Visscher PM, Wray NR, Deary IJ. The epigenetic clock is correlated with physical and cognitive fitness in the Lothian Birth Cohort 1936. Int J Epidemiol. 2015a;44:1388–96.

Marioni RE, Shah S, McRae AF, Chen BH, Colicino E, Harris SE, Gibson J, Henders AK, Redmond P, Cox SR, Pattie A, Corley J, Murphy L, Martin NG, Montgomery GW, Feinberg AP, Fallin MD, Multhaup ML, Jaffe AE, Joehanes R, Schwartz J, Just AC, Lunetta KL, Murabito JM, Starr JM, Horvath S, Baccarelli AA, Levy D, Visscher PM, Wray NR, Deary IJ. DNA methylation age of blood predicts all-cause mortality in later life. Genome Biol. 2015b;16:25.

Martin GM. Epigenetic drift in ageing identical twins. Proc Natl Acad Sci. 2005;102:10413–4.

McCrory C, O'Leary N, Fraga S, Ribeiro AI, Barros H, Kartiosuo N, Raitakari O, Kivimäki M, Vineis P, Layte R, Lifepath Consortium. Socioeconomic differences in children's growth trajectories from infancy to early adulthood: evidence from four European countries. J Epidemiol Community Health. 2017;71(10):981–9.

Meier-Abt F, Bentires-Alj M. How pregnancy at early age protects against breast cancer. Trends Mol Med. 2014;20:143–53.

Nagy R, Sweet K, Eng C. Highly penetrant hereditary cancer syndromes. Oncogene. 2004;23(23):6445–70.

Nevalainen T, Kananen L, Marttila S, Jylhävä J, Mononen N, Kähönen M, Raitakari OT, Hervonen A, Jylhä M, Lehtimäki T, Hurme M. Obesity accelerates epigenetic ageing in middle-aged but not in elderly individuals. Clin Epigenetics. 2017;9:20.

Perna L, Zhang Y, Mons U, Holleczek B, Saum KU, Brenner H. Epigenetic age acceleration predicts cancer, cardiovascular, and all-cause mortality in a German case cohort. Clin Epigenetics. 2016;8:64.

Peto R, Darby S, Deo H, Silcocks P, Whitley E, Doll R. Smoking, smoking cessation, and lung cancer in the UK since 1950: combination of national statistics with two case-control studies. BMJ. 2000;321:323–9.

Peto R, Gray R, Brantom P, Grasso P. Effects on 4080 rats of chronic ingestion of N-nitrosodiethylamine or N-nitrosodimethylamine: a detailed dose-response study. Cancer Res. 1991;51:6415–51.

Quach A, Levine ME, Tanaka T, Lu AT, Chen BH, Ferrucci L, Ritz B, Bandinelli S, Neuhouser ML, Beasley JM, Snetselaar L, Wallace RB, Tsao PS, Absher D, Assimes TL, Stewart JD, Li Y, Hou L, Baccarelli AA, Whitsel EA, Horvath S. Epigenetic clock analysis of diet, exercise, education, and lifestyle factors. Aging. 2017;9:419–46.

Rakyan VK, Down TA, Maslau S, Andrew T, Yang TP, Beyan H, Whittaker P, McCann OT, Finer S, Valdes AM, Leslie RD, Deloukas P, Spector TD. Human ageing-associated DNA hypermethylation occurs preferentially at bivalent chromatin domains. Genome Res. 2010;20:434–9.
Schöllnberger H, Beerenwinkel N, Hoogenveen R, Vineis P. Cell selection as driving force in lung and colon carcinogenesis. Cancer Res. 2010;70(17):6797–803.
Simpkin AJ, Hemani G, Suderman M, Gaunt TR, Lyttleton O, Mcardle WL, Ring SM, Sharp GC, Tilling K, Horvath S, Kunze S, Peters A, Waldenberger M, Ward-Caviness C, Nohr EA, Sørensen TI, Relton CL, Smith GD. Prenatal and early life influences on epigenetic age in children: a study of mother-offspring pairs from two cohort studies. Hum Mol Genet. 2016;25:191–201.
Tan Q, Heijmans BT, Hjelmborg JV, Soerensen M, Christensen K, Christiansen L. Epigenetic drift in the ageing genome: a ten-year follow-up in an elderly twin cohort. Int J Epidemiol. 2016;45:1146–58.
Teschendorff AE, Menon U, Gentry-Maharaj A, Ramus SJ, Weisenberger DJ, Shen H, Campan M, Noushmehr H, Bell CG, Maxwell AP, Savage DA, Mueller-Holzner E, Marth C, Kocjan G, Gayther SA, Jones A, Beck S, Wagner W, Laird PW, Jacobs IJ, Widschwendter M. Age-dependent DNA methylation of genes that are suppressed in stem cells is a hallmark of cancer. Genome Res. 2010;20:440–6.
Teschendorff AE, West J, Beck S. Age-associated epigenetic drift: implications, and a case of epigenetic thrift? Hum Mol Genet. 2013;22:R7–R15.
Trichopoulos D, Lagiou P, Adami HO. Towards an integrated model for breast cancer aetiology: the crucial role of the number of mammary tissue-specific stem cells. Breast Cancer Res. 2005;7:13–7.
Vidal-Bralo L, Lopez-Golan Y, Mera-Varela A, Rego-Perez I, Horvath S, Zhang Y, Del Real Á, Zhai G, Blanco FJ, Riancho JA, Gomez-Reino JJ, Gonzalez A. Specific premature epigenetic ageing of cartilage in osteoarthritis. Aging. 2016;8:2222–31.
Vineis P. Exposomics: mathematics meets biology. Mutagenesis. 2015;30(6):719–22.
Vineis P, Alavanja M, Buffler P, Fontham E, Franceschi S, Gao YT, Gupta PC, Hackshaw A, Matos E, Samet J, Sitas F, Smith J, Stayner L, Straif K, Thun MJ, Wichmann HE, Wu AH, Zaridze D, Peto R, Doll R. Tobacco and cancer: recent epidemiological evidence. J Natl Cancer Inst. 2004;96:99–106.
Vineis P, Schatzkin A, Potter JD. Models of carcinogenesis: an overview. Carcinogenesis. 2010;31(10):1703–9.
Vineis P, Chatziioannou A, Cunliffe VT, Flanagan JM, Hanson M, Kirsch-Volders M, Kyrtopoulos S. Epigenetic memory in response to environmental stressors. FASEB J. 2017;31:2241–51.
Ward-Caviness CK, Nwanaji-Enwerem JC, Wolf K, Wahl S, Colicino E, Trevisi L, Kloog I, Just AC, Vokonas P, Cyrys J, Gieger C, Schwartz J, Baccarelli AA, Schneider A, Peters A. Long-term exposure to air pollution is associated with biological ageing. Oncotarget. 2016;7:74510–25.
Weidner CI, Lin Q, Koch CM, Eisele L, Beier F, Ziegler P, Bauerschlag DO, Jöckel KH, Erbel R, Mühleisen TW, Zenke M, Brümmendorf TH, Wagner W. Ageing of blood can be tracked by DNA methylation changes at just three CpG sites. Genome Biol. 2014;15:R24.
Zannas AS, Arloth J, Carrillo-Roa T, Iurato S, Röh S, Ressler KJ, Nemeroff CB, Smith AK, Bradley B, Heim C, Menke A, Lange JF, Brückl T, Ising M, Wray NR, Erhardt A, Binder EB, Mehta D. Lifetime stress accelerates epigenetic ageing in an urban, African American cohort: relevance of glucocorticoid signaling. Genome Biol. 2015;16:266.
Zykovich A, Hubbard A, Flynn JM, Tarnopolsky M, Fraga MF, Kerksick C, Ogborn D, MacNeil L, Mooney SD, Melov S. Genome-wide DNA methylation changes with age in disease-free human skeletal muscle. Aging Cell. 2014;13:360–6.

Does the Age of Onset Shape the Clinical Picture, Course and Consequences of Schizophrenia? Results from a Long-Term Epidemiological Study

3

Heinz Häfner

3.1 Introduction

Age of onset (AOO) influences the clinical presentation, course and outcome of schizophrenia, thereby probably acting both as a cause and consequence of these aspects of the disorder. For this reason, AOO has been one of the focal points of our research into schizophrenia over a couple of decades. This was explored in a long-term research project into the onset and prodromal stage and in a retrospective and prospective investigation of the course of schizophrenia (Häfner et al. 1998a, b, 2013). The tools used were primarily epidemiological, but we also applied biological–hormonal and genetic approaches in cooperation with our colleagues in Germany and abroad. As the research project unfolded, the initial study objectives became expanded several times as new hypotheses were developed from the results achieved and subsequently tested.

The large-scale epidemiological schizophrenia studies conducted in Europe have used fairly high upper age limits. In 1911 Eugen Bleuler introduced the diagnosis of schizophrenia as a replacement for Emil Kraepelin's term "Dementia praecox". The reason for this was that on the one hand so-called late-onset schizophrenia occurred at remarkable frequencies and on the other an illness course not ending in dementia was quite prevalent. The upper age limit most widely used—if defined at all—in more recent European epidemiological studies is 50–54 years, as was the case in the World Health Organization (WHO) Determinants of Outcome of Severe Mental Disorders (DOSMeD) study (Sartorius et al. 1986; Jablensky et al. 1992). One reason for why an upper age limit was used at all probably had to do with the fact that the symptoms of late- and very-late-onset schizophrenia differ from those of

H. Häfner
Schizophrenia Research Group, Central Institute of Mental Health, Medical Faculty Mannheim, Heidelberg University, Mannheim, Germany
e-mail: heinz.haefner@zi-mannheim.de

G. de Girolamo et al. (eds.), *Age of Onset of Mental Disorders*,
https://doi.org/10.1007/978-3-319-72619-9_3

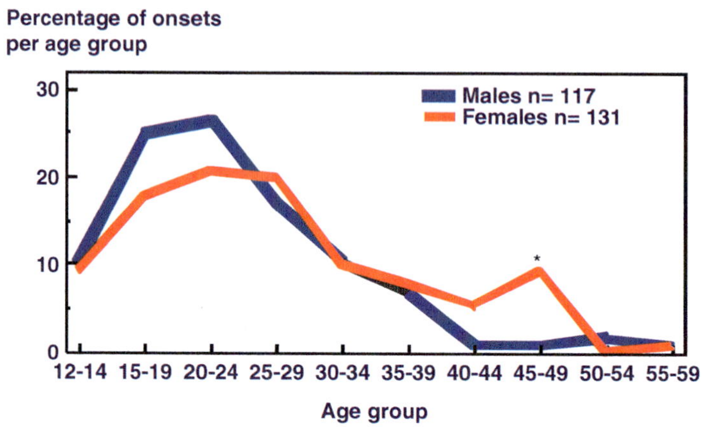

Fig. 3.1 Distribution of age at onset of schizophrenia (first ever sign of mental disorder) by sex; ICD-9: 295, 297, 298.3, 298.4 (ABC Schizophrenia Study). Source: Häfner et al. (1993b). *ICD-9* International Classification of Diseases, Ninth Edition

early-onset schizophrenia (Howard and Jeste 2011). Studies on this topic are rare, and, what is more, systematic studies are lacking.

The traditional graphs depicting the age distribution of schizophrenia onsets give the impression that the main AOO of the disorder lies in adolescence and early adult age (Hambrecht et al. 1992a; Häfner et al. 1993a; Kirkbride et al. 2006) (Fig. 3.1). Thereafter, incidence rates fall continuously along with age, apart from a second peak of female onset at the age of menopause. Reflected in this picture is a widely held belief, which used to play a prominent role in American psychiatry in particular: the *Diagnostic and Statistical Manual of Mental Disorders, Third Edition* (DSM-III) (APA 1980), as well as the related diagnostic research criteria, permitted a restrictively defined diagnosis of schizophrenia only up to the age of 45 years. This was because it was believed that beyond this age schizophrenia onsets no longer occurred, but instead only schizophrenia spectrum disorders such as late-life delusional disorders. The conditions were classified as "late paraphrenias", "involutional psychoses" or coded under other fringe diagnoses from the schizophrenia spectrum. This belief had no empirical foundation, so in subsequent revisions of the classification system this age limit was dropped.

3.2 Age of Onset (AOO) as a Disorder Marker

The belief that the onset of schizophrenia is limited up to the age of 45 years has been proven to be wrong after the results of several epidemiological studies conducted primarily in the Netherlands and Great Britain (Castle and Murray 1993; van Os et al. 1995; Castle et al. 1998): it became clear that beyond age 60 years first-admission rates and, consequently, onset rates for schizophrenia actually continued

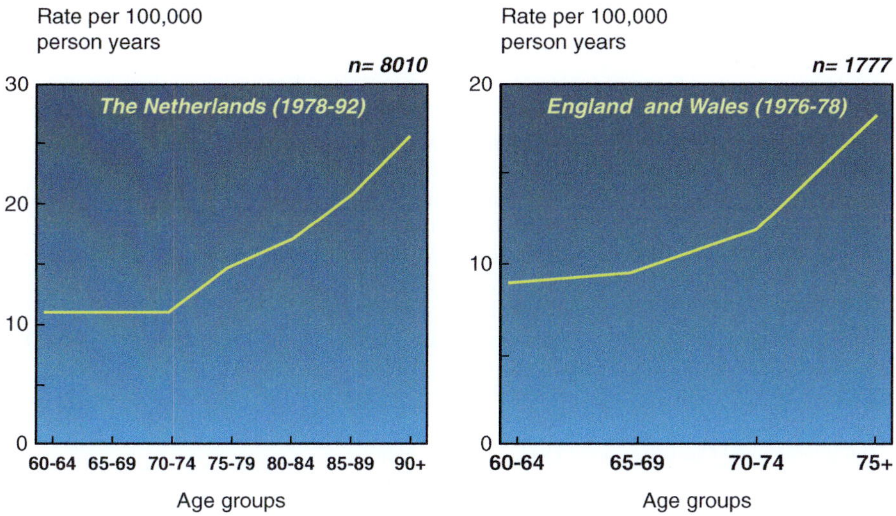

Fig. 3.2 Annual first-contact rates for non-affective psychoses in the elderly population (> 60 years); based on case-register data. Source: van Os et al. (1995), modified

to increase, attaining values in very old age similar to the first-admission rates in younger age groups (Fig. 3.2).

This age distribution prompts the question of whether schizophrenia beginning at a young age and delusional disorder manifesting later in life are the same or two discrete disorders. A further question is whether old age influences a uniform, age-dependent disease process, its aetiology, presentation and consequences to the degree that late-onset schizophrenia becomes perforce distinct from the early-onset schizophrenia of adolescence and early adulthood (see also Castle et al. 1997; Howard et al. 2000; Orr and Castle 2003; Vahia et al. 2010; Howard and Jeste 2011; Maglione et al. 2014; Cohen et al. 2015).

Table 3.1 lists four selected European studies published between 1913 and 1993 that reported percentages of first admissions for schizophrenia and paranoid psychosis beyond the age of 40 years. These studies, ranging from Kraepelin's (1913) analyses to the Camberwell case-register study (Castle and Murray 1993; Howard et al. 1993; Castle et al. 1998), unmistakably show how the percentage of schizophrenia diagnosed in old and very old age rises from study to study. The simultaneous increase in the proportion of the elderly in the populations studied does not fully explain the rise in the frequency of late-onset schizophrenia.

Discussing these phenomena, Lubman and Castle (2002) listed the main risk factors and characteristics of schizophrenia manifesting beyond the age of 60 years: a family history of schizophrenia, although the familial risk in this age span is lower than in early-onset patients (Castle et al. 1998); sensory deficits, especially accumulating hearing and vision loss (in part correctable by hearing aids and spectacles); social isolation; premorbid personality disorder, especially the propensity to be reclusive and suspicious; cognitive deficits similar to those found in patients with an

Table 3.1 Percentages of patients with first admission for schizophrenia and schizophrenia-like psychosis at higher ages according to selected studies

Study, location	Sample size (n)	Sample characteristics	Age (years) >40	>45	>60	>65
Kraepelin (1913), Munich	1054	First admissions with dementia praecox	5.6		0.2	
Bleuler (1943), Zurich	300	First admissions with Bleulerian schizophrenia	15.0		4.0	
Hinterhuber (1973), Innsbruck	157	First admissions with a clinical schizophrenia diagnosis	25.0			
Castle and Murray (1993), London	470	Camberwell case register (1965–1984), schizophrenia (ICD-9: 295)		28.5		12.0

ICD-9 International Classification of Diseases, Ninth Edition

earlier illness onset, but different from the abnormalities observed in psychosis associated with dementia; and female gender (see also Häfner et al. 2001; for discussion of a further risk factor see Wium-Andersen et al. 2014).

The clinical presentation of very-late-onset schizophrenia is characterised by low rates of primary negative symptoms and formal thought disorder, frequently elaborate persecutory delusions, the "partition" delusion in particular, which makes the patients believe that other people or objects can enter their home through walls to cause them harm, and by hallucinations, which may be linked to a delusion (Lubman and Castle 2002). Pronounced social decline over the course of late-onset schizophrenia is rare, because social development and upward social mobility are no longer relevant and socioeconomic status is usually guaranteed by a state pension and/or private pension scheme (Häfner et al. 2001).

3.3 Early- and Late-Onset Schizophrenia: Are They the Same Disorder?

To settle the question of whether early-onset and late-onset schizophrenia are the same disorder, a representative and sufficiently large sample of first-episode cases of schizophrenia spectrum disorder covering the entire lifespan from early youth to advanced age is needed. Our A(ge) B(eginning) C(ourse) Schizophrenia Study cohort was not appropriate to address this question because of its upper age boundary of 59 years, for we, too, had initially made the mistake of limiting the cohort's age. Instead, we explored the age distribution of symptoms in another sample of 1109 consecutive first admissions, not limited by age, to the Central Institute of Mental Health in Mannheim, Germany, for a diagnosis of schizophrenia (Häfner et al. 1998b, 2001). We compared symptomatology on the basis of 5-year age groups across the total life cycle.

Figure 3.3 illustrates prevalence rates of clearly and significantly age-dependent symptoms for men and women across the entire age range: (1) systematised

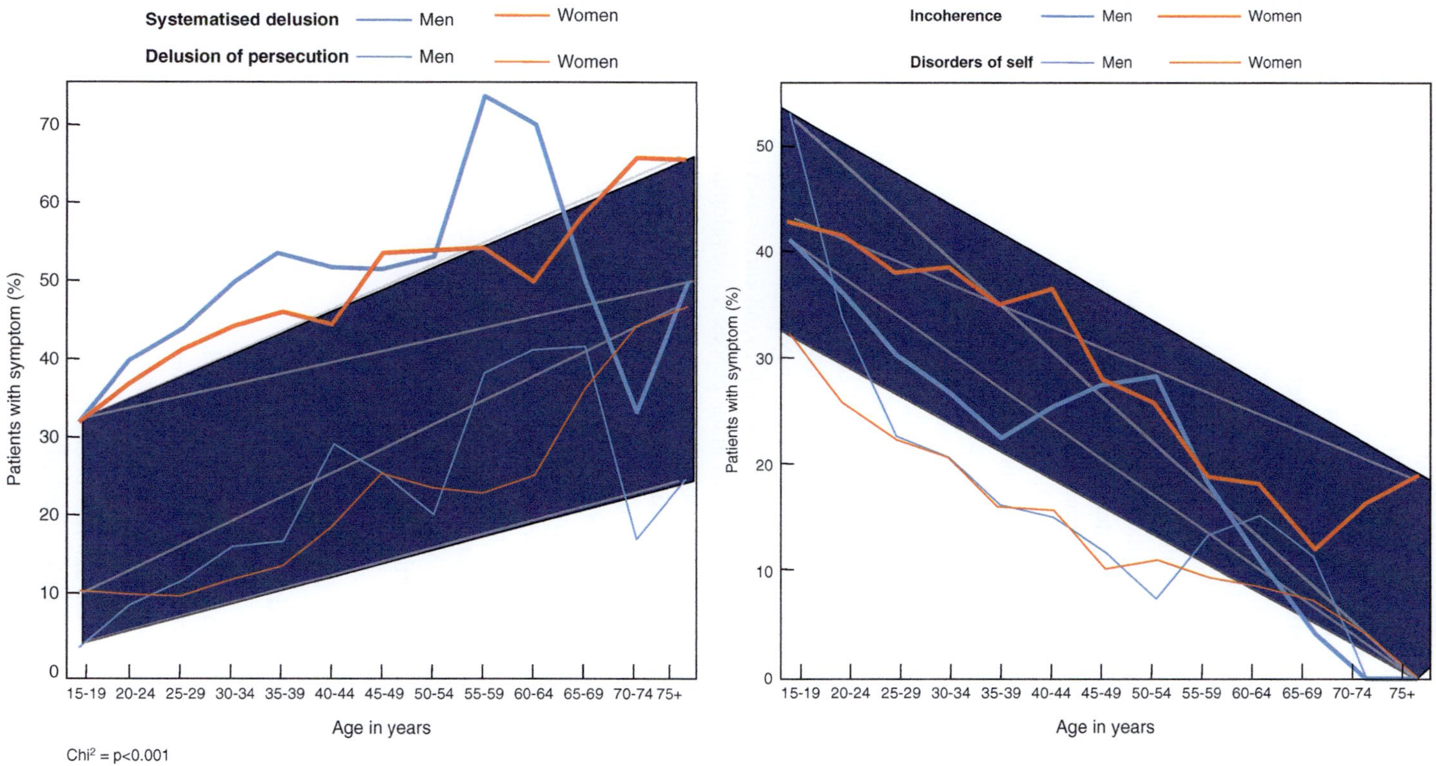

Fig. 3.3 Psychotic symptoms showing significant age trends; based on data from CIMH patient records ($n = 1109$). Source: Häfner et al. (2006). *CIMH* Central Institute of Mental Health

delusions and delusions of persecution; and (2) incoherence and disorders of the self. The picture is remarkable: while all the other symptoms, including most of the Schneiderian first-rank symptoms, exhibited no significant age differences in frequency, only those four depicted in Fig. 3.2 were markedly age-dependent. The prevalence of systematised and paranoid delusions showed a significant, linear increase from low levels in young age groups to a very high level in the oldest group, that of systematised delusions by as much as six-fold (cf. Mason et al. 2013). Incoherence and disorders of the self fell from high prevalences in the youngest group to almost zero in the oldest group.

Systematised delusions contain a cognitive component of coping with primary symptoms. Reflected in the contents of such delusional constructs frequently is a growing tendency to externalisation, i.e. attributing unusual experiences, mishaps or feelings of guilt to outer causes.

The two aspects of delusions are probably influenced by consecutive stages of age-dependent personality development in the sense that they play either a disruptive or a stabilising role. In contrast to paranoid and systematised delusions, incoherence of thought and disordered sense of the self are signs of mental disorganisation. Resulting from incomplete brain maturation and low mental stability, these symptoms are particularly prevalent in childhood- and adolescent-onset schizophrenia (Remschmidt 2009; Eggers 2011). With growing age and increasing mental stability the syndrome shows a steady decline in frequency.

To put it in terms of developmental psychology, an early onset of psychosis hits an immature cognitive personality still in the process of development and not yet in possession of a stable enough structure of the self. This is why childhood- or adolescent-onset psychosis can easily disrupt the basic functions of self-awareness and the cognitive structures. In adult and old age, when personality, the structure of the self and cognitive functions have grown stable, disorganisation symptoms become less prominent and fairly rare. In old age, psychosis no longer has much impact either on the social course and outcome or on the integrative functions of personality. As a result, patients' symptom levels are lower and they present less mental disorganisation and more symptoms of cognitive and projective processing. Having said this, we have not yet directly contributed to analysing the consequences of AOO, but identified a methodological precondition for attaining generally valid results on the topic.

3.4 The ABC Study

Assuming that, despite a certain degree of age-related variation in symptomatology, schizophrenia is a disorder of all ages, we are faced with an unlimited age range of onsets. As a result, age strongly influences the actual state of illness and the amount of pathology, be it biological or psychological in type, as well as the consequences springing directly from the disorder or emerging as a reaction to it.

We explored the associations unfolding on various levels between AOO on the one hand and the primary, secondary and tertiary effects it has on the state and course of illness on the other hand. For this purpose, and to be able to draw generally valid conclusions, in our ABC Schizophrenia Study we studied 232 first-episode cases from a population-based, representative sample of 276 German-speaking first-admission patients aged 12–59 years and diagnosed with schizophrenia spectrum disorder. For a subsample of 130 of these first-admission cases mentally healthy age- and sex-matched controls were randomly drawn from the same population of origin and assessed using the same instruments.

Half of the first-episode sample assessed at first admission ($n = 115$) was reassessed prospectively at seven cross-sections up until the final assessment 12.3 years later and the other half only at the final assessment (an der Heiden and Häfner 2011; Häfner et al. 2013). Age at illness onset and the manifestation of prodromal symptoms were ascertained retrospectively using a multi-level time-grid. To be able to map and compare the course of illness properly and to obtain exact information on the number of relapses and frequently occurring symptoms and other signs of illness, we right-censored the interval between first admission and final assessment by the shortest interval (134 months [11.2 years]) or length of illness course. The empirical illness courses ranged in length from this value to a maximum of 14.6 years (mean 12.3 years), because some patients had to be approached several times before they consented to be interviewed again. Censoring could be performed because the instrument we used, the Interview for the Retrospective Assessment of the Onset and Course of Schizophrenia and Other Psychoses (IRAOS) (Häfner et al. 1999, 2003), allows the illness course to be mapped on a monthly basis.

3.5 Childhood- and Early-Onset Schizophrenia

In a first step we analysed whether an early AOO leads to early consequences and, if it does, what kind of consequences (cf. DeLisi 1992; Rahmati et al. 2015). Childhood onset of schizophrenia is extremely rare and seems to be associated with a particularly poor subsequent illness course (Eggers 1978, 2011; Häfner and Nowotny 1995; Eggers and Bunk 1997; Asarnow et al. 2004; Gillberg 2009; Remschmidt 2009; Hollis and Rapoport 2011; Kendhari et al. 2016; Lin et al. 2016). It affects the core symptoms, produces pronounced negative symptoms, including cognitive deficits, and has a serious impact in the social domain. Since the patients included in our ABC Study sample were at least 12 years old at first admission and one patient was actually 9 years old at illness onset, we have to rely here on results published from child and adolescent psychiatric studies (Fleischhaker et al. 2005; Clemmensen et al. 2012; Steinhausen 2013; Díaz-Caneja et al. 2015) and confine ourselves to concluding that a very early AOO tends to be associated with more severe symptomatology, whereas, as was the case in our sample, a higher AOO has a less detrimental impact on the patients' lives.

Asarnow (1988) reviewed 24 high-risk studies, most of which examined children who had a biological parent diagnosed with schizophrenia, and three were based on samples characterised by behavioural abnormalities indicative of the probands being at risk for schizophrenia. The studies differed in their specifications and quality. Irrespective of their heterogeneity and methodological shortcomings and the resulting differences in the results reported, the studies showed that high-risk children and adolescents tend to show signs of neurointegrative problems, social impairments and early symptoms (especially in middle childhood and adolescence), and deficits in attention and information processing, neuromotor function and social behaviour. Strong evidence also emerged that a family environment characterised by communication deviance, a negative affective style, high expressed emotion and a general disturbance are associated with an increased risk of schizophrenia onset (Asarnow 1988).

In an overview of their studies into childhood-onset schizophrenia based on a sample of 21 patients aged 7–14 years (illness onset 6–11 years) and followed up over a period of 2–7 years ($n = 18$), Asarnow et al. (1994) came to the conclusion that childhood- and later-onset schizophrenia are representations of the same illness. Their data showed that childhood-onset schizophrenia was associated with severe dysfunction and was diagnosable by the same criteria as adult-onset illness. The majority of the sample continued to show symptoms of schizophrenia as they progressed through adolescence, but outcome varied a lot with 56% showing improvement in functioning during the follow-up period and 44% a slightly improved or deteriorating course. Some intrafamilial attributes associated with adult schizophrenia were also found to be associated with schizophrenia in children, but the family environmental correlates differed to some extent between childhood- and later-onset schizophrenia.

Because of the special nature of early-onset schizophrenia, it has become common to distinguish between very-early-onset (< 13 years), early-onset (< 18 years) (Clemmensen et al. 2012, cf. also Lin et al. 2016), late-onset (≥ 40 years) and very-late-onset (> 60 years) schizophrenia (Howard et al. 2000; cf. also Riecher-Rössler et al. 1995, 2003) in clinical terms. These subcategories of schizophrenia, based on age boundaries that tend to vary, differ not only in terms of their symptomatology (e.g. Rajji et al. 2009) and the consequences they lead to, but also in the relevant risk factors.

3.6 Sex Difference in AOO of Schizophrenia

One of the most interesting distinguishing features is the sex difference in the AOO of this disorder. Men are an average of 4.0 years younger than women at first admission (Häfner et al. 1995). This is basically what Emil Kraepelin (1909–1915) had observed already, reporting that women falling ill with schizophrenia tend to be several years older than men at first admission. The finding has since been confirmed several times. For example, Angermeyer and Kühn (1988) in their review of 53 studies on the topic found that 48 of these studies reported a higher age for women than men at first admission. A fundamental question arising in this context is whether it is only age at first admission or perhaps also age at illness onset that differs between the sexes. Angermeyer and Kühn (1988) found that to be the case in only three of the studies included in their analysis.

A direct, prospective assessment of a schizophrenia onset is difficult (i) due to the rarity of the disorder and (ii) to the uncharacteristic nature of the symptoms that illness onset usually occurs with. For this reason we chose a retrospective approach in our ABC Study and assessed AOO in cases already diagnosed with schizophrenia. In the meantime, a few epidemiological studies conducted mainly in the Netherlands, Germany and Great Britain have assessed initial symptoms of incipient schizophrenia prospectively in defined populations (Klosterkötter et al. 2001; Hanssen et al. 2005; van Os et al. 2009; Allardyce and van Os 2010; Dominguez et al. 2011; Yung et al. 2006).

In order to gain reliable information on the onset, initial symptoms and prodromal stage of schizophrenia in our ABC Study, we compiled the IRAOS (Häfner et al. 1999, 2003) on the basis of both existing and internationally tried and tested interview instruments and our own tools and findings. Besides conducting internal validity tests, we also interviewed the significant others of our schizophrenia sample and additionally included in our analyses information drawn from the patients' medical records, school reports and so on. In this way we obtained a highly comprehensive and reliable database to study the onset of schizophrenia and related questions.

The results from the validity tests are depicted in Fig. 3.4, which shows that the mean age at first admission was 28.2 years for men and 32.2 years for women. Age at the maximum of psychotic symptoms, i.e. the climax of the first illness episode, was 27.8 years for men and 32.1 years for women, a difference of 4.3 years. At the

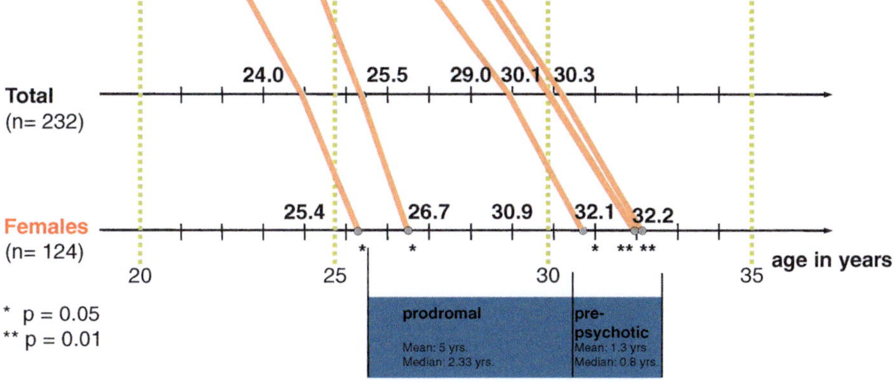

Fig. 3.4 Mean age by 5 definitions of onset until first admission; ABC Study first-episode sample of broadly defined schizophrenia ($n = 232$). Source: Häfner and Gattaz (1995), modified

appearance of the first negative symptom there was a sex difference of 2.6 years and at the appearance of the first sign of illness (illness onset) there was a difference of 2.9 years. What is astonishing about this result is that the sex difference did not emerge gradually with the evolving disorder as a result of the biological disease process interacting with environmental factors, but was already fully there at illness onset. This result strongly indicates that the explanation for the sex difference at illness onset should be looked for in biological factors.

But first we have to establish whether the size of the correlation between AOO and sex in schizophrenia is unique to the German population or a universal phenomenon to be found in all populations and countries. To address this difficult question and to test it as reliably as possible, in cooperation with Sartorius we analysed data from the WHO ten-country study (DOSMeD) (Sartorius et al. 1986; Jablensky et al. 1992). Included in that WHO study were four study sites in developing countries (Agra/India, Chandigarh/India, Cali/Columbia and Ibadan/Nigeria) and seven sites in developed countries (Aarhus/Denmark, Moscow/USSR, Honolulu/USA, Prague/Czech and Slovak Federal Republic, Nagasaki/Japan, Nottingham/England and Dublin/Ireland). We found a 3.4-year higher first-contact age for women than men, which confirmed what we had found based on the German data (Hambrecht et al. 1992a) (Fig. 3.5). The age difference was of about the same size across the study sites. Exceptions to this, for example hardly any difference in Nottingham, turned out mainly to be attributable to shortcomings of data collection and/or

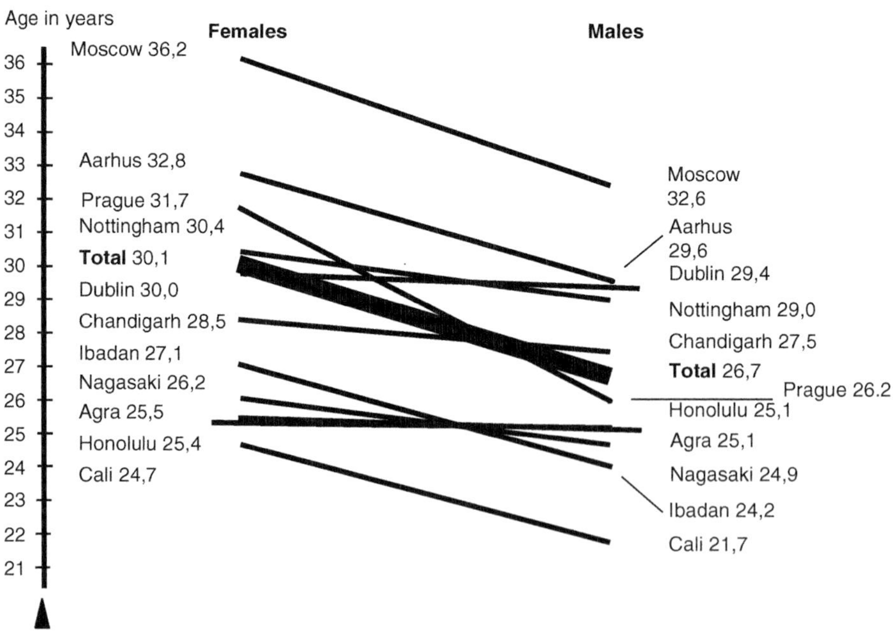

Fig. 3.5 WHO Determinants of Outcome Study: mean ages at onset in the centres and the total sample (n = 1292). Source: Hambrecht et al. (1992a). *WHO* World Health Organization

methodological flaws. A cautious interpretation of these results strongly suggests that sound study designs are bound to yield fairly similar sex differences in schizophrenia AOO all over the world.

A recent British meta-analysis (Eranti et al. 2013) based on 46 newer epidemiological studies on the topic also found a significant, but smaller, sex difference of about 1 year in age at first admission, with males showing an earlier onset. The sex difference in AOO turned out to be greater in studies using the DSM criteria than in studies based on the *International Classification of Diseases* (ICD) criteria. In the latter the difference was non-significant. A sex difference also emerged for developing countries and turned out not to be significantly different in size from the one the authors found for developed countries. Three studies included in the analysis from developing countries (two from India and one from Ethiopia) had in fact reported an earlier age at onset in women than men and one study from India no sex difference at all. However, a closer look at these studies showed that they, especially those conducted in India, were marred by considerable methodological flaws, so their results cannot be considered sound. This fact and the heterogeneity of the studies from developing countries in general call into question the quality of the meta-analysis as such.

A few further studies on the ubiquitous nature of the sex difference in AOO exist (e.g. Hambrecht et al. 1992b; Messias et al. 2007; Ochoa et al. 2012; Morgan et al. 2016). Besides socioeconomic and socio-geographical factors, the influence of latitude has also been discussed (e.g. Shaner et al. 2007), but those analyses, too, fail to yield conclusive results.

Since it seems at least highly reasonable to assume that women are 3–4 years older than men throughout the milestones of incipient schizophrenia, while these milestones follow a fairly parallel course in both men and women, we are faced with the question: what are the biological causes behind this fundamental difference?

3.6.1 Search for the Causes of Sex Difference in the AOO of Schizophrenia

Looking for an answer, we first studied the age distribution of schizophrenia onsets over the life cycle in men and women. We found that the incidence of schizophrenia increases steeply from puberty, i.e. age 12 years in males, with rare onsets occurring before that age, reaches a maximum at age 15–25 years, and subsequently shows a steady decrease until age 40 years to low values, which persist for the rest of the lifespan (Fig. 3.1).

In women the increase in schizophrenia onsets sets in somewhat later, produces a first peak between 15 and 30 years of age and, subsequently, as was the case with male onsets, turns into a continuous decrease, which lasts until age 45–50 years. That age group, which largely coincides with the beginning of menopause, shows a second, lower peak of schizophrenia onsets that is significantly different from male onsets in that age group. After that age female onsets, too, decrease continuously to a permanently low level. After age 55 years incidence rates for both men and women show a plateau.

These age distributions gave us a hint of what might be the underlying cause of the sex difference in AOO, and it is apparently concentrated around the age of beginning menopause.

The Danish case register data on first admissions for schizophrenia over the entire life cycle gave us an opportunity to compare the age distributions. Both the Danish and the Mannheim data yielded a significant sex difference of 4–6 years in age at first admission. The second, lower peak of female onsets emerged in the Danish data also, only an age group later than in Mannheim, i.e. at age 50–55 years (Häfner et al. 1989, 1994; Riecher et al. 1990). Looking for an explanation for the age difference between men and women, we first tested social hypotheses: one explanation might have been that the onset of schizophrenia was perceived later in non-working women in their domestic settings than in men, most of whom went out to work before the initial examination. However, a comparison between working and non-working women using the Mannheim data yielded no difference in age of first admission, whereas both categories of women showed a significant age difference of several years to men (Häfner et al. 1989).

Another hypothesis we tested to explain this unexpected difference was that the Danish women entered menopause at a later age on average than the German women. For this purpose, in cooperation with our Danish colleagues we drew from the Danish case register a representative sample of patients diagnosed with schizophrenia and obtained their hospital records with the consent of the Danish authorities (Häfner et al. 1989; Löffler et al. 1994; cf. also Lützhoft et al. 1995). Using a case note version of the IRAOS we assessed symptoms and age at the first instance of fulfilling the ICD-8 criteria for a diagnosis of schizophrenia. Hence, we had identical definitions of AOO based not only on hospital admission for both sets of case register data, i.e. from Aarhus and Mannheim. The result was surprising: while in Denmark 51% of the men who, on the basis of their symptoms, were clearly classifiable as cases of schizophrenia had actually received that diagnosis at first admission, the corresponding figure for women was only 32%. Danish psychiatrists, who in those days were overwhelmingly men, were apparently less inclined to give their newly admitted female patients the distressing diagnosis of schizophrenia than they were to their male patients (see also Munk-Jörgensen 1985). Instead, they preferred milder and fuzzier diagnoses such as paranoid states, acute paranoid reactions, psychogenic psychosis or borderline. If an objective definition was used, the difference from German women disappeared and the second peak of schizophrenia onsets fell in the age group 45–50 years—the same as in Mannheim.

Now we were ready to test where the sex difference in age of schizophrenia onset actually stemmed from. The way male and female onsets were distributed across the age range, especially the protracted increase at younger age and the second peak at menopausal age in women, suggested that there had to be some kind of protective factor at work that became clearly weaker when women entered menopause and which in some women was capable of delaying the onset of schizophrenia until that point. An alternative explanation would have been that some accelerating factor caused men to fall ill earlier. We tested both hypotheses.

The lower frequency and lower first peak of female onsets, we presumed, might be attributable to oestrogen secretion, which increases in puberty and decreases when menopause sets in. Women's second peak of onsets and markedly higher incidence rates in the second half of life than men's might result from the fact that those women with an elevated genetic load of schizophrenia who in the first half of life used to be protected against the disorder now fall ill when the protective effect of oestrogen wanes.

We tested these hypotheses in animal experiments and found that oestrogen, through its antipsychotic-like effect, is capable of attenuating dopaminergic behaviour by downregulating dopamine D_2-receptor sensitivity (Häfner et al. 1991; Gattaz et al. 1992). In contrast, testosterone had no such effect in an identical test model. Hence, the oestrogen hypothesis can be seen as providing a plausible explanation for the sex difference in AOO.

The oestrogen hypothesis has since been confirmed in an experimental setting, namely through the efficacy of moderate to higher doses of oestrogen administered as an adjunct to antipsychotic therapy in first-episode psychosis and also at later stages of illness (Kulkarni et al. 2002, 2008, 2012, 2014; Akhondzadeh et al. 2003).

DeLisi et al. in 1994 and Albus and Maier in 1995 reported that co-twins and siblings diagnosed with schizophrenia showed no sex difference in AOO. This phenomenon prompted us to test whether genetic factors might be capable of antagonising the protective effect of oestrogen. We compared patients with first-episode schizophrenia who had first-degree relatives diagnosed with schizophrenia in adolescence with patients without familial schizophrenia. And, indeed, patients with familial schizophrenia showed no sex difference in AOO (Fig. 3.6) (Könnecke et al. 2000). In contrast, patients with non-familial schizophrenia exhibited a slightly elevated sex difference of 4.9 years at illness onset. We concluded from this result that the risk-enhancing genetic effect may be slightly more powerful than the risk-reducing hormonal effect.

To conclude, schizophrenia is slightly less frequent in women than men in the first half of life and more frequent in the second half. When the entire lifespan is

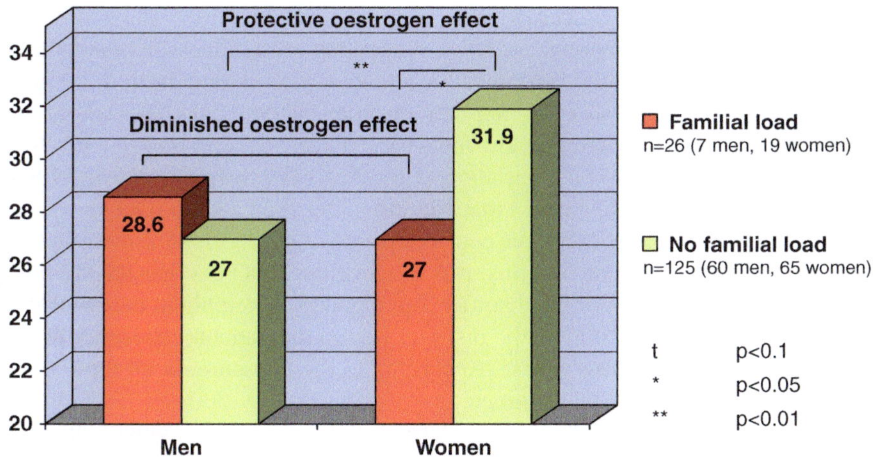

Fig. 3.6 Age at first psychotic symptom by gender and familial load; ABC Study first-episode sample of schizophrenia ($n = 232$). Source: Häfner (2003)

considered, schizophrenia is more or less equally frequent in both sexes. The sequence of milestones of incipient illness and age-related symptom presentation are also essentially the same in men and women. What is remarkable is that, as our study showed, cognitive symptoms associated with delusions, such as systematised delusional ideas and paranoid delusions, clearly increase at a higher age, while in early-onset schizophrenia they are rare (cf. Häfner and Nowotny 1995). This phenomenon has nothing to do with the sex hormone oestrogen, but reflects the normal course of personality development, which during the course of life leads to growing stability and as a result to greater resilience to disruptive pathological events.

3.7 AOO and the Clinical Picture of Schizophrenia

With growing age a familial load of schizophrenia spectrum disorder and pre-, peri- and postnatal brain damage clearly and steadily grow less important as risk factors (Könnecke et al. 2000). But this finding does not explain the reversed tendency of paranoid symptoms, which become more frequent later in life. It is probably due to the clearly greater role that genetic and environmental risk factors play in early-onset schizophrenia that these illnesses tend to be associated with more severe and diffuse pathology, such as diffuse, at times extremely severe, anxiety, fluctuating disorders of attention, severely altered perception of the self and others, elementary distortions of self-experience—such as believing that thoughts are being inserted from outside into one's mind—and confusion (cf. also Stentebjerg-Olesen et al. 2016). This type of pronounced mental disorganisation in combination with incomplete mental development or brain maturation brings forth psychopathology that affects the central areas of personality and is more severe than the psychopathology encountered in later-onset schizophrenia, which acts upon a mental structure that has attained a certain degree of stability in the course of life. This is probably the reason why at a later age the central structures and functions of personality are no longer destabilised to any greater extent.

As already stated, the rational cognitive processing of the illness by way of systematised delusions, paranoid symptoms or a tendency to externalisation, i.e. projecting one's fears and shortcomings to outside factors, can be seen as an age-appropriate way of reacting in old and very old age.

We have so far discussed the variation in the AOO of schizophrenia, and some important factors helping to explain that variation, and shown how AOO across the entire life cycle is associated with the core symptoms of psychosis. A further finding worth adding is that, in relative terms, it is the medium AOO that has the slightest influence on the symptoms of the disorder. But this does not apply to the accompanying phenomena and the impact the disorder has on the patients' lives, nor to the medium- or long-term illness course. According to the literature, in all these three respects men fare less well than women.

If this is true, and indeed the medium-term social course over 5 years following first admission has turned out to be poorer for men than women, the question arises: why is this so? An analysis based on symptom dimensions provides some initial thoughts.

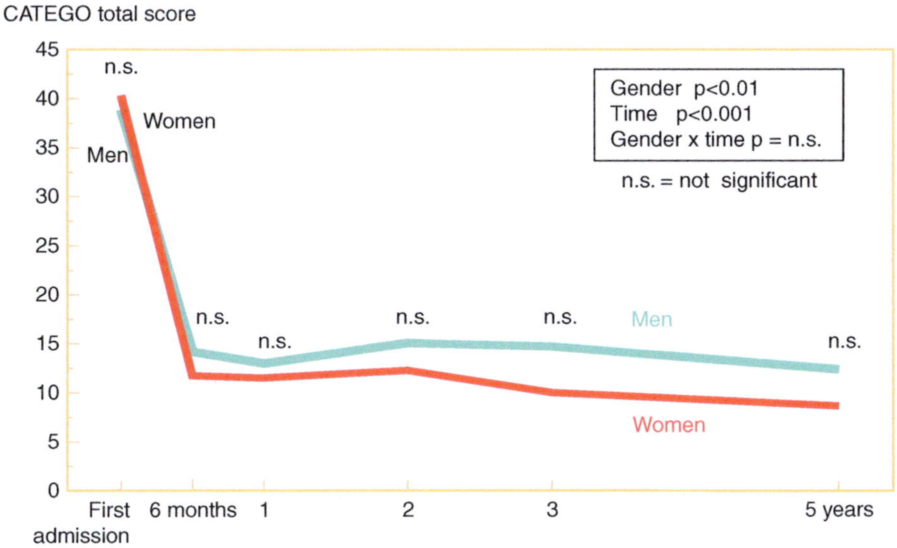

Fig. 3.7 5-Year course of schizophrenia for men and women by the CATEGO total score; ABC Study first-episode follow-up sample (n = 115). Source: Häfner (1998). *CATEGO*: a computer programme for processing Present State Examination data

In the ABC Schizophrenia Study, a representative sample of 115 patients, whose early illness course back to illness onset had been assessed retrospectively at first admission, was re-assessed prospectively 0.5, 1, 2, 3 and 5 years after first admission. As Fig. 3.7 shows, no significant sex difference emerged in the prevalence of positive symptoms typical of the disorder. In view of these results, we concluded that most of the sex difference in the social course could probably be explained by men's younger AOO, as, compared with their female peers, men tend to be at a lower level of social development both in the first psychotic episode and throughout the preceding milestones of the prodromal stage.

Since the main AOO for schizophrenia lies between 15 and 30 years, it coincides with the main period of social development in most societies (Table 3.2). Consequently, differences in AOO or in the age at which the psychosis intrudes in patients' biographies not only have a considerable impact in the socioeconomic domain, but also result in pronounced differences between the sexes. This means that, due to the lower level of social development at illness onset, men's lower age at this point becomes associated with a markedly poorer social course and outcome at least over and after the first few years following this event. This is impressively illustrated by the age of marrying or entering a stable partnership (Fig. 3.8). As Fig. 3.8 shows, the percentages of men—either healthy or suffering from schizophrenia—who are married or in a stable partnership are significantly lower than the corresponding figures for women, who in either category are significantly younger when attaining this milestone (see also Pang et al. 2016). Over the early illness course up until first admission the proportion of married individuals increases steadily among healthy men, while among patients diagnosed with schizophrenia, both male and

Table 3.2 Social-role performance at the emergence of the first sign of mental disorder; ABC Study first-episode sample ($n = 232$) (Source: Häfner 1995)

	Men ($n = 108$)		Women ($n = 124$)	Total ($n = 232$)
Age (years)	22.5		25.4	24.0
School education (%)	70		69	70
Occupational training (%)	41	NS	38	39
Employment (%)	37	*	52	45
Own income (%)	44	NS	55	50
Own accommodation (%)	39	*	54	47
Marriage or stable partnership (%)	28	**	52	41

NS not significant, * $p \leq 0.05$, ** $p \leq 0.01$

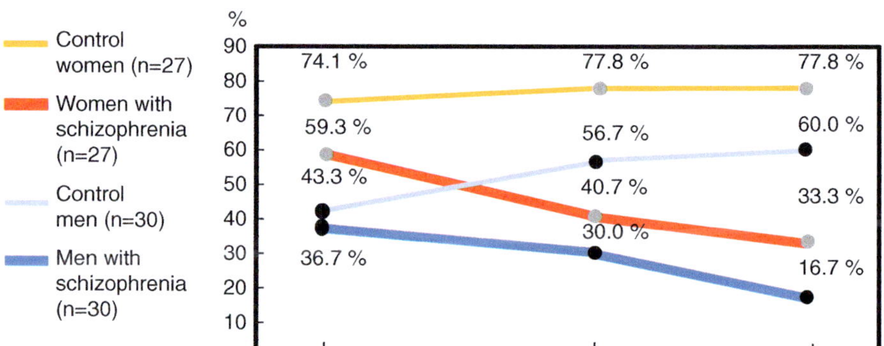

	1st sign	1st psychotic symptom	1st admission
Mean age	24 years	29 years	30 years
Schizo. vs. controls		**	**
Schizo. men vs. women	t		t
Control men vs. women	*	t	t
Schizo. men vs. control men		t	**
Schizo. women vs. control women		**	**

Comparison of means

** = p≤0.01; * = p ≤0.05; t = p ≤0.10

Fig. 3.8 Marriage or stable partnership. Source: Häfner (1996)

female, it shows a steady decline, thus resulting in significant differences between patients and their healthy peers of either sex at the age of first admission.

But, as our analysis showed, the sex difference in AOO turned out not to be the only factor contributing to the finding that men fared less well than women in terms of the medium-term social course. A further highly significant and considerable sex difference operating in that same direction emerged when we compared "normal" social behaviour between young men and women. A comparison of selected behavioural items at first admission in our sample showed that the following nine socially negative items were significantly more frequent among male than female patients: self-neglect, lack of interest in work, poor hygiene, social inattentiveness, reduced

Table 3.3 Behavioural items with significant sex differences (from a total of 303 PSE, PIRS, SANS, DAS and IRAOS items)*; ABC Study first-episode sample ($n = 232$) (Source: Häfner 1998)

More frequent in women	More frequent in men
(a) Cumulative until first admission	
Restlessness	Drug abuse Alcohol abuse
(b) Cross-sectional: at first admission	
Overadaptiveness/conformity	Self-neglect Reduced interest in a job Social inattentiveness Deficits of free-time activities Deficits of communication Social disability (overall estimate) Loss of interests Deficits of personal hygiene

PSE Present State Examination; *PIRS* Psychological Impairments Rating Schedule; *SANS* Scale for the Assessment of Negative Symptoms; *DAS* Disability Assessment Schedule; *IRAOS* Interview for the Retrospective Assessment of the Onset and Course of Schizophrenia and Other Psychoses
*Validated by split-half method for α-correction

leisure activities, deficits in communication, social impairment (global estimate), lack of interests, and frequent alcohol and substance abuse (Table 3.3).

In contrast to these socially very negative behaviours typical of young men with schizophrenia, female patients did not show any pronounced type of socially adverse behaviour, but rather two behavioural items indicative of social adjustment and adaptability, namely overadaptiveness and conformity (Table 3.3).

Since socially adverse illness behaviour tends to be associated with poor therapy adherence, it is reasonable to expect that it will have a detrimental effect on the further social course among male patients, while among females the opposite could be the case. This further hypothesis is still awaiting confirmation.

Looking for the factors explaining this substantial sex difference in behaviour in general, and apparently also in illness behaviour, we should take a look at findings from epidemiological population studies. Indeed, population studies conducted on this topic in developed countries have reported elevated rates of externalising behaviour for males in adolescence and early adulthood, namely asociality, aggressiveness, poor impulse control, and alcohol and substance abuse (Choquet and Ledoux 1994; Döpfner et al. 1997). With growing age, dissocial and aggressive behaviours become clearly less frequent in men and are more or less gone in the second half of life (Fig. 3.9). This normal biological development is of great importance in schizophrenia. As a result, not only does the long-term illness course in male and female patients tend to converge in the core symptoms of the disorder, but also the social course becomes more similar.

To analyse in greater detail how AOO influences the medium-term social course, we divided our sample into three age groups by age at first admission: 12–20, 21–35 and 36–59 years. To measure the patients' socioeconomic status or level of social adaptation we chose as a criterion the ability to earn one's own living. Depicted in Fig. 3.10 are the main stages of early and medium-term illness course. As expected, the oldest group attains the highest socioeconomic status by illness onset and

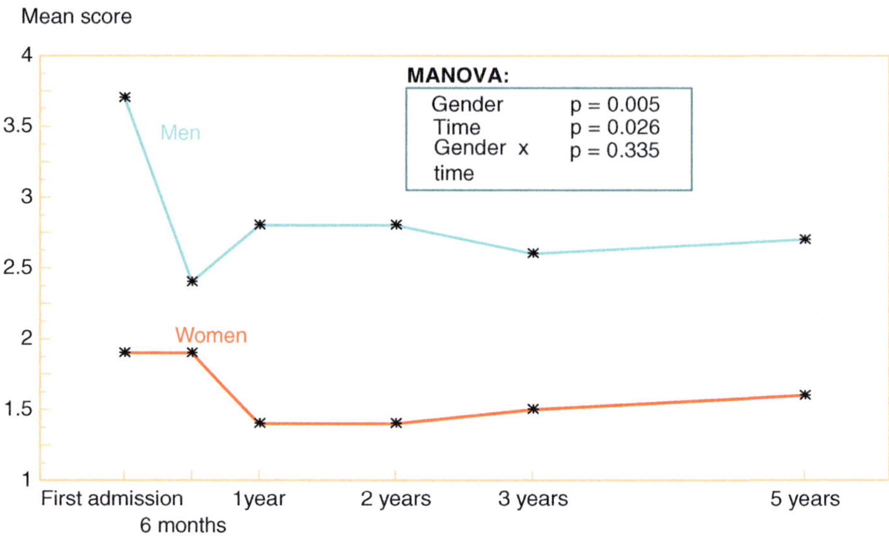

Fig. 3.9 Socially negative behaviour over 5 years after first admission for schizophrenia by sex; ABC Study first-episode follow-up sample ($n = 115$). Source: Häfner et al. (1998c)

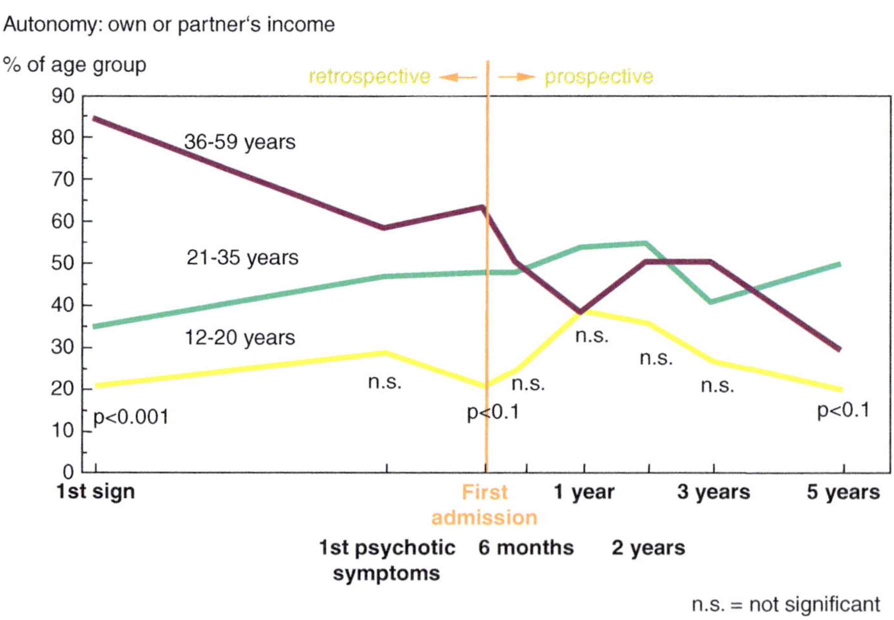

Fig. 3.10 Social course: financial independence; ABC Study follow-up sample ($n = 115$). Source: Häfner et al. (1998b)

consequently also suffers the most pronounced social decline. In contrast, the youngest group, impeded in its social ascent by an early illness onset, does not experience any substantial social decline but rather a kind of social stagnation. The intermediate group, which covers an age period from early adulthood to middle age, occupies a position in between the two extreme groups. This means that, depending on AOO, the medium-term course of schizophrenia is associated either with social decline or with social stagnation.

3.8 AOO and Other Variables Shaping the Course of Schizophrenia

After it had become clear that the medium-term course of the complex disease process called schizophrenia is determined by a variety of factors, we set out to analyse how age, sex and level of social development at illness onset on the one hand and socially adverse illness behaviour on the other hand interact and in doing so shape the medium-term social course. Again, the outcome criterion we chose was the ability to earn one's own living. Adopting path analysis and subsequent stepwise logistic regression we discovered a clear pattern of interaction (Fig. 3.11): patients' socioeconomic status assessed 5 years after first admission and the medium-term social course over that period depended significantly on gender, but the effect came about indirectly via the level of social development at illness onset. But this effect of age of illness onset on social outcome, too, is mediated by the level of social development attained when the first sign of illness and the first psychotic symptom

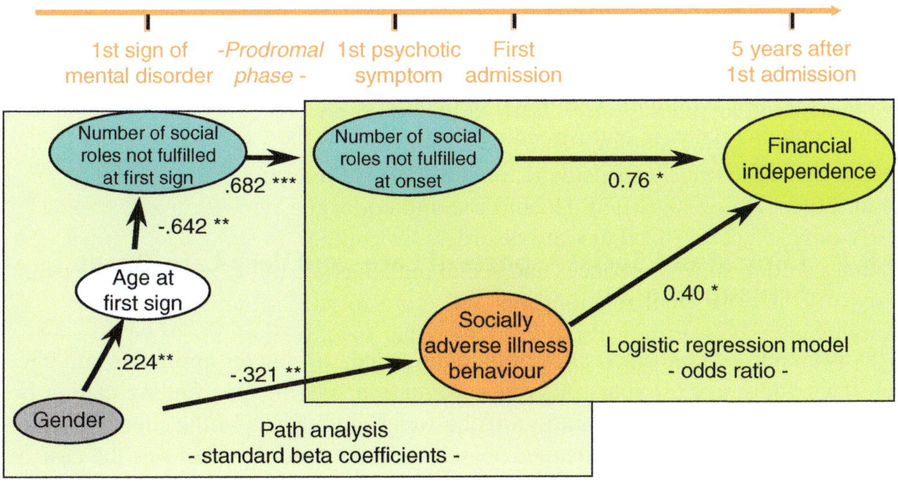

Fig. 3.11 Prediction of 5-year social outcome in schizophrenia: analysis of direct and mediating causal factors; ABC Study first-episode follow-up sample ($n = 115$). Source: Häfner (2000)

manifest. Gender, we found, also influences social outcome directly, namely through men's socially adverse illness behaviour. In old age, these associations become altered, and we come back to these in Sect. 3.8.1.

To conclude, AOO appears to be a polyvalent indicator that provides fundamental access to understanding what is going on in the disorder when other relevant factors are taken into account.

As the above-discussed analyses of the medium-term social course of schizophrenia showed, the disease process as such, i.e. the course of patients' lives and the clinical course of the disorder, is determined by a variety of interacting factors. At the core of this process undoubtedly lies the biologically determined pathology, such as genuine positive symptoms not developed or modified as a way of coping with the disorder. Age and gender, too, must be counted as part of this underlying core biological process and, thus, of the disorder. However, the impact they have is not an isolated one, but is essentially modified in interaction with the personal and social development and the cultural environment. We therefore discuss in the Sect. 3.8.1 whether fundamentally different cultural settings produce other types of social course, perhaps depending on age and gender. In short, social aspects of AOO essentially influence the social course of schizophrenia, except perhaps for childhood-onset and very-late-onset cases.

In our ABC Schizophrenia Study, we assessed first-admission patients with schizophrenia in the age range 12–59 years. We compared three age bands with each other and found that the frequency of hallucinations did not differ significantly between the age groups. In contrast, social course showed marked differences, namely social stagnation in the youngest group, pronounced social decline in the oldest and weak to medium-sized decline in the intermediate group. The factors causing these clear-cut age trends are not to be found in the age-related course of the disorder as such, but in the different socioeconomic starting conditions typical of these age groups. In short, a high socioeconomic status harbours a considerable risk of social decline, while the likelihood of decline associated with a particularly low socioeconomic status is correspondingly smaller, but the expected, normal social ascent is impeded.

3.8.1 Clinical and Social Aspects of Late- and Very-Late-Onset Schizophrenia

This principle of continuous developmental trends no longer applies in old age, i.e. from about age 60 years on, when stagnation sets in. This finding cannot be explained by a sudden termination of the functional trends in the illness course, but rather is attributable to changed socioeconomic conditions, as was the case at a younger age. The risk of experiencing social decline at this later age becomes considerably smaller in Western societies when the majority of the working population enters retirement age and starts to receive an old-age pension or some other type of retirement income. Another aspect of life, namely that of marital status, despite a general trend of decreasing proportions of the populations being married in our culture, still tends to be fairly stable at this age when long-lasting relationships are no longer readily shattered. The socially adverse behaviour typical of young males, a further detrimental effect acting upon the social course of schizophrenia, is long gone at old age. A further characteristic of the disorder at this age, though difficult to measure, is that a mature personality is no longer easily upset and, hence, tends to be spared the experience of such extreme phenomena as severe affective arousal.

Conclusions

The conclusion we can draw from the findings discussed in this chapter is that paranoid symptoms show the highest frequency in late- and very-late-onset schizophrenia spectrum disorder, but that no significant increase in the prevalence of characteristics directly determining the social course occur, such as negative symptoms and pronounced cognitive impairment. An important aspect in this context is that symptomatology may become masked by incipient cognitive decline of different aetiology, such as Alzheimer's disease. The social course is clearly more favourable in late-onset schizophrenia than in early-onset illness, associated as the latter is with a poor illness course in males in particular, or in adolescent-onset and early-adult-onset schizophrenia. In epidemiological terms, late-onset schizophrenia is almost equally prevalent in men and women.

The considerably more favourable social course of late-onset schizophrenia, which can remain free of any major social consequences, is first and foremost a result of the prevailing social conditions in old and very old age. Here a distinction must be made between state and private provisions for retirement and healthcare. Most European countries have comprehensive pension schemes in place. In addition, the prevailing cultural tendencies on the individual level, for example an aspiration to protect and secure one's property and maintain long-standing relationships, have an equally stabilising effect. As a consequence, the social course of late-onset schizophrenia largely depends on the prevailing socioeconomic environment. In contrast, in countries where people in old age are left to scrape a living without any substantial collective or individual socioeconomic security, the social course and outcome of late-onset schizophrenia tends to be the poorest.

This conclusion is confirmed by the results of the Long-Term Chengdu Follow-Up Study, which studied the course of schizophrenia over 14 years in rural China (Ran et al. 2003, 2011, 2015a, b). Since AOO has come to be seen as one of the most important characteristics of schizophrenia (DeLisi 1992), the authors studied 489 persons from an initial sample of 123,572 persons aged 15 years and older in Xinjin County, Chengdu, People's Republic of China from 1994 to 2008 primarily on the basis of a household survey (Ran et al. 2003, 2015a, b). The sample size was large enough to produce valid results. Psychiatric interviews and patient data were additionally collected from hospitals and traditional healers, and for deceased individuals death certificates were obtained, so the data both on the study population and the illness course can be regarded as reliable. In contrast with a majority of epidemiological studies from high-income countries offering more or less ample social security schemes for retirees, the study showed that early-onset psychosis had a more favourable social course than late-onset schizophrenia. Early-onset patients fared better than late-onset patients in terms of functional and occupational outcome. The main factors the authors cite as explaining this finding regarding the social outcome of late-onset schizophrenia were supportive measures offered by the family, community and healthcare institutions, which of course were mostly individual and private in nature and hence differed highly in availability. The authors conclude from their findings that more occupational therapy and support by social workers and generally more age-specific cultural interventions are needed. For obvious reasons they refrain from calling for a political decision to establish a system of social security including a retirement scheme, which would be impossible to implement in a short time. Instead, they call for interventions promoting the individual and social functioning of late-onset patients (Ran et al. 2003, 2015a, b). The authors are aware that their results do not apply to high-income countries. Consequently, the course of schizophrenia with onset in old age depends not only on the intensity of the biological disease process, but also on the familial and the sociopolitical environment.

References

Akhondzadeh S, Nejatisafa AA, Amini H, Mohammadi MR, Rarijani B, Kashani L, et al. Adjunctive estrogen treatment in women with chronic schizophrenia: a double-blind, randomized, and placebo-controlled trial. Prog Neuropsychopharmacol Biol Psychiatry. 2003;27:1007–12.

Albus M, Maier W. Lack of gender differences in age at onset in familial schizophrenia. Schizophr Res. 1995;18:51–9.

Allardyce J, van Os J. The natural history of the course and outcome of schizophrenia. In: Gattaz WF, Busatto G, editors. Advances in schizophrenia research 2009. New York: Springer; 2010. p. 51–66.

an der Heiden W, Häfner H. Course and outcome. In: Weinberger D, Harrison P, editors. Schizophrenia. 3rd ed. Oxford: Blackwell; 2011. p. 104–41.

Angermeyer MC, Kühn L. Gender differences in age at onset of schizophrenia. Eur Arch Psychiatry Neurol Sci. 1988;237:351–64.

APA—American Psychiatric Association. Diagnostic and statistical manual of mental disorders. 3rd ed. Washington, DC: American Psychiatric Press; 1980.

Asarnow JR. Children at risk for schizophrenia. Converging lines of evidence. Schizophr Bull. 1988;14:613–31.

Asarnow JR, Tompson MC, Goldstein MJ. Childhood-onset schizophrenia: a followup study. Schizophr Bull. 1994;20:599–617.

Asarnow JR, Tompson MC, McGrath EP. Annotation: childhood-onset schizophrenia: clinical and treatment issues. J Child Psychol Psychiatry. 2004;45:180–94.

Bleuler E. Dementia praecox oder Gruppe der Schizophrenien. In: Aschaffenburg G, editor. Handbuch der Psychiatrie. Leipzig: Deuticke; 1911. p. 1–420.

Bleuler M. Die spätschizophrenen Krankheitsbilder. Fortschr Neurol Psychiat. 1943;15:259–90.

Castle DJ, Murray RM. The epidemiology of late-onset schizophrenia. Schizophr Bull. 1993;4:691–9.

Castle DJ, Wessely S, Howard R, Murray RM. Schizophrenia with onset at the extremes of adult life. Int J Geriatr Psychiatry. 1997;12:712–7.

Castle DJ, Wessely S, van Os J, Murray RM. Psychosis in the inner city. East Sussex: Psychology Press; 1998.
Choquet M, Ledoux S. Epidémiologie et adolescence. Confrontations psychiatriques. 1994;27(35):287–309.
Clemmensen L, Lammers Vernal D, Steinhausen H-C. A systematic review of the long-term outcome of early onset schizophrenia. BMC Psychiatry. 2012;12:150.
Cohen CI, Meesters PD, Zhao J. New perspectives on schizophrenia in later life: implications for treatment, policy and research. Lancet Psychiatry. 2015;2:340–50.
DeLisi LE. The significance of age of onset for schizophrenia. Schizophr Bull. 1992;18:209–15.
DeLisi LE, Bass N, Boccio A, Shilds G, Morganti C, Vita A. Age of onset in familial schizophrenia. Arch Gen Psychiatry. 1994;51:334–5.
Díaz-Caneja CM, Pina-Camacho L, Rodríguez-Quiroga A, Fraguas D, Parellada M, Arango C. Predictors of outcome in early-onset psychosis: a systematic review. NPJ Schizophr. 2015; https://doi.org/10.1038/npjschz.2014.5.
Dominguez MD, Wichers M, Lieb R, Wittchen H-U, van Os J. Evidence that onset of clinical psychosis is an outcome of progressively more persistent subclinical psychotic experiences: an 8-year cohort study. Schizophr Bull. 2011;37:84–93.
Döpfner M, Pluck J, Berner W, Fegert JM, Huss M, Lenz K, et al. Psychische Auffälligkeiten von Kindern und Jugendlichen in Deutschland – Ergebnisse einer repräsentativen Studie: Methodik, Alters-, Geschlechts- und Beurteilereffekte (Mental disturbances in children and adolescents in Germany. Results of a representative study: age, gender and rater effects). Z Kinder Jugendpsychiatr Psychother. 1997;25:218–33.
Eggers C. Course and prognosis of childhood schizophrenia. J Autism Child Schizophr. 1978;1:21–35.
Eggers C. Schizophrenie des Kindes- und Jugendalters. Berlin: MWV Medizinisch Wissenschaftliche Verlagsgesellschaft; 2011.
Eggers C, Bunk D. The long-term course of childhood-onset schizophrenia: a 42-year follow-up. Schizophr Bull. 1997;23:105–17.
Eranti SV, MacCabe JH, Bundy H, Murray RM. Gender difference in age at onset of schizophrenia: a meta-analysis. Psychol Med. 2013;43:155–67. https://doi.org/10.1017/S003329171200089X.
Fleischhaker C, Schulz E, Tepper K, Martin M, Hennighausen K, Remschmidt H. Long-term course of adolescent schizophrenia. Schizophr Bull. 2005;31:769–80.
Gattaz WF, Behrens S, De Vry J, Häfner H. Östradiol hemmt Dopamin-vermittelte Verhaltensweisen bei Ratten – ein Tiermodell zur Untersuchung der geschlechtsspezifischen Unterschiede bei der Schizophrenie. Fortschr Neurol Psychiatr. 1992;60:8–16.
Gillberg C. Epidemiology of early onset schizophrenia. In: Remschmidt H, editor. Schizophrenia in children and adolescents. Cambridge: Cambridge University Press; 2009. p. 43–59.
Häfner H. Epidemiology of schizophrenia. The disease model of schizophrenia in the light of current epidemiological knowledge. Eur Psychiatry. 1995;10:217–27.
Häfner H. The epidemiology of onset and early course of schizophrenia. In: Häfner H, Wolpert M, editors. New research in psychiatry. Seattle: Hogrefe & Huber; 1996. p. 33–66.
Häfner H. Ist es einzig die Krankheit? - Das Zusammenspiel zwischen Krankheit, biologischen und psychologischen Entwicklungsfaktoren im Verlauf der Schizophrenie - Nachkraepelinsche Perspektiven zum Verlauf der Schizophrenie. In: Möller H-J, Müller N, editors. Schizophrenie - Moderne Konzepte zu Diagnostik, Pathogenese und Therapie. Wien: Springer; 1998. p. 37–60.
Häfner H. Ist es alles nur die Krankheit? Neuere Ergebnisse aus der Schizophrenieforschung. (Schriften der Mathematisch-naturwissenschaftlichen Klasse der Heidelberger Akademie der Wissenschaften, Nr. 7). Berlin: Springer; 2000.
Häfner H. Gender differences in schizophrenia. Psychoneuroendocrinology. 2003;28:17–45.
Häfner H, Gattaz WF. Geschlechtsunterschiede bei der Schizophrenie. Gynäkologe. 1995;6:426–34.
Häfner H, Nowotny B. Epidemiology of early-onset schizophrenia. Eur Arch Psychiatry Clin Neurosci. 1995;245:80–92.
Häfner H, Riecher A, Maurer K, Löffler W, Munk-Jørgensen P, Strömgren E. How does gender influence age at first hospitalization for schizophrenia? A transnational case register study. Psychol Med. 1989;19:903–18.

Häfner H, Behrens S, de Vry J, Gattaz WF. Oestradiol enhances the vulnerability threshold for schizophrenia in women by an early effect on dopaminergic neurotransmission. Eur Arch Psychiatry Clin Neurosci. 1991;241:65–8.
Häfner H, Maurer K, Löffler W, Riecher-Rössler A. The influence of age and sex on the onset and early course of schizophrenia. Br J Psychiatry. 1993a;162:80–6.
Häfner H, Riecher-Rössler A, an der Heiden W, Maurer K, Fätkenheuer B, Löffler W. Generating and testing a causal explanation of the gender difference in age at first onset of schizophrenia. Psychol Med. 1993b;23:925–40.
Häfner H, Maurer K, Löffler W, Fätkenheuer B, an der Heiden W, Riecher-Rössler A, et al. The epidemiology of early schizophrenia. Influence of age and gender on onset and early course. Br J Psychiatry. 1994;164(Suppl 23):29–38.
Häfner H, Maurer K, Löffler W, Bustamante S, an der Heiden W, Riecher-Rössler A, et al. Onset and early course of schizophrenia. In: Häfner H, Gattaz WF, editors. Search for the causes of schizophrenia III. Berlin: Springer; 1995. p. 43–66.
Häfner H, Maurer K, Löffler W, an der Heiden W, Munk-Jφrgensen P, Hambrecht M, et al. The ABC schizophrenia study: a preliminary overview of the results. Soc Psychiatry Psychiatr Epidemiol. 1998a;3:380–6.
Häfner H, Hambrecht M, Löffler W, Munk-Jørgensen P, Riecher-Rössler A. Is schizophrenia a disorder of all ages? A comparison of first episodes and early course across the life-cycle. Psychol Med. 1998b;28:351–65.
Häfner H, an der Heiden W, Löffler W, Maurer K, Hambrecht M. Beginn und Frühverlauf schizophrener Erkrankungen. In: Klosterkötter J, editor. Frühdiagnostik und Frühbehandlung psychischer Störungen. Heidelberg: Springer; 1998c. p. 1–29.
Häfner H, Löffler W, Maurer K, Riecher-Rössler A, Stein A. Interview für die retrospektive Erfassung des Erkrankungsbeginns und -verlaufs bei Schizophrenie und anderen Psychosen. Bern: Huber; 1999.
Häfner H, Löffler W, Riecher-Rössler A, Häfner-Ranabauer W. Schizophrenie und Wahn im höheren und hohen Lebensalter. Nervenarzt. 2001;72:347–57.
Häfner H, Löffler W, Maurer K, Riecher-Rössler A, Stein A. IRAOS. Interview for the Retrospective Assessment of the Onset and Course of Schizophrenia and Other Psychoses. Hogrefe & Huber: Göttingen; 2003.
Häfner H, Ehrenreich H, Gattaz WF, Louza MR, Riecher-Rössler A, Kulkarni J. Oestrogen – a protective factor in schizophrenia? Curr Psychiatry Rev. 2006;2:339–52.
Häfner H, Maurer K, an der Heiden W. ABC Schizophrenia study: an overview of results since 1996. Soc Psychiatry Psychiatr Epidemiol. 2013;48:1021–31. https://doi.org/10.1007/s00127-013-0700-4.
Hambrecht M, Maurer K, Sartorius N, Häfner H. Transnational stability of gender differences in schizophrenia? An analysis based on the WHO Study on Determinants of Outcome of Severe Mental Disorders. Eur Arch Psychiatry Clin Neurosci. 1992a;242:6–12.
Hambrecht M, Maurer K, Häfner H. Gender differences in schizophrenia in three cultures. Results from the collaborative WHO Disability Study. Soc Psychiatry Psychiatr Epidemiol. 1992b;27:117–21.
Hanssen M, Bak M, Bijl R, Vollebergh W, van Os J. The incidence and outcome of subclinical psychotic experiences in the general population. Br J Clin Psychol. 2005;44:181–91.
Hinterhuber H. Zur Katamnese der Schizophrenien. Fortschr Neurol Psychiatr. 1973;41:527–58.
Hollis C, Rapoport J. Child and adolescent schizophrenia. In: Weinberger DR, Harrison PJ, editors. Schizophrenia. 3rd ed. Oxford: Blackwell; 2011. p. 24–46.
Howard R, Jeste D. Late-onset schizophrenia. In: Weinberger DR, Harrison PJ, editors. Schizophrenia. 3rd ed. Oxford: Blackwell; 2011. p. 47–61.
Howard R, Castle DJ, Wessely S, Murray RM. A comparative study of 470 cases of early-onset and late-onset schizophrenia. Br J Psychiatry. 1993;163:352–7.
Howard R, Rabins PV, Seeman MV, Jeste DV. Late-onset schizophrenia and very-late-onset schizophrenia-like psychosis: an international consensus. The International Late-Onset Schizophrenia Group. Am J Psychiatry. 2000;157:172–88.

Jablensky A, Sartorius N, Ernberg G, Anker M, Korten A, Cooper JE, et al. Schizophrenia: manifestations, incidence and course in different cultures. A World Health Organization ten-country study. Psychological Medicine Monograph Suppl 20. Cambridge: Cambridge University Press; 1992.

Kendhari J, Shankar R, Young-Walker L. A review of childhood-onset schizophrenia. Focus. 2016;14:328–32.

Kirkbride JB, Fearon P, Morgan C, Dazzan P, Morgan K, Tarrant J, et al. Heterogeneity in incidence rates of schizophrenia and other psychotic syndromes: findings from the 3-center AeSOP study. Arch Gen Psychiatry. 2006;63:250–8.

Klosterkötter J, Hellmich M, Steinmeyer EM, Schultze-Lutter F. Diagnosing schizophrenia in the initial prodromal phase. Arch Gen Psychiatry. 2001;58:158–64.

Könnecke R, Häfner H, Maurer K, Löffler W, an der Heiden W. Main risk factors for schizophrenia: increased familial loading and pre- and peri-natal complications antagonize the protective effect of oestrogen in women. Schizophr Res. 2000;44:81–93.

Kraepelin E. Psychiatrie. 8. Aufl. (Bd. 1-4). Leipzig: Barth; 1909-1915.

Kraepelin E. Psychiatrie. 8. Aufl. (Bd. 3, Teil 2). Leipzig: Barth; 1913.

Kulkarni J, de Castella A, Downey M, Hammond J, Reidel A, Ward S, et al. Results of two controlled studies on estrogen: avenue to neuroprotection in schizophrenia. In: Häfner H, editor. Risk and protective factors in schizophrenia—towards a conceptual model of the disease process. Darmstadt: Steinkopff; 2002. p. 271–84.

Kulkarni JA, de Castella PB, Fitzgerald PB, Gurvich CT, Bailey M, Bartholomeusz C, et al. Estrogen in severe mental illness: a potential new treatment approach. Arch Gen Psychiatry. 2008;65:955–60.

Kulkarni J, Gavrilidis E, Hayes E, Heaton V, Worsley R. Special biological issues in the management of women with schizophrenia. Expert Rev Neurother. 2012;12:823–33.

Kulkarni J, Gavrilidis E, Wang W, Gurvich C, van Rheenen T, Berk K, et al. Estradiol for treatment-resistant schizophrenia: a large-scale randomized-controlled trial in women of child-bearing age. Mol Psychiatry. 2014;20:695–702.

Lin A, Wardenaar KJ, Pontillo M, De Crescenzo F, Mazzone L, Vicari S, et al. Is it still correct to differentiate between early and very early onset psychosis? Schizophr Res. 2016;170:211–6. https://doi.org/10.1016/j.schres.2015.11.020.

Löffler W, Häfner H, Fätkenheuer B, Maurer K, Riecher-Rössler A, Lützhoft J, et al. Validation of Danish case-register diagnosis for schizophrenia. Acta Psychiatr Scand. 1994;90:196–203.

Lubman DI, Castle DJ. Late-onset schizophrenia: make the right diagnosis when psychosis emerges after age 60. Curr Psychiatry. 2002;1(12):35–44.

Lützhoft JH, Skadhede S, Fätkenheuer B, Häfner H, Löffler W, Riecher-Rössler A, et al. Symptom assessment in casenotes and the clinical diagnosis of schizophrenia. Psychpathology. 1995;28:131–9.

Maglione JE, Thomas SE, Jeste DV. Late-onset schizophrenia: do recent studies support categorizing LOS as a subtype of schizophrenia? Curr Opin Psychiatry. 2014;27:173–8.

Mason O, Stott J, Sweeting R. Dimensions of positive symptoms in late versus early onset psychosis. Int Psychogeriatr. 2013;25:320–7.

Messias E, Chen C-X, Eaton WW. Epidemiology of schizophrenia: review of findings and myths. Psychiatr Clin North Am. 2007;30:323–38.

Morgan C, John S, Esan O, Hibben M, Patel V, Weiss H, et al. The incidence of psychoses in diverse settings, INTREPID (2): a feasibility study in India, Nigeria, and Trinidad. Psychol Med. 2016;46:1923–33.

Munk-Jørgensen P. The schizophrenia diagnosis in Denmark. A register-based investigation. Acta Psychiatr Scand. 1985;72:266–73.

Ochoa S, Usall J, Cobo J, Labad X, Kulkarni J. Gender differences in schizophrenia and first-episode psychosis: a comprehensive literature review. Schizophr Res Treat. 2012:916198. https://doi.org/10.1155/2012/916198.

Orr KGD, Castle DJ. Schizophrenia at the extremes of life. In: Murray RM, Jones PB, Susser E, van Os J, Cannon M, editors. The epidemiology of schizophrenia. Cambridge: Cambridge University Press; 2003. p. 167–90.

van Os J, Howard R, Takei N, Murray R. Increasing age is a risk factor for psychosis in the elderly. Soc Psychiatry Psychiatr Epidemiol. 1995;30:161–4.

van Os J, Linscott R, Myin-Germeys I, Delespaul P, Krabbendam L. A systematic review and meta-analysis of the psychosis continuum: evidence for a psychosis proneness-persistence-impairment model of psychotic disorder. Psychol Med. 2009;39:179–95.

Pang S, Subramaniam M, Abdin E, Poon LY, Chong SA, Verma S. Gender differences in patients with first-episode psychosis in the Singapore Early Psychosis Intervention Programme. Early Interv Psychiatry. 2016;10:528–34. https://doi.org/10.1111/eip.12208.

Rahmati M, Rahgozar M, Fadaei F, Bakhshi E, Cheraghi L. Identifying some risk factors of time to relapses in schizophrenic patients using Bayesian approach with Event-Dependent Frailty Model. Iran J Psychiatry. 2015;10:123–7.

Rajji TK, Ismail Z, Mulsant BH. Age at onset and cognition in schizophrenia: meta-analysis. Br J Psychiatry. 2009;195:286–93.

Ran MS, Xiang MZ, Chan CL, Leff J, Simpson P, Huang MS, et al. Effectiveness of psychoeducational intervention for rural Chinese families experiencing schizophrenia—a randomised controlled trial. Soc Psychiatry Psychiatr Epidemiol. 2003;38:69–75.

Ran MS, Chen S, Chen EY, Ran BY, Tang CP, Lin FR, et al. Risk factors for poor work functioning of persons with schizophrenia in rural China. Soc Psychiatry Psychiatr Epidemiol. 2011;46:1087–93.

Ran MS, Weng X, Chan CL, Chen EY, Tang CP, Lin FR, et al. Different outcomes of never-treated and treated patients with schizophrenia: 14-year follow-up study in rural China. Br J Psychiatry. 2015a;207:495–500. https://doi.org/10.1192/bjp.bp.114.157685.

Ran MS, Chan CL, Ng SM, Guo LT, Xiang MZ. The effectiveness of psychoeducational family intervention for patients with schizophrenia in a 14-year follow-up study in a Chinese rural area. Psychol Med. 2015b;45:2197–204. https://doi.org/10.1017/S0033291715000197.

Remschmidt H, editor. Schizophrenia in children and adolescents. Cambridge: Cambridge University Press; 2009.

Riecher A, Maurer K, Löffler W, Fätkenheuer B, an der Heiden W, Munk-Jörgensen P, et al. Gender differences in age at onset and course of schizophrenic disorders. In: Häfner H, Gattaz W, editors. Search for the causes of schizophrenia, vol. II. Berlin: Springer; 1990. p. 14–33.

Riecher-Rössler A, Rössler W, Förstl H, Meise U. Late-onset schizophrenia and late paraphrenia. Schizophr Bull. 1995;21:343–54.

Riecher-Rössler A, Häfner H, Häfner-Ranabauer W, Löffler W, Reinhard I. Late-onset schizophrenia versus paranoid psychoses. A valid distinction? Am J Geriatr Psychiatry. 2003;11:595–604.

Sartorius N, Jablensky A, Korten A, Ernberg G, Anker M, Cooper JE, et al. Early manifestations and first-contact incidence of schizophrenia in different cultures. Psychol Med. 1986;16:909–28.

Shaner A, Miller G, Mintz J. Evidence of a latitudinal gradient in the age at onset of schizophrenia. Schizophr Res. 2007;94:58–63.

Steinhausen H-C. What happens to children and adolescents with mental disorders? Findings from long-term outcome research (in German). Z Kinder Jugendpsychiatr Psychother. 2013;41:419–31.

Stentebjerg-Olesen M, Pagsberg AK, Fink-Jensen A, Correll CU, Jeppesen P. Clinical characteristics and predictors of outcome of schizophrenia spectrum psychosis in children and adolescents: a systematic review. J Child Adolesc Psychopharmacol. 2016;26:410–27.

Vahia IV, Palmer BW, Depp C, Fellows I, Golshan S, Kraemer HC, et al. Is late-onset schizophrenia a subtype of schizophrenia? Acta Psychiatr Scand. 2010;122:414–26.

Wium-Andersen MK, Orsted DD, Nordestgaard BG. Elevated C-reactive protein associated with late- and very-late-onset schizophrenia in the general population: a prospective study. Schizophr Bull. 2014;40:1117–27.

Yung AR, Stanford C, Cosgrave E, Killackey E, Phillips L, Nelson B, et al. Testing the ultra high risk (prodromal) criteria for the prediction of psychosis in a clinical sample of young people. Schizophr Res. 2006;84:57–66.

4 The Age of Onset of Schizophrenia Spectrum Disorders

Jouko Miettunen, Johanna Immonen, John J. McGrath, Matti Isohanni, and Erika Jääskeläinen

4.1 Introduction

Schizophrenia spectrum disorders are complex, often chronic and severe psychiatric disorders and are one of the leading causes of disability worldwide (WHO 2008). They usually start early and may cause marked lifelong impairments in social,

J. Miettunen (✉) · J. Immonen
Center for Life Course Health Research, University of Oulu, Oulu, Finland

Medical Research Center Oulu, Oulu University Hospital and University of Oulu, Oulu, Finland
e-mail: jouko.miettunen@oulu.fi; johanna.immonen@student.oulu.fi

J. J. McGrath
Queensland Centre for Mental Health Research, The Park Centre for Mental Health, Wacol, QLD, Australia

Queensland Brain Institute, University of Queensland, St Lucia, QLD, Australia

National Centre for Register-Based Research, Aarhus BSS, Aarhus University, Aarhus, Denmark
e-mail: j.mcgrath@uq.edu.au

M. Isohanni
Center for Life Course Health Research, University of Oulu, Oulu, Finland
e-mail: matti.isohanni@oulu.fi

E. Jääskeläinen
Center for Life Course Health Research, University of Oulu, Oulu, Finland

Medical Research Center Oulu, Oulu University Hospital and University of Oulu, Oulu, Finland

Department of Psychiatry, Research Unit of Clinical Neuroscience, University of Oulu, Oulu, Finland

Department of Psychiatry, Oulu University Hospital, Oulu, Finland
e-mail: erika.jaaskelainen@oulu.fi

G. de Girolamo et al. (eds.), *Age of Onset of Mental Disorders*,
https://doi.org/10.1007/978-3-319-72619-9_4

occupational and cognitive functioning, increased mortality and somatic co-morbidity, as well as stigma. The age of onset (AOO) of schizophrenia spectrum disorders, i.e. schizophrenia and related disorders, is often in early adulthood (Häfner et al. 1993; Thorup et al. 2007), but it can also occur during childhood or adolescence (Hollis and Rapoport 2011) or even in late adulthood and old age (Howard et al. 2000; Howard and Jeste 2011).

AOO has been considered the single most important characteristic of schizophrenia that could help when examining its origin and genetic mechanism (DeLisi 1992; Goldberg et al. 2011). Onset age is also a crucial determinant of an affected individual's future and socioeconomic costs of the illness to society (Stepniak et al. 2014). For example, schizophrenia is an important contributor to the burden of disease (Whiteford et al. 2013) - this not only reflects the disability associated with this disorder, and the suboptimal recovery proportions (13.5% in meta-analysis by Jääskeläinen et al. 2013), but also the high prevalence of relatively early AOO cases. Understanding the onset distribution of long-lasting psychotic disorders can be used in planning preventive and early intervention services (Jones 2013).

Studies on AOO in schizophrenia spectrum disorders, mainly in schizophrenia, have provided variable results. One reason for this is likely to be the variability in the study designs and in the definition of AOO. Regarding schizophrenia, it is reasonable to assume that most patients receive treatment, and thereby their onset age can be estimated at least retrospectively (Jones 2013). Due to this, some studies have defined AOO from the start of positive or other psychotic symptoms, some from first treatment contact and some from the first hospitalisation (Eranti et al. 2013). How accurately AOO is estimated may vary by treatment services, culture, duration of untreated psychosis and type of symptoms (Eranti et al. 2013; Penttilä et al. 2014). There are also untreated individuals who are missed in clinical studies but less often in studies based on community surveys. AOO has been dichotomised in many studies, but it can also be studied with a continuous variable. Often, for example, only early-onset schizophrenia (EOS; e.g. onset age below 18 years) or late-onset schizophrenia (LOS; e.g. onset age after 40 or 55 years) cases have been studied. Also, other terms and definitions are commonly used, such as very-early- or very-late-onset schizophrenia. Onset age is thought to be a useful phenotype marker and studies have attempted to found the best cut-offs for AOO to differentiate patient groups, with varying results. Regarding symptomatology, both EOS (Armando et al. 2015) and LOS (Howard and Jeste 2011) patients have been characterised as having more auditory hallucinations than patients with "regular" AOO. EOS is also characterised by higher levels of negative symptoms and bizarre behaviour (Armando et al. 2015), whereas LOS is characterised as having more delusions (Howard and Jeste 2011).

Previous general systematic reviews have focused on either on EOS (Nicolson and Rapoport 1999; Hollis and Rapoport 2011) or LOS (Howard et al. 2000; Howard and Jeste 2011) cases. The systematic review by Rajji et al. (2009) of cognition and onset age included both EOS and LOS cases, whereas other specific reviews have studied only EOS or LOS cases. Different predictors for earlier onset age have also been studied (Verdoux et al. 1997; Esterberg et al. 2010; Large et al. 2011; Eranti et al. 2013). In previous studies, earlier AOO of schizophrenia has been found to be associated with poorer outcome of illness both in adults (Immonen et al. 2017) and in EOS (Clemmensen et al. 2012). However, most factors related to AOO in schizophrenia have not been studied systematically.

More recently, attention has also been focused on isolated psychotic-like symptoms such as hallucinations and delusions (i.e. psychotic experiences [PEs]) (Kelleher et al. 2012; McGrath et al. 2016, 2017). While most people with these experiences do not develop the full clinical disorder, it is informative to compare the AOO of PEs with the AOO of the full clinical disorder.

The aim of this chapter is to characterise the AOO of schizophrenia spectrum disorders, factors associated with early onset, and how AOO is associated with clinical and social outcome, cognition, brain structure and mortality.

4.2 Incidence by Age and Sex

The review by van der Werf et al. (2014) presents incidence rates by gender for different age bands: males had higher risk until the age of 40 years and after that females were at higher risk. In both genders the highest risk was in the age group of 20–29 years, in which the estimated incidence among males and females was 4.15 and 1.71 per 10,000 person-years, respectively. Males have earlier onset than females; however, the difference is not as large as previously thought. A large register-based Danish study (Thorup et al. 2007) found that the difference between males and females in median onset age (27 vs. 29 years) in schizophrenia that met *International Classification of Diseases* (ICD) criteria was not as large as in mean onset age (29 vs. 33 years), indicating different AOO distribution in the two sexes. The incidence rates by age and sex from their study are presented in the Fig. 4.1 (reprinted from Thorup et al. 2007). Of the other schizophrenia spectrum disorders, delusional disorder (Peralta and Cuesta 2016) and schizoaffective disorder (Cotton et al. 2013) typically have a later AOO than schizophrenia.

A recent meta-analysis estimated the difference in mean onset age between men and women to be about 1 year, sex difference was found only in studies using *Diagnostic and Statistical Manual of Mental Disorders* (DSM) criteria, not in studies based on broader ICD criteria (Eranti et al. 2013). The small gender difference in onset age seems to be present also in other non-affective psychoses (Eranti et al. 2013). Interestingly, the gender differences in AOO do not seem to exist among those with a family history of psychosis (Esterberg et al. 2010), with advanced paternal age (Rosenfield et al. 2010) or who are using cannabis (Donoghue et al. 2014). Early studies have suggested a second peak in onset age among females (Häfner et al. 1993; Castle et al. 1995); however, the review by van der Werf et al. (2014) was not able to detect such a peak. AOO of schizophrenia could be earlier now than in previous studies, as found by Di Maggio et al. (2001) in their medical record review of three different birth cohorts. AOO of schizophrenia may also vary

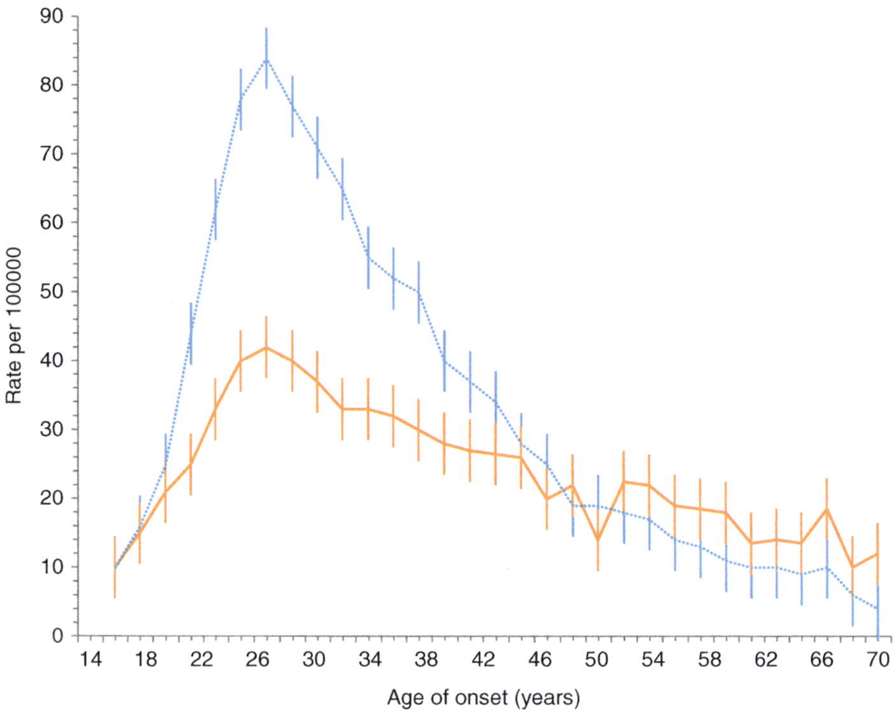

Fig. 4.1 Adjusted incidence rates of schizophrenia by age and gender (baseline is the ICD-10 period, 1995–2001). Orange line: females; blue line: males (reprinted from Thorup et al. (2007) with permission from Cambridge University Press). *ICD-10* International Classification of Diseases, Tenth Edition

by country and culture. This is suggested, for example, by the WHO Mental Health Survey of AOO of PEs, in which the median AOO of PEs varied from 15 to 37 years (McGrath et al. 2016).

Community-based surveys have identified that a substantial proportion of individuals who do not have a confirmed psychotic disorder endorse items related to the presence of hallucinations and delusions (PEs). Based on 31,261 adults (aged 18 years and older) across 18 countries, the mean lifetime prevalence of ever having a lifetime PE was 5.8%, with hallucinatory experiences (5.2%) being more common than delusional experiences (1.3%) (McGrath et al. 2015). With respect to the AOO of PEs, the median (interquartile range) AOO based on projected lifetime estimates was 26 (17–41) years, indicating that PEs commence across a wider age range than schizophrenia. In addition, in contrast to schizophrenia, the AOO distributions for PEs did not differ by sex. Curiously, community members who only reported delusional symptoms had a significantly later AOO than those who only reported hallucination (McGrath et al. 2016). It can be also noted that early onset of symptoms predicts conversion to psychosis among ultra-high-risk individuals (Amminger et al. 2006).

4.3 Risk Factors for Early Onset

4.3.1 Genetic Influence and Family History

Genetic data and family history have been studied frequently in relation to the onset age of schizophrenia spectrum disorders. Esterberg et al. (2010) performed a meta-analysis on family history in 15 studies. They found that those with a family history of psychosis have significantly younger onset age, with a small effect size (Cohen's $d = 0.17$). In the individual studies the highest effect sizes were up to 0.54, but in some studies there was no significant effect and in some of these the effect was even the opposite. Likewise, high familial loading has been linked with earlier AOO (Suvisaari et al. 1998; Goldberg et al. 2011).

The studies looking at genetic influence have not found any clear evidence. For instance, Stepniak et al. (2014) did not find any direct or indirect effect of polygenic risk score on onset age. On the other hand, Nicolson and Rapoport (1999) reported that childhood-onset cases (onset below age 12 years) had more severe premorbid neurodevelopmental abnormalities and a seemingly higher rate of familial schizophrenia spectrum disorders than later-onset cases.

4.3.2 Early Risk Factors

Various pregnancy- and birth-related factors have been studied in association with AOO. Subjects with onset of schizophrenia before age 22 years were 2.7 times more likely than those with onset at a later age to have had a history of an abnormal presentation at birth and ten times more likely to have had a history of complicated caesarean birth in a meta-analysis of 11 studies (Verdoux et al. 1997). Studies published after this meta-analysis have also found a similar association (Castle et al. 1997; Scherr et al. 2012; Stepniak et al. 2014). In the study by Kirov et al. (1996), obstetric complications were associated with earlier onset in males but not in females. Pre-eclampsia, the use of forceps and the need for an incubator at birth have been found to be associated with early AOO in a sample including all psychoses (Rubio-Abadal et al. 2015). There also seemed to be an association between advanced paternal age and earlier onset age (Stepniak et al. 2014). Individuals with EOS (<25 years) had been found to have higher rate of developmental delays than late-onset (>60 years) cases (11.9% vs. 0%; relative risk 0.88; 95% confidence interval 0.83–0.94) (Castle et al. 1997).

4.3.3 Premorbid Factors

Cannabis use and poor premorbid adjustment have been found to be associated with early AOO. Regarding cannabis use, a meta-analysis of 41 studies found that the age at onset of psychosis for cannabis users was on average 2.7 years younger than for non-users (Large et al. 2011). This has also been found in later studies (Scherr et al. 2012;

Donoghue et al. 2014). Stepniak et al. (2014) found that cannabis users not only had an earlier mean onset age of schizophrenia (23.2 vs. 25.3 years) but also an earlier onset of the prodromal phase (20.2 vs. 22.4 years). It has been also found that earlier onset age among cannabis users may be especially true among females (Compton et al. 2009). The meta-analysis by Large et al. (2011) also found earlier onset age among other substance users. Gunnell et al. (2002) has found lower premorbid IQ to be linked with earlier onset age in a large Swedish conscript study. In addition, regarding premorbid adjustment, several studies have found poorer premorbid adjustment among early-onset cases than late-onset cases (Foerster et al. 1991; Gupta et al. 1995; Vourdas et al. 2003; Goldberg et al. 2011).

Interestingly, the number of environmental factors can be associated with early AOO, as there is an earlier mean onset age of schizophrenia (22.6 vs. 30.7 years) and of prodromal phase (19.4 vs. 28.3 years) among those with four or more environmental risk factors than in those without environmental risk factors (Stepniak et al. 2014). However, many single risk factors studied were not associated with AOO (Stepniak et al. 2014). The study by Scherr et al. (2012) looked at several predictors for AOO and noted that factors such as obstetric complications and cannabis use predict AOO in non-familial but not in familial schizophrenia.

To summarise, various risk factors have been identified for earlier onset in schizophrenia spectrum disorders; statistically significant findings are summarised in Table 4.1. Few studies have looked for factors relating especially to LOS, but sensory deficits and premorbid personality characteristics have been found to be associated with the onset of schizophrenia at a later age (Howard and Jeste 2011). Late-onset patients are also more often married than those with earlier AOO (Vahia et al. 2010).

4.4 Age of Onset (AOO) and Outcome

AOO is one of the most commonly analysed predictors of outcome in schizophrenia spectrum disorders, but the results obtained in different original studies are far from conclusive. To overcome this issue, there have been systematic reviews on the effect of AOO on the long-term outcome of schizophrenia. Yet, there are no meta-analyses or systematic reviews which have simultaneously analysed the outcomes of all schizophrenia cases, as childhood-onset schizophrenia and LOS tend to be studied independently.

The recent meta-analysis from our group (Immonen et al. 2017) studied onset age and long-term (at least 2-year follow-up) outcome among schizophrenia patients. The results of this study concern mainly adult- and adolescent-onset schizophrenia even though no upper or lower age limits were applied as such. This is because psychiatric research and treatment tend to be done in either adult, adolescent or children settings and, hence, the samples of many studies typically include only these particular patients. Original studies were excluded from the meta-analysis

Table 4.1 Statistically significant predictors for early onset of schizophrenia found in previous meta-analyses and original studies

Predictors
Family history and genetic influence
• Meta-analysis of 15 studies found that those with family history of psychosis have significantly younger onset age (Cohen's $d = 0.17$) (Esterberg et al. 2010)
• Those with parental history of psychosis and paternal history of psychosis had earlier onset age (Rubio-Abadal et al. 2015)
• Family history of affective disorders and any psychiatric disorder associated with earlier onset of schizophrenia (Kendler and MacLean 1990; Byrne et al. 2002)
• Higher familial loading associated with earlier onset age (Suvisaari et al. 1998; Goldberg et al. 2011)
• Combination of met-containing genotypes of *BDNF* gene and Ser/Ser D_3 receptor predicted earlier mean onset age of schizophrenia and of prodromal phase (Gourion et al. 2005)
Early factors
• History of abnormal presentation at birth and caesarean birth associated with earlier onset age in a meta-analysis of 11 studies (Verdoux et al. 1997). Obstetric complications have been associated with earlier onset also in later studies (Castle et al. 1997; Scherr et al. 2012)
• Perinatal complications associated with earlier onset age of schizophrenia and of prodromal phase (Stepniak et al. 2014)
• Lower birth weight associated significantly with earlier onset age even after other significant predictors were taken into account (Rubio-Abadal et al. 2015)
• Developmental difficulties and delays have been associated with earlier onset of schizophrenia (Castle et al. 1997; Scherr et al. 2012)
• Those with pre-eclampsia had earlier mean onset age in schizophrenia (Rubio-Abadal et al. 2015).
• Use of forceps at birth associated with earlier mean onset of psychosis even after other significant predictors were taken into account (Rubio-Abadal et al. 2015).
• Need for incubator at birth associated with earlier mean onset of psychosis (Rubio-Abadal et al. 2015).
• Enuresis/encopresis predicted earlier onset of schizophrenia (Scherr et al. 2012)
Premorbid factors
• Meta-analysis of 41 studies published found that the age at onset of psychosis for cannabis users was on average 2.7 years younger than for non-users (Large et al. 2011)
• Also in later studies, cannabis users have had an earlier age of first symptoms than non-users (Donoghue et al. 2014; Scherr et al. 2012). The gender difference in age of onset was diminished in cannabis smokers compared with non-cannabis smokers (Donoghue et al. 2014)
• Earlier mean onset age of schizophrenia and of prodromal phase has been found among those using cannabis (Stepniak et al. 2014)
• Meta-analysis of 41 studies found that the age at onset of psychosis for those using any substances (alcohol, cannabis or other) was on average 2.0 years earlier than for non-users (Large et al. 2011)
• Stimulant drug use previous to psychosis onset associated with earlier onset of psychosis (Rubio-Abadal et al. 2015)
• Earlier onset age of schizophrenia and of prodromal phase was found among those with ≥ 4 environmental risk factors when compared with those without environmental risk factors (Stepniak et al. 2014)

(continued)

Table 4.1 (continued)

Predictors
• Poorer childhood and adolescent premorbid adjustment significantly associated with earlier age of onset (Gupta et al. 1995)
• Early-onset patients showed more deviant premorbid social adjustment and higher premorbid schizoid and schizotypal traits than late-onset patients (Vourdas et al. 2003)
• Earlier mean onset age of schizophrenia and of prodromal phase was found among those with neurotrauma (Stepniak et al. 2014)

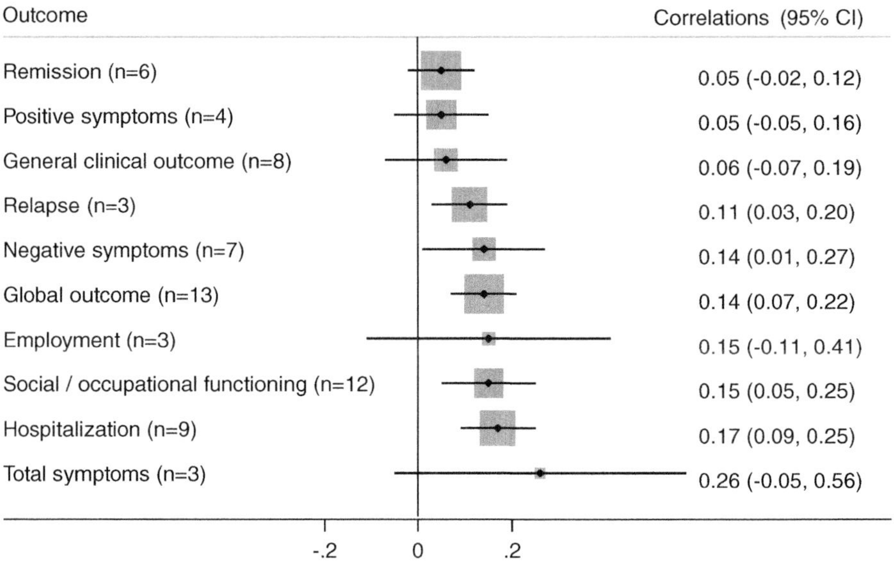

Fig. 4.2 Correlations between age of onset and outcomes (reprinted from Immonen et al. 2017). *CI* conference interval, *n* number of studies. Positive correlation indicates that younger age of onset associates with poorer outcome

if the sample was biased based on the AOO (i.e. it included only early- or late-onset patients) as comparability of the effect sizes was required.

Outcomes included clinical outcomes (remission, relapse, hospitalisation, positive symptoms, negative symptoms, total symptoms and general clinical outcome), social/occupational capacity, employment status and global outcome. There was a statistically significant correlation between younger age at onset and more hospitalisations, more negative symptoms, more relapses, poorer social/occupational functioning and poorer global outcome. Other relationships were not significant. The effect of age at onset on the outcomes was small as significant correlations ranged from 0.11 to 0.17. Figure 4.2 shows correlations between age at onset and the included outcome categories (reprinted from Immonen et al. 2017). Positive correlation indicates that an earlier AOO results in poorer outcome. Male gender had a confounding effect on the clinical outcome, as in the samples with a higher proportion of males, the correlation between earlier AOO and poorer general clinical outcome became significant (Immonen et al. 2017). The effect of AOO is mostly independent of gender, but it is possible that males with an early onset have a poorer clinical outcome. This has not been directly studied, but first-episode psychosis studies have found that males have greater symptom severity and more substance use problems at treatment entry (Cotton et al. 2009). AOO can be important also in relation to hallucinations as it is the only feature distinguishing hallucinations in schizophrenia from hallucinations in other disorders (Waters and Fernyhough 2017).

Clemmensen et al. (2012) summarised studies on the long-term outcome on EOS and samples including also individuals with later AOO (MIX samples). The sample mean age was restricted to below 18 years in the included studies. They found that EOS samples had worse outcomes than MIX samples. The outcome was defined as good, moderate or poor based on the Global Functioning Score or a study-specific outcome. Only 15.4% of the EOS patients had a good outcome versus 19.6% of the MIX samples. A poor outcome was experienced by 60.1% in EOS studies versus 46.8% in MIX studies. This shows that early manifestation of schizophrenia is connected with a particularly poor prognosis.

Duration of untreated psychosis (DUP) may vary by onset age, with late-onset patients having a shorter DUP (Sato et al. 2004). This indicates that the effect of AOO on the outcome may be even larger as a longer DUP has been linked with a worse outcome (Penttilä et al. 2014). However, AOO did not affect the relationship between DUP and outcome in a recent meta-analysis (Penttilä et al. 2014). Regarding occupational outcome, it is clear that earlier onset age affects education. For example, the Northern Finland Birth Cohort 1966 study those with onset age before 22 years had six-fold odds for stagnating at the basic educational level compared with cases having an onset between 22 and 31 years of age (Isohanni et al. 2001). Factors related to local services are also associated with length of DUP, for instance due to clinicians missing or being reluctant to use schizophrenia or psychosis as a diagnosis in children. Not only the AOO but also the mode of onset may affect outcome in schizophrenia. For instance, when the AOO and mode of onset have been studied simultaneously, both earlier AOO and more gradual mode of onset was associated with more severe general psychopathology (Compton et al. 2017).

4.5 AOO and Cognition

Cognitive deficits occur in about 80% of schizophrenia patients (Palmer et al. 2009). There are several factors that have been found to be associated with the cognitive deficit, such as negative symptoms (Aleman et al. 1999), poor premorbid school marks (Rannikko et al. 2015b), low education (Ekerholm et al. 2012), higher doses of antipsychotics (Husa et al. 2017) and genetic factors (Shafee et al. 2017). Cognitive dysfunctions rather than positive symptoms are considered to be core features of schizophrenia, since they are strongly correlated with poor functional outcomes as well as being predictors of general outcome and rehabilitation effectiveness (Keefe et al. 2011).

When compared with adult-onset schizophrenia, there are considerable fewer studies on cognition in EOS and LOS (Rajji et al. 2009). The meta-analysis by Rajji et al. (2009) included studies on onset age and cognition in schizophrenia published between 1980 and 2008. They found that individuals with youth-onset schizophrenia demonstrate larger deficits than those with first-episode schizophrenia in several areas of cognition (arithmetic, executive function, IQ, psychomotor speed of processing and verbal memory). In contrast, those with late-onset schizophrenia demonstrate larger deficits only on attention, fluency, global cognition, IQ and visuospatial construction. They conclude that the cognitive pattern of people with late-onset schizophrenia suggests that their deficits are specific rather than being solely as a result of ageing and related factors. It may be good to note that at the time of measuring the cognition, the duration of illness was considerably longer among studies on LOS (weighted mean 7.7 years) and somewhat longer in youth-onset schizophrenia (mean 2.3 years) than first-episode schizophrenia (7.7 years). On the other hand, most marked cognitive decline happened around psychosis, a few years before and after onset, and remains relatively stable thereafter (Vyas et al. 2011; Bora and Murray 2014). A review of intelligence scores reported that scores in EOS often range between 80 and 90, which are lower than those of adult-onset patients (Vyas et al. 2011). An interesting form of schizophrenia is schizophrenia in people with a learning disability. In this subgroup, average AOO is non-significantly later than among other schizophrenia cases (Doody et al. 1998). This can be due to difficulties in correctly diagnosing schizophrenia among these individuals, as co-morbid learning disability has been linked with false negative clinical diagnosis when compared with the research diagnosis of schizophrenia (Moilanen et al. 2003).

Based on meta-analysis, cognition does not deteriorate after psychosis onset in first-episode psychosis or in ultra-high-risk samples based on follow-up studies; instead, there are improvements in cognitive abilities in both groups and this may be due to practice effects and improvement on symptoms (Bora and Murray 2014). There is no evidence of the loss of acquired cognitive skills after the onset of psychosis. Change of verbal learning and memory was analysed in a population-based schizophrenia sample around early middle age. Compared with non-psychotic controls, there was no evidence of greater decline in verbal episodic memory between ages 34 and 43 years in schizophrenia, though the schizophrenia sample had an overall lower cognitive performance at the baseline (Rannikko et al. 2015a).

Cognitive deficits observed in schizophrenia seem to at least partially develop long before the onset of psychosis. They appear to be a consequence of an abnormal neurodevelopment, and may be best explained by problems in acquisition on certain skills during neurodevelopment. This can partly explain the associations found between earlier onset age and poorer functioning in some cognitive tasks.

4.6 AOO and Brain Morphometry

AOO has also been linked with brain alterations. Fraguas et al. (2016) have reviewed studies on progression of brain changes in early-onset psychosis when compared with controls. Early-onset patients showed greater progressive frontal grey matter loss over the first few years after illness onset; age at baseline magnetic resonance

Table 4.2 Statistically significant associations between onset age of schizophrenia and brain morphometry found in original studies

• Larger thalamic volume in late-onset schizophrenia (>45 years) than in earlier onset ($t = 2.90$, degrees of freedom [df] = 56, $p < 0.05$) (Corey-Bloom et al. 1995)
• Earlier age of onset correlated with larger volumes of caudate ($r = -0.29$) and lenticular nuclei ($r = 0.24$) (Jeste et al. 1998)
• Younger age at first hospitalisation associated with greater reduction in right temporal lobe size over time ($r = 0.44$, $p = 0.02$) (DeLisi and Hoff 2005)
• Younger age at first symptoms associated with decrease in left caudate ($r = 0.46$, $p < 0.05$) in a 4-year follow-up (DeLisi et al. 1995)
• Younger age at first hospitalisation associated with less reduction in right lateral ventricle size over time ($r = 0.45$, $p = 0.02$) (DeLisi et al. 1995). The rate of ventricular change during the first 5 years was significantly correlated (left ventricle: $r = 0.58$; right ventricle: $r = 0.42$) with age at first hospitalisation (DeLisi et al. 2004).
• More frequent moderate to severe ventricular abnormalities (29% vs. 0%, $P = 0.004$) and cortical atrophy (23% vs. 0%, $P = 0.01$) in early-onset paranoid psychosis cases than in late-onset cases (Tonkonogy and Geller 1999)

imaging (MRI) scan was associated with greater loss of temporal grey matter volume over time in patients than in controls (Fraguas et al. 2016).

The studies including adult samples have also looked at the effect of AOO on brain volumes (for review, see Hahn et al. 2014). Previous studies have found earlier onset age to be associated with, for example, lower volumes in the thalamus (Corey-Bloom et al. 1995) and temporal lobe (DeLisi and Hoff 2005) and larger ventricular volumes (DeLisi et al. 1995, 2004; Tonkonogy and Geller 1999). Table 4.2 summarises the statistically significant findings on AOO and brain morphometry in schizophrenia. There are only a few Diffusion Tensor Imaging (DTI) or functional neuroimaging studies, and these have had mixed results (Hahn et al. 2014). In one DTI study, a differential effect of age at onset was noted bilaterally in medial prefrontal white matter ($p = 0.002$); these regions included parts of the superior fronto-occipital fasciculus, corticopontine tract, anterior thalamic radiation and corpus callosum (Kyriakopoulos et al. 2009).

4.7 AOO and Mortality

In their comprehensive review on risk factors for suicide in schizophrenia, Popovic et al. (2014) found that older AOO was associated with suicide among schizophrenia patients; however, this was based only on two studies. On the other hand, Panariello et al. (2010) reported that EOS cases (AOO below 22 years) made more suicide attempts (30% vs. 20%) than LOS cases (AOO above 22 years). A meta-analysis looking at factors associated with either suicide attempts or deliberate self-injury found that these were predicted by, for instance, younger AOO and younger age at first treatment (Challis et al. 2013).

Regarding mortality due to natural causes, there are not many studies looking at AOO. In a Dutch study among older patients, mortality compared to the general population was still high, but AOO was not associated with higher mortality risk (Meesters et al. 2016). In a Finnish register study among older patients, AOO after 60 years, especially among males, was associated with a higher risk of death than in those with an earlier AOO. This finding was mostly explained as being related to physical co-morbidities and accidents (Talaslahti et al. 2015).

Regarding reasons for high mortality due to natural causes, somatic co-morbidities are common in schizophrenia. EOS cases in adulthood and in old age may have a higher somatic burden, for example due to higher cumulative antipsychotic use and smoking. Studies on the topic are quite rare, but a study of the Northern Finland Birth Cohort 1966 indicates that EOS cases could be at higher risk of insulin resistance (Timonen et al. 2009). On the other hand, LOS cases (onset after age 40 years) have two to three times higher risk of subsequently getting a diagnosis of dementia than patients with osteoarthritis or the general population (Kørner et al. 2009).

4.8 Discussion

We have reviewed research on AOO in schizophrenia regarding clinical and social outcomes, cognition, brain structure and mortality. A summary of our findings is presented in Box 4.1.

The findings are consistent with the view that earlier onset of schizophrenia is associated with poor outcome. Adolescence includes rapid brain development but also unique and critical psychosocial alterations: a separation from original family and independence, education, occupational decisions, and the start of dyadic and family relations. EOS may prevent these critical developmental steps; for example, it may stop the educational path (Isohanni et al. 2001). Missing the achievement of adult identity may also jeopardise coping with the disease and collaboration with treatment systems. It has been shown that both brain alterations (Rossi et al. 2000; Mitelman et al. 2007; Jääskeläinen et al. 2014) and poor premorbid social adjustments (Alvarez-Jimenez et al. 2012) are associated with poor outcome. It has also been found that AOO and premorbid functioning may act as mediators between

Box 4.1 Summary of Findings on Age of Onset in Schizophrenia Spectrum Disorders

- The peak age of onset (AOO) for schizophrenia is between 20 and 29 years, with males having an earlier AOO.
- Cannabis use, family history of psychosis and poor premorbid adjustment are associated with earlier AOO.
- Earlier onset has been found to be associated with poorer clinical and social outcome and larger deficits in cognition than later onset.
- Later AOO has been linked with more suicides.
- Studies on AOO have heterogeneous methods.

gender, familial history of psychosis and clinical outcome (Goldberg et al. 2011). Thus, AOO may determine the degree to which brain structural change and cognitive impairments lead to a poor outcome.

Treatment adherence can be poor, especially in EOS cases; for instance, individuals with an AOO of schizophrenia under 23 years participated less often in psychosocial therapies in therapeutic community wards (Isohanni and Nieminen 1990). Response to treatment in the first episode has also been reported as being poorer among those with earlier AOO. In one study, after a 10-year follow-up, 84% of treatment-resistant psychosis cases were treatment resistant from illness onset, and younger age at onset and longer DUP predicted treatment resistance from illness onset (Demjaha et al. 2017). Patients with EOS are likely to have larger cumulative exposure to antipsychotic medications if they survive to old age, and this may relate to a poorer long-term outcome in terms of cognition (Husa et al. 2017), brain changes (Huhtaniska et al. 2017) and somatic outcomes such as those due to weight gain and insulin resistance (Newcomer and Leucht 2011).

Because of the poor outcome, there are several different types of interventions targeted at these patients (Penn et al. 2005; Claxton et al. 2017; Fusar-Poli et al. 2017). Family interventions, for instance, have been suggested as early psychosis can have a negative impact on service users and their families (Onwumere et al. 2011). Early interventions are potentially useful, as young people with psychosis have, for instance, smaller social networks than their peers (Macdonald et al. 2000). According to a recent review, cognitive–behavioural therapy, cognitive remediation and family intervention have also shown some good results in EOS patients (Armando et al. 2015). Alvarez-Jimenez et al. (2011) suggest that benign and cost-effective treatment approaches, including adequate social and family support, are optimal for young first-onset patients and minimise the side effects of prolonged exposure to antipsychotic medications. The results of this review indicate that, while prevention may not be achievable, if we can delay AOO for schizophrenia, this could reduce the burden of the disease, and thus would be a suitable interim outcome (van der Gaag et al. 2013).

Schizophrenia can start at any age, as about half of the patients have AOO before and half after age 30 years (Kirkbride et al. 2006; Thorup et al. 2007). The diagnostic criteria for schizophrenia are the same regardless of onset age, but there has been discussion regarding whether there should be subtypes based on AOO (Tonkonogy and Geller 1999). Regarding current at-risk and psychotic-onset criteria there has also been discussion about their validity, especially in children compared with adults (Armando et al. 2015). The onset age has been defined and categorised differently in the included studies and samples have been selected partly based on AOO, and this may have affected these findings. Also, in general, the results on AOO in schizophrenia studies may be biased as studies often include patients in different phases of illness. A first-episode study would be preferable, as those with EOS surviving to old age are also likely to have better outcomes regarding all aspects of illness than those who are deceased. Due to gender differences in onset age, this would mean that more males are included if these cases are excluded. Many studies also exclude those with late AOO due to study methodology, and because of this the studies may include fewer female patients than otherwise would be the case (van der Werf et al. 2014). Gender differences were not present among patients with various risk factors (cannabis use, family history and advanced paternal age), perhaps indicating that these factors have potential to override the sex differences in AOO.

More good-quality studies on AOO in schizophrenia are needed that include patients without restriction due to the onset age. There is a lack of research on certain topics relating, for example, to differences in AOO in different cultures and varying rates of maturation between people living in different parts of the world should be studied further. Family history has been associated with earlier onset of psychosis; thus, further study could examine whether the effect is similar if the child is reared with a parent with schizophrenia or apart from them. There have been relatively few studies focusing on LOS, and these patients samples could be further utilised to study factors protecting from earlier AOO.

Conclusions

AOO is an important characteristic of schizophrenia that could help when examining the origin, genetic mechanism and care of schizophrenia. In this chapter we have reviewed a lot of research on various topics relating to AOO in schizophrenia, but more good-quality studies are needed that include patients without restriction due to the onset age. Understanding factors that influence AOO in schizophrenia may offer clues to preventing or at least delaying the onset and milden the severity of this debilitating group of disorders.

Acknowledgments This work was supported by grants from the NARSAD (National Alliance for Research on Schizophrenia & Depression): Brain and Behavior Research Fund and the Academy of Finland (#268 336, #278 286). The funders had no role in the writing of the manuscript.

References

Aleman A, Hijman R, De Haan EHF, Kahn RS. Memory impairment in schizophrenia: a meta-analysis. Am J Psychiatry. 1999;156:1358–66.

Alvarez-Jimenez M, Gleeson JF, Henry LP, Harrigan SM, Harris MG, Amminger GP, Killackey E, Yung AR, Herrman H, Jackson HJ, McGorry PD. Prediction of a single psychotic episode: a 7.5-year, prospective study in first-episode psychosis. Schizophr Res. 2011;125:236–46.

Alvarez-Jimenez M, Priede A, Hetrick SE, Bendall S, Killackey E, Parker AG, McGorry PD, Gleeson JF. Risk factors for relapse following treatment for first episode psychosis: a systematic review and meta-analysis of longitudinal studies. Schizophr Res. 2012;139:116–28.

Amminger GP, Leicester S, Yung AR, Phillips LJ, Berger GE, Francey SM, Yuen HP, McGorry PD. Early onset of symptoms predicts conversion to non-affective psychosis in ultra-high risk individuals. Schizophr Res. 2006;84:67–76.

Armando M, Pontillo M, Vicari S. Psychosocial interventions for very early and early-onset schizophrenia: a review of treatment efficacy. Curr Opin Psychiatry. 2015;28:312–23.

Bora E, Murray RM. Meta-analysis of cognitive deficits in ultra-high risk to psychosis and first-episode psychosis: do the cognitive deficits progress over, or after, the onset of psychosis? Schizophr Bull. 2014;40:744–55.

Byrne M, Agerbo E, Mortensen PB. Family history of psychiatric disorders and age at first contact in schizophrenia: an epidemiological study. Br J Psychiatry. 2002;181(Suppl 43):19–25.

Castle DJ, Abel K, Takei N, Murray RM. Gender differences in schizophrenia: hormonal effect or subtypes? Schizophr Bull. 1995;21:1–12.
Castle DJ, Wessely S, Howard R, Murray RM. Schizophrenia with onset at the extremes of adult life. Int J Geriatr Psychiatry. 1997;12:712–7.
Challis S, Nielssen O, Harris A, Large M. Systematic meta-analysis of the risk factors for deliberate self-harm before and after treatment for first-episode psychosis. Acta Psychiatr Scand. 2013;127:442–54.
Claxton M, Onwumere J, Fornells-Ambrojo M. Do family interventions improve outcomes in early psychosis? A systematic review and meta-analysis. Front Psychol. 2017;8:371.
Clemmensen L, Vernal DL, Steinhausen HC. A systematic review of the long–term outcome of early onset schizophrenia. BMC Psychiatry. 2012;12:150. https://doi.org/10.1186/1471-244X-12-150.
Compton MT, Kelley ME, Ramsay CE, Pringle M, Goulding SM, Esterberg ML, Stewart T, Walker EF. Association of pre–onset cannabis, alcohol, and tobacco use with age at onset of prodrome and age at onset of psychosis in first–episode patients. Am J Psychiatry. 2009;166:1251–7.
Compton MT, Berez C, Walker EF. The relative importance of family history, gender, mode of onset, and age at onset in predicting clinical features of first-episode psychotic disorders. Clin Schizophr Relat Psychoses. 2017;11(3):143–50. https://doi.org/10.3371/CSRP.COBE.103114.
Corey-Bloom J, Jernigan T, Archibald S, Harris MJ, Jeste DV. Quantitative magnetic resonance imaging of the brain in late-life schizophrenia. Am J Psychiatry. 1995;152:447–9.
Cotton SM, Lambert M, Schimmelmann BG, Foley DL, Morley KI, McGorry PD, Conus P. Gender differences in premorbid, entry, treatment, and outcome characteristics in a treated epidemiological sample of 661 patients with first episode psychosis. Schizophr Res. 2009;114:17–24.
Cotton SM, Lambert M, Schimmelmann BG, Mackinnon A, Gleeson JF, Berk M, Hides L, Chanen AM, Scott J, Schöttle D, McGorry PD, Conus P. Differences between first episode schizophrenia and schizoaffective disorder. Schizophr Res. 2013;147:169–74.
DeLisi LE. The significance of age of onset for schizophrenia. Schizophr Bull. 1992;18:209–15.
DeLisi LE, Hoff AL. Failure to find progressive temporal lobe volume decreases 10 years subsequent to a first episode of schizophrenia. Psychiatry Res Neuroimaging. 2005;138:265–8.
DeLisi LE, Tew W, Xie S, Hoff AL, Sakuma M, Kushner M, Lee G, Shedlack K, Smith AM, Grimson R. A prospective follow-up study of brain morphology and cognition in first-episode schizophrenic patients: preliminary findings. Biol Psychiatry. 1995;38:349–60.
DeLisi LE, Sakuma M, Maurizio AM, Relja M, Hoff AL. Cerebral ventricular change over the first 10 years after the onset of schizophrenia. Psychiatry Res Neuroimaging. 2004;130:57–70.
Demjaha A, Lappin JM, Stahl D, Patel MX, MacCabe JH, Howes OD, Heslin M, Reininghaus UA, Donoghue K, Lomas B, Charalambides M, Onyejiaka A, Fearon P, Jones P, Doody G, Morgan C, Dazzan P, Murray RM. Antipsychotic treatment resistance in first-episode psychosis: prevalence, subtypes and predictors. Psychol Med. 2017;47:1981–9.
Di Maggio C, Martinez M, Ménard JF, Petit M, Thibaut F. Evidence of a cohort effect for age at onset of schizophrenia. Am J Psychiatry. 2001;158:489–92.
Donoghue K, Doody GA, Murray RM, Jones PB, Morgan C, Dazzan P, Hart J, Mazzoncini R, Maccabe JH. Cannabis use, gender and age of onset of schizophrenia: data from the ÆSOP study. Psychiatry Res. 2014;215:528–32.
Doody GA, Johnstone EC, Sanderson TL, Owens DG, Muir WJ. 'Pfropfschizophrenie' revisited. Schizophrenia in people with mild learning disability. Br J Psychiatry. 1998;173:145–53.
Ekerholm M, Waltersson SF, Fagerberg T, Söderman E, Terenius L, Agartz I, Jönsson EG, Nyman H. Neurocognitive function in long-term treated schizophrenia: a five-year follow-up study. Psychiatry Res. 2012;200:144–52.
Eranti SV, MacCabe JH, Bundy H, Murray RM. Gender difference in age at onset of schizophrenia: a meta–analysis. Psychol Med. 2013;43:155–67.
Esterberg ML, Trotman HD, Holtzman C, Compton MT, Walker EF. The impact of a family history of psychosis on age–at–onset and positive and negative symptoms of schizophrenia: a meta–analysis. Schizophr Res. 2010;120:121–30.
Foerster A, Lewis SW, Owen MJ, Murray RM. Low birth weight and a family history of schizophrenia predict poor premorbid functioning in psychosis. Schizophr Res. 1991;5:13–20.

Fraguas D, Díaz-Caneja CM, Pina-Camacho L, Janssen J, Arango C. Progressive brain changes in children and adolescents with early–onset psychosis: a meta–analysis of longitudinal MRI studies. Schizophr Res. 2016;173:132–9.

Fusar-Poli P, McGorry PD, Kane JM. Improving outcomes of first-episode psychosis: an overview. World Psychiatry. 2017;16:251–65.

Goldberg X, Fatjó-Vilas M, Penadés R, Miret S, Muñoz MJ, Vossen H, Fañanás L. Neurodevelopmental liability to schizophrenia: the complex mediating role of age at onset and premorbid adjustment. Schizophr Res. 2011;133:143–9.

Gourion D, Goldberger C, Leroy S, Bourdel MC, Olié JP, Krebs MO. Age at onset of schizophrenia: interaction between brain-derived neurotrophic factor and dopamine D3 receptor gene variants. Neuroreport. 2005;16:1407–10.

Gunnell D, Harrison G, Rasmussen F, Fouskakis D, Tynelius P. Associations between premorbid intellectual performance, early-life exposures and early-onset schizophrenia. Cohort study. Br J Psychiatry. 2002;181:298–305.

Gupta S, Rajaprabhakaran R, Arndt S, Flaum M, Andreasen NC. Premorbid adjustment as a predictor of phenomenological and neurobiological indices in schizophrenia. Schizophr Res. 1995;16:189–97.

Häfner H, Maurer K, Löffler W, Riecher-Rössler A. The influence of age and sex on the onset and early course of schizophrenia. Br J Psychiatry. 1993;162:80–6.

Hahn C, Lim HK, Lee CU. Neuroimaging findings in late-onset schizophrenia and bipolar disorder. J Geriatr Psychiatry Neurol. 2014;27:56–62.

Hollis C, Rapoport J. Child and adolescent schizophrenia. In: Weinberger DR, Harrison PJ, editors. Schizophrenia. 3rd ed. Chichester: Blackwell Publishing Ltd; 2011. p. 24–46.

Howard R, Jeste DV. Late–onset schizophrenia. In: Weinberger DR, Harrison PJ, editors. Schizophrenia. 3rd ed. Chichester: Blackwell Publishing Ltd; 2011. p. 47–61.

Howard R, Rabins PV, Seeman MV, Jeste DV. Late–onset schizophrenia and very-late-onset schizophrenia-like psychosis: an international consensus. The International Late-Onset Schizophrenia group. Am J Psychiatry. 2000;157:172–8.

Huhtaniska H, Jääskeläinen E, Hirvonen N, Remes J, Murray GK, Veijola J, Isohanni M, Miettunen J. Long-term antipsychotic use and brain changes in schizophrenia—a systematic review and meta-analysis. Hum Psychopharmacol. 2017;32:e2574. https://doi.org/10.1002/hup.2574.

Husa A, Moilanen J, Murray G, Marttila R, Haapea M, Rannikko I, Barnett JH, Jones P, Isohanni M, Remes AM, Koponen H, Miettunen J, Jääskeläinen E. Lifetime antipsychotic medication and cognitive performance in schizophrenia at age 43 years in a general population birth cohort. Psychiatry Res. 2017;247:130–8.

Immonen J, Jääskeläinen E, Korpela H, Miettunen J. Age at onset and the outcomes of schizophrenia: systematic review and meta–analysis. Early Interv Psychiatry. 2017;11(6):453–60. https://doi.org/10.1111/eip.12412.

Isohanni M, Nieminen P. The determinants of therapeutic community activity at an acute patients' psychiatric ward. Int J Ther Commun. 1990;11:139–48.

Isohanni I, Jones PB, Järvelin M-R, Nieminen P, Rantakallio P, Jokelainen J, Croudace TJ, Isohanni M. Educational consequences of mental disorders treated in hospital. A 31-year follow-up of the Northern Finland 1966 Birth Cohort. Psychol Med. 2001;31:339–49.

Jääskeläinen E, Juola P, Hirvonen N, McGrath JJ, Saha S, Isohanni M, Veijola J, Miettunen J. A systematic review and meta-analysis of recovery in schizophrenia. Schizophr Bull. 2013;39:1296–306.

Jääskeläinen E, Juola P, Kurtti J, Haapea M, Kyllönen M, Miettunen J, Tanskanen P, Murray GK, Huhtaniska S, Barnes A, Veijola J, Isohanni M. Associations between brain morphology and outcome in schizophrenia in a general population sample. Eur Psychiatry. 2014;29:456–62.

Jeste DV, McAdams LA, Palmer BW, Braff D, Jernigan TL, Paulsen JS, Stout JC, Symonds LL, Bailey A, Heaton RK. Relationship of neuropsychological and MRI measures to age of onset of schizophrenia. Acta Psychiatr Scand. 1998;98:156–64.

Jones PB. Adult mental health disorders and their age at onset. Br J Psychiatry Suppl. 2013;54:s5–10.

Keefe RS, Vinogradov S, Medalia A, Silverstein SM, Bell MD, Diskinson D, Ventura J, Marder SR, Stroup T. Report from the working group conference on multisite trial design for cognitive remediation in schizophrenia. Schizophr Bull. 2011;37(Suppl 5):1057–65.

Kelleher I, Keeley H, Corcoran P, Lynch F, Fitzpatrick C, Devlin N, Molloy C, Roddy S, Clarke MC, Harley M, Arseneault L, Wasserman C, Carli V, Sarchiapone M, Hoven C, Wasserman D, Cannon M. Clinicopathological significance of psychotic experiences in non–psychotic young people: evidence from four population–based studies. Br J Psychiatry. 2012;201:26–32.

Kendler KS, MacLean CJ. Estimating familial effects on age at onset and liability to schizophrenia. I. Results of a large sample family study. Genet Epidemiol. 1990;7:409–17.

Kirkbride JB, Fearon P, Morgan C, Dazzan P, Morgan K, Tarrant J, Lloyd T, Holloway J, Hutchinson G, Leff JP, Mallett RM, Harrison GL, Murray RM, Jones PB. Heterogeneity in incidence rates of schizophrenia and other psychotic syndromes: findings from the 3-center AeSOP study. Arch Gen Psychiatry. 2006;63:250–8.

Kirov G, Jones PB, Harvey I, Lewis SW, Toone BK, Rifkin L, Sham P, Murray RM. Do obstetric complications cause the earlier age at onset in male than female schizophrenics? Schizophr Res. 1996;20:117–24.

Kørner A, Lopez AG, Lauritzen L, Andersen PK, Kessing LV. Late and very-late first-contact schizophrenia and the risk of dementia—a nationwide register based study. Int J Geriatr Psychiatry. 2009;24:61–7.

Kyriakopoulos M, Perez-Iglesias R, Woolley JB, Kanaan RA, Vyas NS, Barker GJ, Frangou S, McGuire PK. Effect of age at onset of schizophrenia on white matter abnormalities. Br J Psychiatry. 2009;195:346–53.

Large M, Sharma S, Compton MT, Slade T, Nielssen O. Cannabis use and earlier onset of psychosis: a systematic meta-analysis. Arch Gen Psychiatry. 2011;68:555–61.

Macdonald EM, Hayes RL, Baglioni AJ. The quantity and quality of the social networks of young people with early psychosis compared with closely matched controls. Schizophr Res. 2000;46:25–30.

McGrath JJ, Saha S, Al-Hamzawi A, Alonso J, Bromet EJ, Bruffaerts R, Caldas-de-Almeida JM, Chiu WT, de Jonge P, Fayyad J, Florescu S, Gureje O, Haro JM, Hu C, Kovess-Masfety V, Lepine JP, Lim CC, Mora ME, Navarro-Mateu F, Ochoa S, Sampson N, Scott K, Viana MC, Kessler RC. Psychotic experiences in the general population: a cross-national analysis based on 31261 respondents from 18 Countries. JAMA Psychiatry. 2015;72:697–705.

McGrath JJ, Saha S, Al-Hamzawi AO, Alonso J, Andrade L, Borges G, Bromet EJ, Oakley Browne M, Bruffaerts R, Caldas de Almeida JM, Fayyad J, Florescu S, de Girolamo G, Gureje O, Hu C, de Jonge P, Kovess-Masfety V, Lepine JP, Lim CC, Navarro-Mateu F, Piazza M, Sampson N, Posada-Villa J, Kendler KS, Kessler RC. Age of onset and lifetime projected risk of psychotic experiences: cross-national data from the world mental health survey. Schizophr Bull. 2016;42:933–41.

McGrath JJ, McLaughlin KA, Saha S, Aguilar-Gaxiola S, Al-Hamzawi A, Alonso J, Bruffaerts R, de Girolamo G, de Jonge P, Esan O, Florescu S, Gureje O, Haro JM, Hu C, Karam EG, Kovess-Masfety V, Lee S, Lepine JP, Lim CC, Medina-Mora ME, Mneimneh Z, Pennell BE, Piazza M, Posada-Villa J, Sampson N, Viana MC, Xavier M, Bromet EJ, Kendler KS, Kessler RC. The association between childhood adversities and subsequent first onset of psychotic experiences: a cross-national analysis of 23 998 respondents from 17 countries. Psychol Med. 2017;47:1230–45.

Meesters PD, Comijs HC, Smit JH, Eikelenboom P, de Haan L, Beekman AT, Stek ML. Mortality and its determinants in late-life schizophrenia: a 5-year prospective study in a Dutch catchment area. Am J Geriatr Psychiatry. 2016;24:272–7.

Mitelman SA, Brickman AM, Shihabuddin L, Newmark RE, Hazlett EA, Haznedar MM, Buchsbaum MS. A comprehensive assessment of gray and white matter volumes and their relationship to outcome and severity in schizophrenia. Neuroimage. 2007;37:449–62.

Moilanen K, Veijola J, Läksy K, Mäkikyrö T, Miettunen J, Kantojärvi L, Kokkonen P, Karvonen J, Herva A, Joukamaa M, Järvelin M-R, Moring J, Jones P, Isohanni M. Reasons for the diagnostic discordance between clinicians and researchers in schizophrenia in the Northern Finland 1966 Birth Cohort. Soc Psychiatry Psychiatr Epidemiol. 2003;38:305–10.

Newcomer JW, Leucht S. Metabolic adverse effects associated with antipsychotic medications. In: Weinberger DR, Harrison PJ, editors. Schizophrenia. 3rd ed. Oxford: Wiley-Blackwell; 2011. p. 588–97.

Nicolson R, Rapoport JL. Childhood–onset schizophrenia: rare but worth studying. Biol Psychiatry. 1999;46:1418–28.

Onwumere J, Bebbington P, Kuipers E. Family interventions in early psychosis: specificity and effectiveness. Epidemiol Psychiatr Sci. 2011;20:113–9.

Palmer BW, Dawes SE, Heaton RK. What do we know about neuropsychological aspects of schizophrenia? Neuropsychol Rev. 2009;19:365–84.

Panariello F, O'Driscoll L, de Souza RP, Tiwari A, Manchia M, Kennedy J, DeLuca V. Age at onset in Canadian schizophrenia patients: admixture analysis. Schizophr Res. 2010;122:278–9.

Penn DL, Waldheter EJ, Perkins DO, Mueser KT, Lieberman JA. Psychosocial treatment for first-episode psychosis: a research update. Am J Psychiatry. 2005;162:2220–32.

Penttilä M, Jääskeläinen E, Hirvonen N, Isohanni M, Miettunen J. Duration of untreated psychosis as predictor of long–term outcome in schizophrenia. A systematic review and meta–analysis. Br J Psychiatry. 2014;205:88–94.

Peralta V, Cuesta MJ. Delusional disorder and schizophrenia: a comparative study across multiple domains. Psychol Med. 2016;46:2829–39.

Popovic D, Benabarre A, Crespo JM, Goikolea JM, González-Pinto A, Gutiérrez-Rojas L, Montes JM, Vieta E. Risk factors for suicide in schizophrenia: systematic review and clinical recommendations. Acta Psychiatr Scand. 2014;130:418–26.

Rajji TK, Ismail Z, Mulsant BH. Age at onset and cognition in schizophrenia: meta–analysis. Br J Psychiatry. 2009;195:286–93.

Rannikko I, Haapea M, Miettunen J, Veijola J, Murray GK, Barnett JH, Husa AP, Jones PB, Isohanni M, Jääskeläinen E. Changes in verbal learning and memory in schizophrenia and non-psychotic controls in midlife: a nine-year follow-up in the Northern Finland Birth Cohort study 1966. Psychiatry Res. 2015a;228:671–9.

Rannikko I, Murray GK, Juola P, Salo H, Haapea M, Miettunen J, Veijola J, Barnett JH, Husa AP, Jones PB, Järvelin M-R, Isohanni M, Jääskeläinen E. Poor premorbid school performance, but not severity of illness, predicts cognitive decline in schizophrenia in midlife. Schizophr Res Cogn. 2015b;2:120–6.

Rosenfield PJ, Kleinhaus K, Opler M, Perrin M, Learned N, Goetz R, Stanford A, Messinger J, Harkavy-Friedman J, Malaspina D. Later paternal age and sex differences in schizophrenia symptoms. Schizophr Res. 2010;116:191–5.

Rossi A, Bustini M, Prosperini P, Marinangeli MG, Splendiani A, Daneluzzo E, Stratta P. Neuromorphological abnormalities in schizophrenic patients with good and poor outcome. Acta Psychiatr Scand. 2000;101:161–6.

Rubio-Abadal E, Ochoa S, Barajas A, Baños I, Dolz M, Sanchez B, Del Cacho N, Carlson J, Huerta-Ramos E, GENIPE Group, Usall J. Birth weight and obstetric complications determine age at onset in first episode of psychosis. J Psychiatr Res. 2015;65:108–14.

Sato T, Bottlender R, Schröter A, Möller HJ. Psychopathology of early-onset versus late–onset schizophrenia revisited: an observation of 473 neuroleptic-naive patients before and after first-admission treatments. Schizophr Res. 2004;67:175–83.

Scherr M, Hamann M, Schwerthöffer D, Froböse T, Vukovich R, Pitschel-Walz G, Bäuml J. Environmental risk factors and their impact on the age of onset of schizophrenia: comparing familial to non-familial schizophrenia. Nord J Psychiatry. 2012;66:107–14.

Shafee R, Nanda P, Padmanabhan JL, Tandon N, Alliey-Rodriguez N, Keefe RSE, Hill SK, Bishop JR, Clementz BA, Tamminga CA, Gershon ES, Pearlson GD, Keshavan MS, Sweeney JA, Robinson EB, McCarroll SA. Higher genetic risk of schizophrenia is associated with lower cognitive performance in healthy individuals. bioRxiv. 2017;103622. https://doi.org/10.1101/103622.

Stepniak B, Papiol S, Hammer C, Ramin A, Everts S, Hennig L, Begemann M, Ehrenreich H. Accumulated environmental risk determining age at schizophrenia onset: a deep phenotyping-based study. Lancet Psychiatry. 2014;1:444–53.

Suvisaari JM, Haukka J, Tanskanen A, Lönnqvist JK. Age at onset and outcome in schizophrenia are related to the degree of familial loading. Br J Psychiatry. 1998;173:494–500.

Talaslahti T, Alanen HM, Hakko H, Isohanni M, Häkkinen U, Leinonen E. Patients with very-late-onset schizophrenia-like psychosis have higher mortality rates than elderly patients with earlier onset schizophrenia. Int J Geriatr Psychiatry. 2015;30:453–9.

Thorup A, Waltoft BL, Pedersen CB, Mortensen PB, Nordentoft M. Young males have a higher risk of developing schizophrenia: a Danish register study. Psychol Med. 2007;37:479–84.

Timonen MJ, Saari KM, Jokelainen JJ, Meyer-Rochow VB, Räsänen PK, Koponen HJ. Insulin resistance and schizophrenia: results from the Northern Finland 1966 Birth Cohort. Schizophr Res. 2009;113:107–8.

Tonkonogy JM, Geller JL. Late-onset paranoid psychosis as a distinct clinicopathologic entity: magnetic resonance imaging data in elderly patients with paranoid psychosis of late onset and schizophrenia of early onset. Neuropsychiatry Neuropsychol Behav Neurol. 1999;12:230–5.

Vahia IV, Palmer BW, Depp C, Fellows I, Golshan S, Kraemer HC, Jeste DV. Is late-onset schizophrenia a subtype of schizophrenia? Acta Psychiatr Scand. 2010;122:414–26.

van der Gaag M, Smit F, Bechdolf A, French P, Linszen DH, Yung AR, McGorry P, Cuijpers P. Preventing a first episode of psychosis: meta-analysis of randomized controlled prevention trials of 12 month and longer-term follow-ups. Schizophr Res. 2013;149:56–62.

van der Werf M, Hanssen M, Köhler S, Verkaaik M, Verhey FR, RISE Investigators, van Winkel R, van Os J, Allardyce J. Systematic review and collaborative recalculation of 133,693 incident cases of schizophrenia. Psychol Med. 2014;44:9–16.

Verdoux H, Geddes JR, Takei N, Lawrie SM, Bovet P, Eagles JM, Heun R, McCreadie RG, McNeil TF, O'Callaghan E, Stöber G, Willinger MU, Wright P, Murray RM. Obstetric complications and age at onset in schizophrenia: an international collaborative meta-analysis of individual patient data. Am J Psychiatry. 1997;154:1220–7.

Vourdas A, Pipe R, Corrigall R, Frangou S. Increased developmental deviance and premorbid dysfunction in early onset schizophrenia. Schizophr Res. 2003;62:13–22.

Vyas NS, Patel NH, Puri BK. Neurobiology and phenotypic expression in early onset schizophrenia. Early Interv Psychiatry. 2011;5:3–14.

Waters F, Fernyhough C. Hallucinations: a systematic review of points of similarity and difference across diagnostic classes. Schizophr Bull. 2017;43:32–43.

Whiteford HA, Degenhardt L, Rehm J, Baxter AJ, Ferrari AJ, Erskine HE, Charlson FJ, Norman RE, Flaxman AD, Johns N, Burstein R, Murray CJ, Vos T. Global burden of disease attributable to mental and substance use disorders: findings from the Global Burden of Disease Study 2010. Lancet. 2013;382:1575–86.

WHO. The global burden of disease: 2004 update. Geneva: World Health Organization Press; 2008. http://www.who.int/healthinfo/global_burden_disease/. Accessed 29 Jun 2017.

5 The Age of Onset of Bipolar Disorders

Jessica Dagani, Ross J. Baldessarini, Giulia Signorini, Olav Nielssen, Giovanni de Girolamo, and Matthew Large

5.1 Introduction

Bipolar disorder (BD) usually is a lifelong, episodic disorder that is often associated with significant disability and cost to the community, both for treatment and from loss of economic output because of disability. In 2013 there were nearly 50 million cases of BD globally, accounting for the loss of nearly ten million disability-adjusted life years (DALYs). BD is responsible for 0.4% of total DALYs and 1.3% of total years lived with disability (YLDs) due to all diseases (Ferrari et al. 2016). Based on a recent meta-analysis of 38 studies from 26 countries, the pooled, age-standardized

J. Dagani · G. Signorini · G. de Girolamo (✉)
Unit of Psychiatric Epidemiology and Evaluation, IRCCS St John of God Clinical Research Center, Brescia, Italy
e-mail: jdagani@fatebenefratelli.eu; gsignorini@fatebenefratelli.eu; gdegirolamo@fatebenefratelli.eu

R. J. Baldessarini
Harvard Medical School, Boston, MA, USA

International Consortium for Bipolar and Psychotic Disorder Research, Mailman Research Center, McLean Hospital, Belmont, MA, USA
e-mail: rbaldessarini@mclean.harvard.edu

O. Nielssen
Macquarie University, Sydney, NSW, Australia

School of Psychiatry, University of New South Wales, Sydney, NSW, Australia

St Vincents Hospital, Sydney, NSW, Australia

M. Large
School of Psychiatry, University of New South Wales, Sydney, NSW, Australia

Prince of Wales Hospital Sydney, Sydney, NSW, Australia
e-mail: Matthew.Large@health.nsw.gov.au

G. de Girolamo et al. (eds.), *Age of Onset of Mental Disorders*,
https://doi.org/10.1007/978-3-319-72619-9_5

prevalence of BD was 0.7% (CI 0.6–0.8%), with a ratio of females to males of 1.25 (95% CI, 0.91–2.0) (Ferrari et al. 2016).

Estimates of the prevalence of BD have been as high as 5%, depending on the diagnostic criteria used (Yildiz et al. 2015). Even at a prevalence of less than 1% (estimated for type I BD or BD-I), BD represents a major public health challenge, because of the lifelong course of the illness and associated disability, morbidity, all-cause mortality, and high rates of both suicide attempts and completed suicide (Oswald et al. 2007; Tondo and Baldessarini 2015; Tondo et al. 2016). BD also presents challenges for diagnosis, in distinguishing the illness from unipolar major depression and from normal fluctuations in mood, and for maintaining needed, sustained treatment (Evans 2000; Baldessarini 2013).

Younger AoO in BD has been associated with longer delay in the initiation of treatment (Baldessarini et al. 1999; Post et al. 2010; Joslyn et al. 2016; Dagani et al. 2017), greater severity of subsequent morbidity (Post et al. 2010), and more frequent co-occurring anxiety and substance abuse (Joslyn et al. 2016). The overall latency from onset of BD to sustained mood-stabilizing treatment has been estimated at 6–9 years, may be longer among women with type II BD (BD-II), and is as long as 16–18 years following adolescent onset BD (Baldessarini et al. 1999; Post et al. 2010; Dagani et al. 2017).

Despite evidence that earlier treatment is associated with better clinical outcomes for some disorders, notably schizophrenia and other psychotic disorders (Marshall et al. 2005; Large et al. 2008), early intervention in BD has only recently received attention and its long-term clinical impact remains uncertain. Nevertheless, the typically prolonged latency from illness onset to correct diagnosis and appropriate treatment of BD, as noted above, strongly encourages research on the AoO of BD in order to support early case identification and development of effective and earlier interventions.

The growing interest in the age of onset (AoO) of diseases is because knowing when illnesses develop might improve our understanding of the underlying causes of diseases and facilitate earlier interventions aimed at reducing long-term morbidity, disability, and mortality. It is likely that earlier intervention improves the outcome of mental disorders (Conus et al. 2014; Herrman 2014; Malhi et al. 2014). Early intervention in BD is a less developed field, and effects of earlier diagnosis and treatment on the prognosis of BD are not securely established (Baethge et al. 2003a, b, 2017; Bratti et al. 2003).

Epidemiological studies of AoO of mental disorders are complicated by the variety of clinical presentations and lack of agreed definitions of illness onset. Onset of BD is particularly difficult to define, even in prospective studies, because early illness often includes depression, whereas an episode of mania-like illness (mania, hypomania, or mixed state) is required to establish a diagnosis of BD (Ratheesh et al. 2017). Attenuated or sub-syndromal forms of depression and hypomania are commonly encountered in BD patients and can be difficult to distinguish from ordinary fluctuations of mood. Moreover, the antecedents of BD can present as behavioural disturbances in childhood and adolescence, or with substance abuse, panic attacks, or other anxiety syndromes (Faedda et al. 2018). Retrospective studies of AoO are subject to recall error (Montlahuc et al. 2016), which may be further complicated by effects of the illness itself. Despite these methodological difficulties, a better understanding of the onset of BD would support efforts to develop and evaluate early interventions that might improve some of the adverse outcomes associated with chronic and commonly relapsing forms of BD.

We conducted a systematic review and meta-analysis aimed at providing a reliable, pooled estimate of AoO in BD based on a large, comprehensive sample of studies meeting critical inclusion criteria, and explored effects of selected demographic, clinical, and methodological factors for association with AoO and on the variation in its reported estimates.

5.2 Methods

Data acquisition was based on the Preferred Reporting Items for Systematic Reviews and Meta-Analyses (PRISMA) guidelines (Moher et al. 2010).

5.2.1 Searches

We conducted a systematic search of English, French, German, and Italian language publications indexed in the electronic databases PubMed, Web of Science, and Psychology and Behavioral Science Collection, from their inception to 31 December 2014. The search string was "onset AND bipolar" in titles or abstracts. We also hand-searched reference lists of identified reports to identify additional citations.

5.2.2 Inclusion and Exclusion Criteria

Two investigators independently screened article titles and abstracts to exclude irrelevant studies, duplicate or overlapping reports, meta-analyses, or reviews, and reports of fewer than ten subjects. Potentially relevant reports were independently examined in full text by two investigators to apply predetermined eligibility criteria and extract required data. When two or more reports involved overlapping samples, the report with the largest sample was selected. An assessment of investigator inter-rater reliability was made by calculating agreement (Cohen's kappa [κ] statistic) in AoO data in 10% of randomly screened abstracts and full texts that were then reviewed by at least two additional investigators.

Studies were included if they (a) reported on cohorts of patients with BD, including BD-I, BD-II, and BD–not otherwise specified (BD-NOS), or cyclothymia and (b) provided data on mean AoO of BD (defined as age at first mood symptoms [including depression if followed by mania or hypomania], mood syndromes, mood episodes, or based on undefined AoO of the disorder). Exclusion criteria were

(a) specialized samples (based on particular selection criteria such as genetic or other biological characteristics); (b) age-specific samples, particularly paediatric populations; and (c) samples including disorders other than BD without separate reporting on BD subjects.

5.2.3 Data Extraction

Two authors independently recorded reported AoO and data for a predetermined list of potential moderating variables, using a data recording form designed for this purpose. Disagreements were resolved by consensus after further joint examination. The following data were extracted:

(a) Sample size
(b) Mean AoO of BD, with standard deviation (SD), using the definitions in the primary research report. When a report included multiple estimates of AoO, our first choice was age at first symptoms, second was first episode of mood disorder (including depression followed later by mania, hypomania, or a manic-depressive mixed state), and third was undefined "AoO". When multiple indications of the polarity of first lifetime episodes of BD were reported (e.g. first depressive and first [hypo]manic episode), the earliest type was selected
(c) Country where the study was conducted
(d) Proportion of women in each study sample
(e) Proportion of BD diagnostic subtypes
(f) Proportion of first episodes with depressive versus (hypo)manic polarity
(g) Year of publication
(h) Study design (retrospective, cross-sectional, or prospective)
(i) Assessment of each report based on a "strength of reporting" scale score

5.2.4 Assessment of Strength of Reporting

We developed a four-point strength-of-reporting rating scale from items of the Newcastle-Ottawa Scale for assessing the quality of non-randomized studies (Deeks et al. 2003). For each study, a point was awarded for each of the following:

1. Defined onset of initial symptoms or a first lifetime episode of mood disorder later proved to be BD
2. Used the life chart method or other specific chronological methods for ascertaining AoO systematically
3. Used a structured interview rather than clinical assessment alone to confirm the diagnosis of BD
4. Had a sample size ≥ 50
5. Resulting in an overall reporting strength score of between 0 and 4

5.2.5 Meta-analysis

Meta-analytic pooled estimates of AoO were calculated using random-effects modelling, chosen a priori, as we assumed that differences in sampling and in definitions of AoO would result in high between-study heterogeneity. Heterogeneity was examined using the Q-value and I^2 statistic derived from Q. Publication bias was assessed using an Egger's regression test and the Duval and Tweedie trim-and-fill method. Analyses were conducted using *Comprehensive Meta-Analysis.3*® (Biostat Corp., Englewood, NJ).

The contribution to between-study heterogeneity that might be explained by definitions of AoO and other categorical differences in study characteristics or methods were examined with subgroup analyses. Subgroups included the proportions of females in study samples, BD-I and BD-II diagnostic types, the nation and geographic region of the study, and definition of AoO (age at first symptoms, first episode of mood disorder, or undefined AoO). We also examined the contribution of strength-of-reporting scores to between-study heterogeneity.

We used mixed effects meta-regression modelling to assess the contribution to between-study heterogeneity in estimates of AoO and selected modifier variables. Candidate variables were (a) current mean age of the sample, (b) proportion of female subjects, (c) proportion of participants diagnosed with BD-I, (d) proportion with depressive polarity at onset, (e) proportion of subjects with a family history of mood disorder (in first-degree relatives), and (f) year of publication. Moderator variables that contributed to between-study heterogeneity at an α of 0.05 were then included in random-effects meta-regression models.

5.3 Results

5.3.1 Searches and Data Extraction

The systematic literature search and report-selection process yielded 264 studies with a total of 65,565 subjects (averaging 248/study), from an initial set of 8,735 potentially relevant publications (Fig. 5.1). There was a high level of agreement in search results at the level of abstracts (Cohen's $\kappa = 0.90$) and full texts ($\kappa = 0.83$) as sources of estimates of mean AoO ± SD, for inclusion in further analyses. For the full list of papers included in the meta-analysis, please refer to the Appendix at the end of the book (Table 5.6 and related references). Minor between-investigator differences in data extraction arose in 12 of the 264 included studies and were resolved by further joint examination of the text.

5.3.2 Average AoO

The pooled AoO across the 264 studies analysed was 25.3 years (95% confidence interval [CI], 24.4–26.2 years; 95% prediction interval [PI], 11.1–39.5 years;

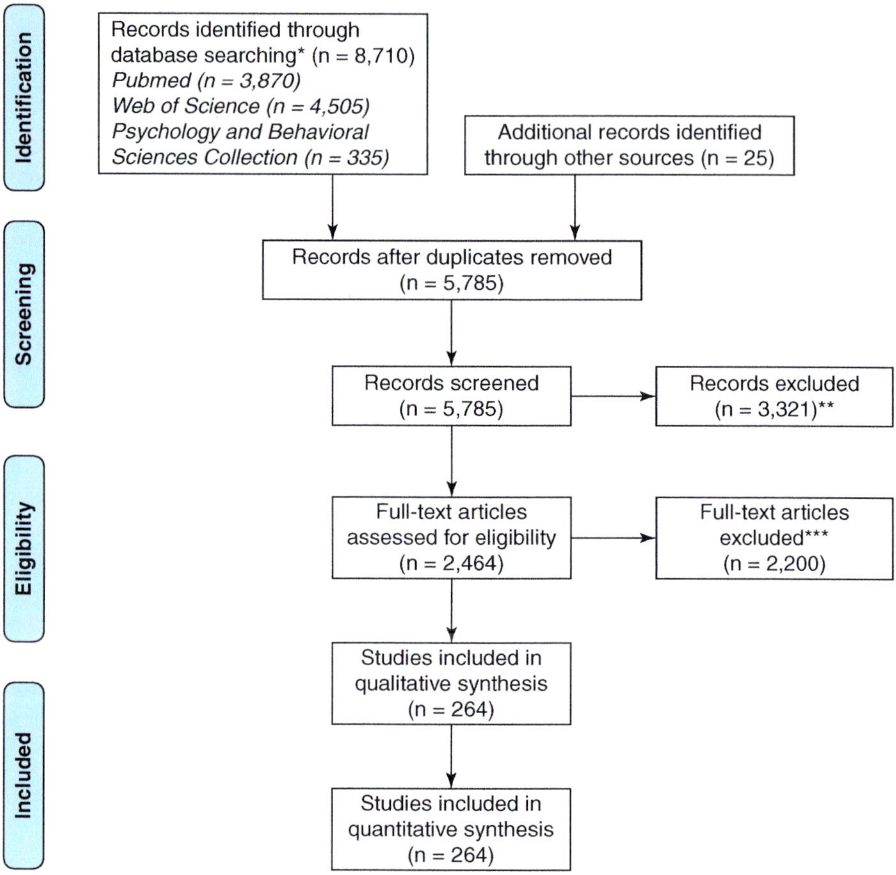

Fig. 5.1 PRISMA flow chart for selection of studies for analysis. * Search performed on 31 December 2014, using the search string "onset AND bipolar". ** Excluded: meta-analyses, reviews, not concerning BD, not reporting original findings, commentaries, case reports, and small case series. *** Not reporting mean AoO, SD, and sample size, multiple reports of the same study, reporting preselected or age-specific samples, reporting mixed samples of BD plus other disorders without data regarding only BD

median AoO = 25.6 years; interquartile range [IQR], 22.4–28.1). There was very high between-sample heterogeneity ($I^2 = 99.6$), reflected in the wide range of AoO estimates among individual studies, from 12.7 to 45.0 years (Table 5.6).

There was evidence of publication bias towards studies reporting younger AoO (Egger's regression, intercept = 8.77; $t = 7.96$ [df=262], $p = <0.001$). Trim-and-fill analysis (51 studies) filled to the left of mean and adjusted value of 23.8 (CI = 23.1–24.6) years indicated that publication bias reduced the pooled AoO estimate by approximately 6%.

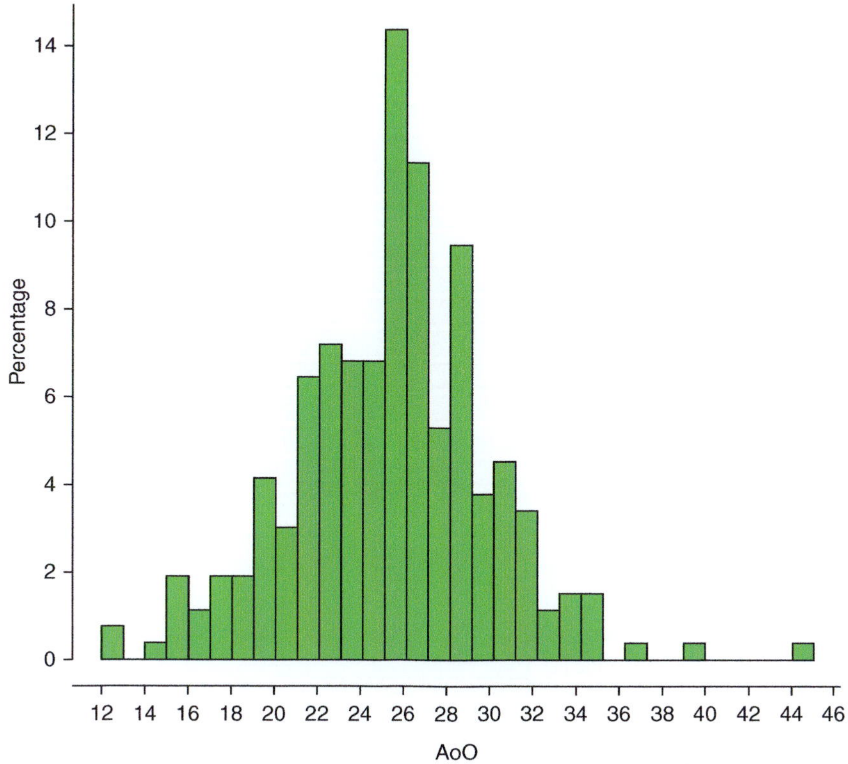

Fig. 5.2 Histogram of mean AoO. Histogram of mean AoO (bars) in 264 studies (from Table 5.1), as the proportion (%) of studies at reported mean onset ages

A graphic representation of the empirical mean AoO of the 264 included studies is reported in Fig. 5.2.

5.3.3 International Differences

Pooled AoO estimates for specific countries, based on 1–62 studies per country, also yielded a wide range of values with high heterogeneity (Q = 736 [df = 40], $I^2 = 99.6\%$, $p < 0.001$). These national estimates of AoO ranged from a low value of 19.9 (CI, 17.8–22.0) years in Hungary to a high value of 45.0 (CI, 41.8–48.2) years in nearby Croatia, based on single studies (Fig. 5.3).

There was very high statistical heterogeneity between the ten major geographic regions with ($Q = 73$ [df = 9], $I^2 = 99.6\%$, $p < 0.001$; Table 5.1, Fig. 5.3). Heterogeneity within each region was also >80% except in South and Central America (68.4%; Table 5.1). The youngest regional average AoO estimate was 15.2 years in Australasia, and the oldest was 31.8 years in East Asia.

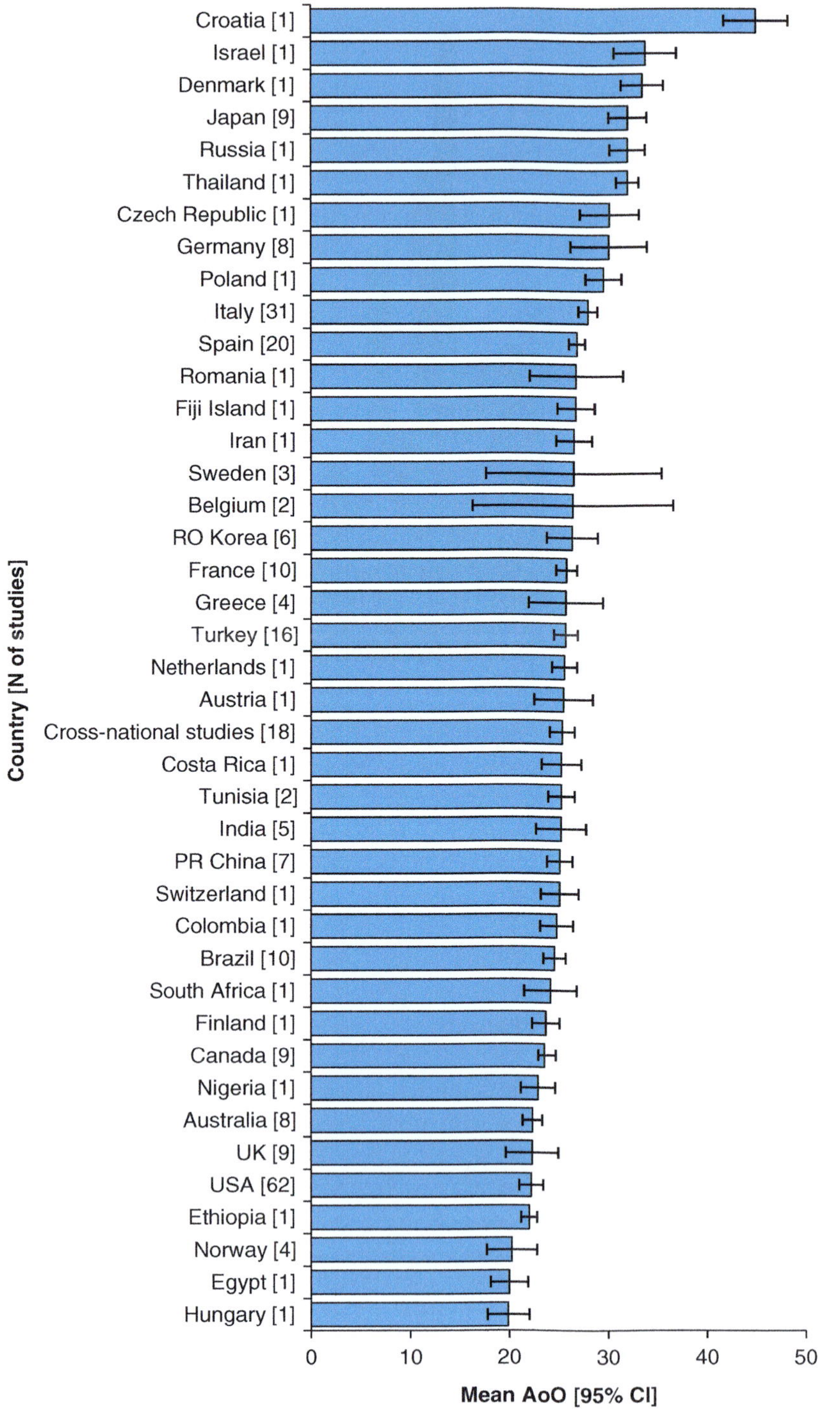

Fig. 5.3 International differences in pooled AoO estimates. Mean (± 95% CI) AoO of BD by country [with a number of studies], ranked from highest to lowest estimates

Table 5.1 Mean age at onset of bipolar disorder in world regions

Regions	Studies (n)	Mean onset age (years)	95% CI	Heterogeneity I^2 (%)
Australasia	9	21.7	18.1–25.3	99.4
North America	71	22.4	21.4–23.4	97.9
Africa	6	23.2	21.6–24.8	81.8
Nordic Europe	11	24.6	21.8–27.5	96.6
South and Central America	12	24.7	23.7–25.6	68.4
South Asia	5	25.3	22.7–27.8	89.1
Cross-national	18	25.4	24.1–62.7	98.8
Mainland Europe	107	26.9	26.2–27.5	95.8
East Asia	23	28.2	26.0–30.5	99.0
Middle East	2	30.1	23.0–37.1	93.4
Total	**264**	**25.2**	**24.8–25.7**	**99.6**

Average AoO estimates for each region were based on meta-analytic pooling of data shown in this table

Table 5.2 Factors associated with onset age in bipolar disorder subjects: univariate meta-regressions

Covariate	Regression coefficient	Coefficient p-value	Explanatory value (r^2 [%])	Heterogeneity (I^2 [%])
Mean current age	+0.355	<0.001	27.16	99.5
Depressive onset (%)	+0.026	0.45	14.14	98.7
Bipolar I (%)	+0.015	0.42	7.35	99.6
Females (%)	+0.007	0.86	4.73	99.6
Family history of mood disorder (%)	−0.074	0.06	0.00	94.9
Publication year	−0.102	0.10	3.64	99.5

5.3.4 Family History

Based on the meta-regression of a limited number of studies reporting the proportion of subjects with a family history of mood disorder among first-degree relatives, we found a trend towards a younger AoO among people with a positive family history (meta-regression coefficient = −0.07, $p = 0.06$; Table 5.2). This finding indicates that an increase of 10% in the proportion of patients with a family history of mood disorder reduced the mean AoO by almost 1 year.

5.3.5 Comparison of Type I Versus Type II BD

We found no significant differences in pooled AoO estimates between samples of BD-I and BD-II subjects, in either the 91 separate samples of BD-I and 28 of BD-II subjects, and among the 18 studies that included both BP-I and BP-II subgroups (Table 5.3), or in a meta-regression assessing the effect of the proportion of BP-I subjects on AoO.

Table 5.3 Mean AoO in bipolar I and II disorders

Diagnosis	Studies (*n*)	Mean onset age (years)	95% CI	Heterogeneity I^2 (%)
		100% bipolar I or bipolar II samples		
Bipolar I	91	25.8	25.2–26.5	96.6
Bipolar II	28	25.5	23.4–27.5	97.2
Total	**119**	**25.8**	**25.2–26.4**	**96.9**
		Matched samples		
Bipolar I	18	26.7	25.1–28.3	94.4
Bipolar II	18	30.0	24.5–29.4	95.5
Total	**36**	**26.8**	**25.4–28.2**	**94.9**

Mean AoO estimates did not differ between BD-I and BD-II subjects

Table 5.4 Mean AoO among female and male bipolar disorder patients in matched samples

Sex	Samples (*n*)	Mean onset age (years)	95% CI	Heterogeneity I^2 (%)
Females	15	25.3	23.9–26.6	94.5
Males	15	26.4	24.4–28.5	97.0
Total	**30**	**26.0**	**24.6–27.4**	**96.3**

5.3.6 Cyclothymia

Five of the 264 studies included small proportions of patients (46/427; 10.8%) diagnosed with cyclothymia (Zhang et al. 1997; Ohara et al. 1998; Gutiérrez-Rojas et al. 2008; Feinman and Dunner 1996; Harnic et al. 2013). The pooled AoO of this subgroup of studies was 27.3 (CI, 23.7–30.9) years, which did not differ significantly from the studies that excluded patients with cyclothymia (pooled AoO, 25.3 years; 95% CI, 24.4–26.2 years; $Q = 1.14$, $p = 0.30$).

5.3.7 Sex Differences

Sex was not a statistically significant moderator of AoO considering either the proportion of females in an overall univariate meta-regression ($p = 0.86$; Table 5.2) or the 15 studies reporting on both men (26.4 [CI, 24.4–28.5] years) and women (25.3 [CI, 23.9–26.6] years; Table 5.4).

5.3.8 Current Age, Publication Year, Polarity of Onset, and Definitions of AoO

Older *current age* (meta-regression coefficient = 0.35) was associated with older estimates of AoO, and this variable accounted for 27.2% of observed between-study heterogeneity (Table 5.2). In addition, more recent *year of publication of the study* was associated with non-significantly lower AoO (Table 5.2).

Depressive versus manic or hypomanic *first lifetime episode polarity* of BD was associated with non-significantly older estimated AoO in a small subset of studies (depressive onset, $n = 5$, AoO = 21.9, CI = 18.5–25.4 years; [hypo]manic onset, $n = 5$, AoO = 23.8, CI = 21.4–26.2 years; Q = 0.76, $p = 0.38$). An overall univariate meta-regression considering the proportion of patients whose first episode of mood disorder was an episode of depression confirmed that the polarity at onset was not a statistically significant moderator ($p = 0.45$; Table 5.2).

Finally, differences in the definition of AoO made a non-significant contribution to between-sample heterogeneity ($Q = 1.1$, $p = 0.57$).

5.3.9 Strength of Reporting

Between-study heterogeneity in estimates of AoO was not significantly associated with any of the following indicators of reporting strength:

(a) Definition of AoO by initial symptoms or first episode of mood disorder, rather than clinically ascertained, but unspecified, "illness onset" ($p = 0.82$)
(b) Whether or not AoO was estimated using life charts or other chronological methods ($p = 0.41$)
(c) Use of structured interviews or rating scales to support the diagnosis of BD ($p = 0.09$)
(d) Sample size ≥50 subjects versus fewer ($p = 0.39$)
(e) Overall reporting strength score (0–4; $p = 0.91$) (Table 5.5)

Table 5.5 Subgroup analysis of study quality

Subgroups	Studies (n)	Point estimate	95% CI	Heterogeneity I^2 (%)
Reporting quality item 1 (*AoO based on initial symptoms or episode*)				
No	163	25.4	24.7–26.1	97.5
Yes	101	25.2	23.6–26.8	99.8
Reporting quality item 2 (*life chart method or other chronological method*)				
No	246	25.4	24.4–26.3	99.6
Yes	18	24.5	22.5–26.4	96.9
Reporting quality item 3 (*structured interview or scale to confirm diagnosis*)				
No	67	26.2	25.2–27.3	98.1
Yes	197	25.0	23.9–26.0	99.6
Reporting quality item 4 (*sample size ≥50*)				
No	63	24.7	23.2–26.2	96.2
Yes	201	25.5	24.5–26.5	99.7
Reporting strength global score				
Score 0	13	24.8	21.3–28.4	97.8
Score 1	64	25.8	24.6–26.9	97.0
Score 2	115	25.4	24.5–26.2	98.0
Score 3	65	24.8	22.8–26.9	99.9
Score 4	7	24.7	21.7–27.7	97.3

Among all 264 studies, meta-analytically averaged AoO was 25.3 (CI, 24.4–26.2) years

5.4 Discussion

5.4.1 General Considerations

We report the largest and most up-to-date meta-analysis of the AoO of BD, based on 264 studies with 65,565 subjects from most regions of the world, including countries with a wide range of health systems and levels of economic development. The main finding is a meta-analytically pooled overall AoO of BD of 25.3 (95% CI, 24.4–26.2; median 25.6) years, with high levels of heterogeneity among individual studies ($I^2 = 99.6\%$), and a wide range of AoO values (12.7–32.3 years; Table 5.6; Fig. 5.2). The extreme heterogeneity of the data is also evident in the 95% PI of 11.1–39.5 years, suggesting that any future studies will have a 95% chance of finding a mean AoO between these two values.

We found marked differences in AoO between countries, from a low for Hungary of 19.9 to a high in Croatia of 45.0 years, and between world regions, from 15.2 years in Australasia to 31.8 years in East Asia (Table 5.1). These differences suggest that some of the observed heterogeneity might be due to social, cultural, or biological factors that vary between nations and geographic regions or to differences in ascertainment methods that are not clear from the published reports.

The association between a history of mood disorder among first-degree relatives and a younger AoO of BD, reported in several large, well-designed studies (Johnson et al. 2000, Baldessarini et al. 2012b; Ratheesh et al. 2017), was not confirmed by this meta-analysis, although there was a trend towards significance ($p = 0.06$) (Table 5.3). The finding of younger AoO in studies of patients with strong family histories of mood disorder, especially with multiple cases of BD, suggests a familial or genetic association with clinical expression of BD at a younger age, and possibly a worse long-term prognosis (Thesing et al. 2015; Carlson and Pataki 2016). However, the association was not confirmed by other research studies (e.g. Grigoroiu-Serbanescu et al. 2005), and the finding might be due to increased awareness of the disorder, resulting in earlier assessment and treatment.

We expected to find between-study differences in AoO with respect to variables such as sex, BD diagnostic type (BD-I vs. BD-II), and depressive versus [hypo] manic polarity of onset (Tables 5.3 and 5.4). However, none of these factors was found to contribute significantly to between-study heterogeneity.

The finding of no difference in AoO between female and male subjects (Table 5.4) is consistent with findings of some investigators (Hendrick et al. 2000; Diflorio and Jones 2010). However, other studies have reported younger AoO of BD among males, especially those presenting in the manic phase (Arnold 2003; Kawa et al. 2005; Kennedy et al. 2005; Holtzman et al. 2016).

The absence of a significant difference between AoO of BD-I and BD-II also contrasts with the findings of large, primary studies (Baldessarini et al. 2012b; Tondo et al. 2010). A later AoO in BD-II is expected, given the greater difficulty in making this diagnosis in many patients, and its clinical similarity to unipolar major depressive disorder, in which an even later onset has been reported (Baldessarini et al. 2010;

Tondo et al. 2010; Dervic et al. 2015). However, the present meta-analysis of all available studies did not find an overall difference in AoO for BD-I compared to BD-II, nor in a subgroup analysis of 18 studies that included both BD-I and BD-II patients evaluated under matched conditions (Table 5.2), consistent with the findings of a number of primary studies (Vieta and Suppes 2008; Dell'Osso et al. 2016; Vinberg et al. 2017).

In addition to the negative findings with respect to potential demographic and clinical moderators of AoO, we found little evidence that the high degree of heterogeneity among studies was accounted for by differences in the methods used in the primary research. More generally, methodological quality ratings in the primary studies, as measured by our strength-of-reporting scale, did not explain between-study heterogeneity (Table 5.5). Finally, we found an older AoO in studies of subjects with older current age, which made a significant contribution to the overall variation in the results. The association may reflect a bias towards young onset among younger subjects who had not passed through the entire range of time at risk for developing BD, or may reflect recall bias among older subjects.

5.4.2 Clinical Implications

Interest in AoO of BD and other mental disorders arises in part from emerging efforts to improve prediction, earlier recognition, and more timely intervention in order to reduce morbidity, disability, and mortality from inadequately treated illness. There is a particular interest in the prediction and early recognition of BD in juveniles and young adults (Faedda et al. 2018). Nevertheless, it has yet to be established that early intervention in BD does improve the course of the illness. Several studies report better outcomes with early intervention (Franchini et al. 1999; Colom et al. 2010; Joyce et al. 2016), whereas others have found that delay in initial treatment or the number of previous episode recurrences in BD did not predict response to treatment or outcome, even after years of illness and multiple episodes (Baethge et al. 2003a, b, 2017; Bratti et al. 2003). Nevertheless, the lack of any difference in response to treatment associated with the duration of untreated BD does not consider the potentially devastating effect on morbidity and disability of long periods of untreated BD (Baethge et al. 2017).

The expectation that earlier, better treatment might alter the course of BD stems from the hypothesis that BD is a progressive illness, first proposed by Kraepelin more than a century ago (Oepen et al. 2004), with shortening cycles of illness, and in which more frequent and severe episodes would be expected to result in greater morbidity and declining treatment response over time. However, the impression of a progressive course in BD might be an artefact of not matching research subjects by the total number of episodes of illness, along with the considerable variation in the course of BD and the exclusion of less severe and single episode patients from clinical samples. At this point, we do not have conclusive evidence of progression or acceleration of BD in patients with untreated episodes or longer duration of illness (Oepen et al. 2004; Baldessarini et al. 2012a).

5.4.3 Strengths and Limitations

The main limitation of this study arises from the nature of meta-analytic data-pooling itself, which involves averaging a large number of studies, each of which reports average results from a variety of subjects. Unless they are relatively large, differences may not be detected in the process of averaging averages. For example, *averaged* proportions of female subjects or subjects with a family history of mood disorder in samples that have a high level of heterogeneity might overlook potentially important differences that could be detected by meta-analysis of individual patient data gathered under matched conditions in single studies. In addition, the extraordinary range of reported estimates of AoO of BD across individual studies and between geographic regions remains largely unexplained. Nevertheless, the strength of this meta-analysis is the very large number of large samples, and the representative nature of the primary studies that were included.

Conclusions

This meta-analytic review of 264 primary research studies with nearly 66,000 subjects yielded a pooled value for the AoO of BD of 25.3 years. There were large differences in AoO for BD among individual countries and regions of the world, for which there was no obvious explanation and which requires further research. We did not find differences in AoO due to sex, diagnostic subtype, or the methods employed in the primary research, and meta-analysis did not confirm that the presence of a family history of mood disorder was associated with earlier AoO although there was a trend towards significance.

Early and effective clinical intervention has the potential to reduce the burden of BD and the morbidity associated with delay in treatment. The comparatively early mean AoO, which shows that many cases of BD occur in adolescence and early adult life, confirms the need for more accessible and effective systems of care for young persons with emerging BD (Berk et al. 2007; McGorry et al. 2007, 2010; Patton et al. 2007; Lambert et al. 2016). AoO is an important statistic to guide future mental health policies for the care of those who have or might develop BD.

Acknowledgements Supported in part by a grant from the Bruce J. Anderson Foundation and by the McLean Private Donors Psychiatry Research Fund (to RJB). We are grateful to Drs. Clarissa Ferrari, Moira Marizzoni, Fabiana Faustini, Giulia Oliosi, and Sabina Moro for valuable contributions to the preparation of the manuscript.

Disclosures: No author or immediate family member has financial relationships with commercial organizations that might appear to represent conflicts of interest with the material presented here.

Appendix

Table 5.6 Studies of AoO of BD ($N = 264$)

Authors (year)	Country	Subjects (n)	Mean age	% Females	% Bipolar I	Onset age ±SD
Aghanwa (2001)	Fiji	82	–	47.6	–	26.8 ± 8.7
Akdeniz et al. (2003)	Turkey	49	50.1	100	–	34.1 ± 9.0
Akiskal et al. (1983)	USA	41	–	61.0	100	26.1 ± 13.3
Aldana et al. (2009)	Spain	67	42.2	–	70.2	26.4 ± 10.9
Altamura et al. (2010)	Italy	320	46.0	56.2	40.0	30.0 ± 10.8
Altindag et al. (2006)	Turkey	70	34.1	42.9	100	23.5 ± 7.5
Altshuler et al. (1995)	USA	55	40.8	47.3	52.7	24.0 ± 9.3
Ancın et al. (2010)	Spain	141	44.1	58.8	80.1	26.8 ± 10.2
Andersson et al. (2008)	Norway	25	36.3	80.0	–	22.0 ± 10.3
Andreazza et al. (2009)	Cross-national	60	31.8	63.3	–	23.7 ± 6.0
Arai et al. (2007)	Japan	148	48.9	46.0	64.0	33.5 ± 11.4
Atkinson et al. (1997)	Canada	37	42.3	48.7	–	28.7 ± 9.9
Atmaca et al. (2006)	Turkey	12	28.2	50.0	100	28.2 ± 6.5
Azorin et al. (2008)	France	958	44.4	59.0	100	28.0 ± 10.3
Baldessarini et al. (2010)	Cross-national	1566	–	54.3	69.6	28.8 ± 12.1
Baldessarini et al. (2012b)	Cross-national	1315	43.8	56.4	100	26.8 ± 8.9
Baldessarini et al. (2014)	Italy	1081	44.2	58.1	59.8	28.5 ± 12.4
Baron et al. (1982)	USA	142	–	57.0	–	26.3 ±11.7
Basso et al. (2002)	USA	86	35.6	75.6	100	25.4 ± 13.7
Bauer et al. (1994)	USA	37	41.0	67.6	35.1	24.0 ± 16.0
Bauer et al. (2010)	USA	270	37.6	75.9	65.6	19.1 ± 6.9
Bauer et al. (2014)	Cross-national	4037	48.1	58.8	100	25.4 ± 10.7
Beckmann and Goodwin (1980)	USA	18	–	–	50.0	28.9 ± 12.8
Bellantuono et al. (2007)	Italy	559	45.8	54.6	–	29.7 ± 11.1
Bellivier et al. (2003)	Cross-national	579	–	–	100	26.3 ± 7.0
Bellivier et al. (2014)	Cross-national	3616	44.0	55.7	100	28.8 ± 10.9
Benazzi (1999)	Italy	144	40.1	72.9	0	26.1 ± 10.8
Benazzi (2008)	Italy	441	40.9	67.5	0	22.7 ± 10.7
Benedetti et al. (2008)	Italy	20	34.6	55	100	25.6 ± 12

(continued)

Table 5.6 (continued)

Authors (year)	Country	Subjects (*n*)	Mean age	% Females	% Bipolar I	Onset age ±SD
Benedetti et al. (2012)	Italy	122	46.7	73.8	100	32.2 ± 10.0
Benedetti et al. (2014)	Italy	136	46.5	68.4	100	29.1 ± 9.6
Beyer et al. (2008)	USA	146	45.0	66.4	–	24.1 ± 14.1
Biffin et al. (2009)	Australia	162	42.6	61.1	100	23.2 ± 4.5
Birmaher et al. (2010)	USA	83	32.9	90.4	61.4	17.4 ± 6.2
Blumberg et al. (2003)	USA	36	31.0	56.0	100	17.4 ± 8.0
Bora et al. (2007)	Australia	65	38.0	53.9	100	23.4 ± 7.1
Bozikas et al. (2006)	Greece	19	39.0	57.9	100	26.0 ± 7.0
Brambilla et al. (2001)	USA	22	36.0	40.9	77.3	20.0 ± 7.0
Braunig et al. (2009)	Germany	155	–	60.0	100	22.8 ± 2.7
Brugue et al. (2008)	Spain	264	35.4	58.0	69.7	24.4 ± 7.4
Carballo et al. (2008)	USA	152	–	–	–	19.8 ± 10.0
Cardoso et al. (2008)	Brazil	178	42.8	70.8	–	25.6 ± 11.5
Carlson et al. (2012)	USA	126	29.3	48.4	100	25.4 ± 8.8
Casas-Barquero et al. (2007)	Spain	40	46.1	75.0	77.5	27.6 ± 8.0
Cervantes et al. (2001)	Canada	18	43.2	38.9	–	28.8 ± 10.6
Cha et al. (2009)	Korea	258	33.6	54.2	–	25.7 ± 9.3
Chen and Dilsaver (1995)	USA	168	–	69	–	20.6 ± 9.4
Cichon et al. (1995)	Germany	99	49.8	–	100	28.4 ± 11.4
Col et al. (2014)	Turkey	78	37.9	64.1	100	27.7 ± 9.8
Colom et al. (2006)	Spain	224	42.3	58.9	62.5	27.3 ± 10.9
Conus et al. (2010)	Australia	87	22.1	44.8	100	22.1 ± 3.6
Dawson et al. (2014)	USA	94	31	45.8	100	19 ± 8
Del Grande et al. (2012)	Italy	98	40.7	53.1	87.1	25.7 ± 9.8
Demirel et al. (2014)	Turkey	109	35.0	11.0	100	24.8 ± 7.4
Derntl et al. (2009)	Germany	62	42.9	59.7	41.9	39.2 ± 9.6
DeRosse et al. (2013)	USA	269	36.7	50.9	100	22.3 ± 8.1
Dias et al. (2009)	Spain	65	37.8	63.1	100	24.1 ± 8.6
Di Florio et al. (2014)	UK	1212	47.8	100	77.1	23.1 ± 8.2
Ehnvall and Agren (2002)	Sweden	10	48.2	40.0	40.0	31.2 ± 17.0
El Kissi et al. (2013)	Tunisia	60	43.0	–	80.0	26.2 ± 9.0
El-Hadidy et al. (2013)	Egypt	90	34.3	51.5	100	20.0 ± 9.1
Engström et al. (2003)	Sweden	100	55.8	60.0	75.0	30.4 ± 10.1

Table 5.6 (continued)

Authors (year)	Country	Subjects (*n*)	Mean age	% Females	% Bipolar I	Onset age ±SD
Ernst and Goldberg (2004)	USA	56	40.8	44.6	82.1	21.7 ± 9.6
Eryilmaz et al. (2014)	Turkey	69	32.1	65.2	–	22.3 ± 12.7
Etain et al. (2007)	France	351	42.6	59.3	74.1	26.5 ± 11.1
Etain et al. (2013)	Cross-national	587	40.6	60.1	72.4	24.2 ± 10.1
Fagiolini et al. (2007)	USA	261	44.5	60.2	–	21.8 ± 14.0
Feinman and Dunner (1996)	USA	188	41.8	47.3	22.3	22.1 ± 12.0
Forbes et al. (2005)	USA	38	–	–	68.0	12.7 ± 3.0
Fornaro et al. (2010)	Italy	148	46.8	100	23.0	25.2 ± 9.7
Francis and Gasparo (1994)	USA	100	37.7	67.0	100	27.3 ± 11.9
Frangou (2002)	UK	63	42.0	58.7	100	25.5 ± 10.2
Frey et al. (2008)	USA	36	35.4	61.1	80.6	20.0 ± 6.9
Gan et al. (2011)	China	169	–	59.2	21.3	24.4 ± 9.4
Gao et al. (2008)	USA	144	36.1	52.8	68.8	12.7 ± 6.3
Garcia-Amador et al. (2009)	Spain	305	42.0	56.1	64.9	27.2 ± 11.2
Gasperini et al. (1993)	Italy	113	45.6	63.0	–	30.5 ± 12.3
Gassab et al. (2002)	Tunisia	96	–	57.3	81.2	24.8 ± 8.2
Ghaemi et al. (2004)	USA	36	39.5	63.9	72.2	15.5 ± 8.1
Glenn et al. (2006)	Cross-national	49	38.0	71.4	91.8	21.5 ± 11.4
Goghari and Sponheim (2008)	USA	31	43.6	22.6	–	22.1 ± 8.1
Gogos et al. (2010)	Australia	40	42.4	60.0	–	22.2 ± 8.8
Goldberg et al. (1998)	USA	184	40.5	53.8	100	27.0 ± 12.3
Goldberg and Garno (2009)	USA	100	–	–	–	17.5 ± 9.4
Goldstein and Levitt (2006)	USA	1298	39.5	59.4	100	31.1 ± 17.3
Grande et al. (2014)	Brazil	115	44.0	70.4	68.7	27.3 ± 12.1
Grigoroiu-Serbanescu et al. (2014)	Cross-national	1857	44.0	59.7	100	27.2 ± 9.0
Gruber et al. (2008)	USA	26	24.4	26.9	–	23.8 ± 5.0
Gulseren et al. (2006)	Turkey	12	30.9	33.3	100	24.8 ± 3.6
Gutiérrez-Rojas et al. (2008)	Spain	108	48.0	69.0	74.0	30.4 ± 13.7
Harnic et al. (2013)	Italy	60	47.7	53.0	50.0	28.8 ± 8.3
Haro et al. (2006)	Cross-national	3536	44.6	55.2	100	29.9 ± 11.0

(continued)

Table 5.6 (continued)

Authors (year)	Country	Subjects (*n*)	Mean age	% Females	% Bipolar I	Onset age ±SD
Hauser et al. (2000)	USA	47	40.7	57.5	53.2	21.0 ± 9.8
Hays et al. (1998)	USA	74	42.4	62.2	–	25.7 ± 13.1
Henry et al. (2008)	France	179	39.2	62.6	78.8	25.6 ± 10.7
Horesh et al. (2011)	Israel	50	–	60.0	–	33.8 ± 11.4
Hosang et al. (2012a)	UK	512	48.0	66.0	89.8	21.8 ± 18.6
Hosang et al. (2012b)	UK	96	51.2	72.0	–	20.8 ± 16.4
Kanske et al. (2013)	Germany	22	39.4	63.6	100	25.2 ± 7.7
Kato et al. (1998)	Cross-national	220	31.4	67.3	–	21.9 ± 9.7
Kato et al. (2000)	Japan	145	49.2	62.1	71.0	34.5 ± 12.9
Kauer-Sant'Anna et al. (2007)	Brazil	163	42.6	71.8	–	25.3 ± 12.3
Keck Jr et al. (1995)	USA	71	35.0	54.9	100	26.0 ± 13.0
Kesebir et al. (2012)	Turkey	100	39.0	59.0	–	23.3 ± 6.1
Khess et al. (1997)	India	32	–	12.5	100	28.0 ± 9.7
Kim et al. (2007)	USA	41	35.4	61.0	63.4	18.8 ± 7.1
Kim et al. (2014)	Korea	128	33.7	54.7	100	28.5 ± 10.5
Kim et al. (2008)	Korea	179	33.1	49.2	100	27.5 ± 11.2
Koc and Kesebir (2014)	Turkey	146	44.0	60.3	–	30.1 ± 12.0
Kucukali et al. (2010)	Turkey	184	42.8	62.0	–	25.9 ± 9.4
Kudo et al. (2001)	Japan	13	52.2	38.5	100	31.3 ± 8.7
Kumar et al. (2010)	UK	47	46.3	55.3	100	26.2 ± 8.7
Kunugi et al. (2004)	Japan	519	49.3	53.0	66.9	36.7 ± 14.1
Kurumaji et al. (2014)	Japan	128	46.0	54.7	0	34.2 ± 1.2
Lagerberg et al. (2014)	Norway	324	34.9	63.6	63.3	22.2 ± 9.0
Latalova et al. (2011)	Czech Republic	41	44.1	51.2	–	30.2 ± 9.7
Lee and Dunner (2008)	USA	44	42.2	59.1	27.3	17.2 ± 9.8
Lee et al. (2010)	Korea	260	35.5	57.3	76.2	21.2 ± 8.8
Levin et al. (2014)	USA	86	40.8	67.4	–	26.8 ± 11.9
Lev-Ran et al. (2013)	USA	1905	–	–	–	24.0 ± 15.3
Levy et al. (2011)	USA	82	38.8	47.0	100	26.1 ± 9.1
Lex et al. (2011)	Austria	41	47.1	63.4	100	25.5 ± 9.7
Li et al. (2011)	China	24	28.4	37.5	100	22.4 ± 5.8
Li et al. (2014)	China	16	30.3	56.0	–	25.0 ± 5.8
Li et al. (2015)	China	33	23.6	51.5	100	22.8 ± 5.1
Licht et al. (1994)	Denmark	111	43.1	60.4	100	33.5 ± 11.5
Lopez et al. (2001)	Spain	169	–	58.0	100	29.0 ± 13.2
Lopez-Jaramillo et al. (2010)	Colombia	98	38.6	34.7	–	24.8 ± 8.4

Table 5.6 (continued)

Authors (year)	Country	Subjects (*n*)	Mean age	% Females	% Bipolar I	Onset age ±SD
Loranger and Levine (1978)	USA	200	–	50.0	100	32.3 ± 13.7
Maina et al. (2007)	Italy	142	43.6	54.9	63.4	28.3 ± 9.0
Maina et al. (2013)	Italy	309	52.2	63.1	32.4	30.5 ± 12.1
Martínez-Arán et al. (2004)	Spain	108	41.5	53.7	–	25.7 ± 8.8
Martínez-Arán et al. (2005)	Spain	60	38.4	60.0	81.7	25.7 ± 6.6
Mathieu et al. (2014)	France	310	42.4	58.3	75.2	24.9 ± 9.8
Matsuo et al. (2009)	USA	42	35.7	78.6	81.0	16.6 ± 6.7
Mazza et al. (2012)	Italy	114	45.2	55.3	41.2	28.7 ± 7.9
Mazzarini et al. (2010)	Spain	164	48.5	56.1	0	31.8 ± 13.7
McCraw et al. (2014)	Australia	173	38.1	61.8	14.5	14.9 ± 0.5
McElroy et al. (1991)	USA	17	39.6	–	100	26.7 ± 13.8
McElroy et al. (2011)	Cross-national	875	41.1	56.0	81.0	20.8 ± 10.9
McIntyre et al. (2007)	Canada	377	37.8	56.2	–	22.6 ± 10.6
McIntyre et al. (2010)	Cross-national	176	38.7	–	67.6	18.3 ± 9.3
Medda et al. (2010)	Italy	96	44.9	56.3	100	25.9 ± 10.3
Miklowitz et al. (2003)	USA	101	35.6	63.4	98.0	24.4 ± 9.6
Miller et al. (2013)	USA	80	46.6	63.7	53.8	19.8 ± 9.4
Min et al. (2012)	Korea	184	41.5	65.2	–	29.0 ± 11.6
Mitchell et al. (2009)	Australia	217	38.6	55.3	89.7	21.0 ± 7.9
Morselli et al. (2003)	Cross-national	1041	–	–	–	25.6 ± 10.8
Mosolov et al. (2014)	Russia	147	47.0	78.9	0	32.0 ± 11.0
Mrad et al. (2007)	France	130	37.6	37.7	100	23.8 ± 8.9
Mula et al. (2008)	Italy	121	44.2	57.0	57.9	30.5 ± 9.7
Mula et al. (2010)	Italy	91	42.4	60.4	47.3	28.2 ± 11.4
Nardi et al. (2005)	Brazil	57	35.0	47.4	100	22.1 ± 10.2
Negash et al. (2005)	Ethiopia	295	29.5	44.8	100	22.0 ± 7.0
Nehra et al. (2006)	India	46	33.5	32.6	–	29.2 ± 10.5
Nery et al. (2014)	Brazil	482	40.6	71.2	89.9	24.7 ± 11.0
Neves et al. (2009)	Brazil	168	42.2	70.2	29.2	23.8 ± 10.4
Neves et al. (2010)	Brazil	198	42.1	70.0	67.7	23.5 ± 11.3
Nguyen and Low (2013)	Canada	888	37.3	49.9	–	21.8 ± 12.2
Nivoli et al. (2014)	Spain	470	46.1	53.2	70.6	25.2 ± 8.8
Ohara et al. (1998)	Japan	40	40.4	42.5	55.0	28.2 ± 11.7
Okan Ibiloglu and Caykoylu (2011)	Turkey	96	38.7	69.8	52.1	25.1 ± 4.0

(continued)

Table 5.6 (continued)

Authors (year)	Country	Subjects (*n*)	Mean age	% Females	% Bipolar I	Onset age ±SD
Onyeama et al. (2010)	Nigeria	89	–	–	–	22.9 ± 8.3
Oquendo et al. (2000a)	USA	44	33.7	50.0	–	25.5 ± 11.5
Ortiz et al. (2011)	Canada	379	50.1	63.3	70.0	25.1 ± 10.6
Ostacher et al. (2010)	USA	2109	–	–	–	16.8 ± 8.6
Ozerdem et al. (2001)	Turkey	108	36.1	63.0	82.4	27.6 ± 11.4
Ozgürdal et al. (2009)	Germany	20	43.9	65.0	100	32.6 ± 7.1
Ozyildirim et al. (2010)	Turkey	97	39.8	75.3	100	23.5 ± 9.0
Pacheco et al. (2010)	Costa Rica	84	42.0	66.7	100	25.3 ± 9.4
Pae et al. (2007)	Korea	151	33.3	51.0	100	26.8 ± 9.7
Paholpak et al. (2014)	Thailand	424	42.7	60.9	95.3	32.0 ± 11.9
Papadimitriou et al. (1998)	Greece	48	–	–	–	26.3 ± 2.0
Pardoen et al. (1996)	Belgium	27	–	–	59.0	32.0 ± 14.6
Parmentier et al. (2012)	France	652	42.4	58.0	–	25.4 ± 10.5
Patrick et al. (1978)	USA	148	47.5	52.7	53.4	29.0 ± 10.7
Pavlickova et al. (2014)	UK	21	48.9	61.9	66.7	25.6 ± 8.7
Perich et al. (2014)	Australia	157	38.6	64		22 ± 9.6
Perron et al. (2012)	France	87	43.8	–	–	26.5 ± 10.0
Perroud et al. (2014)	Switzerland	138	42.0	55.1	34.1	25.1 ± 11.5
Perugi et al. (1997)	Italy	261	38.2	58.6	100	26.3 ± 10.3
Perugi et al. (2000)	Italy	320	38.4	55.9	100	26.5 ± 10.4
Piccardi et al. (2002)	Italy	101	–	54.5	–	22.6 ± 6.5
Pinto et al. (2011)	Canada	91	–	–	0	20.2 ± 7.6
Pope et al. (2007)	UK	77	42.1	57.1	88.3	26.1 ± 10.2
Popescu et al. (1991)	Romania	24	35.4	62.5	–	26.8 ± 11.8
Porcelli et al. (2014)	Italy	21	53.4	76.1	–	28.3 ± 10.4
Primavera et al. (2013)	Italy	18	46.2	–	100	27.7 ± 6.9
Radonic et al. (2011)	Croatia	15	54.0	66.6	–	45.0 ± 6.4
Ram and Ram (2010)	India	97	31.5	23.7	–	26.0 ± 9.3
Ramacciotti et al. (2005)	Italy	51	40.6	43.1	100	27.4 ± 10.7
Ravizza et al. (1982)	Italy	100	–	–	–	31.8 ± 13.9
Reinares et al. (2013)	Spain	106	41.0	49.1	–	25.8 ± 8.2
Rinieris et al. (1979)	Greece	87	44.4	67.8	–	30.9 ± 11.8
Robb et al. (1998)	Canada	69	36.0	60.9	78.0	24.3 ± 1.0
Robertson et al. (2012)	Australia	113	38.5	69.0	0	20.0 ± 10.6

Table 5.6 (continued)

Authors (year)	Country	Subjects (*n*)	Mean age	% Females	% Bipolar I	Onset age ±SD
Roiser et al. (2009)	USA	49	33.6	73.5	22.5	15.8 ± 6.2
Rosa et al. (2008)	Brazil	92	44.5	76.1	85.9	26.7 ± 8.4
Rydén et al. (2009)	Sweden	159	39.2	62.3	50.3	19.7 ± 10.7
Safari et al. (2014)	Turkey	66	37	56.1	97	26.6 ± 10.1
Sassi et al. (2002)	USA	29	33.7	41.4	82.8	19.1 ± 7.0
Sato et al. (2002)	Germany	576	38.6	50.7	100	28.9 ± 10.7
Saus et al. (2010)	Spain	189	48.3	64.0	77.3	30.0 ± 12.7
Savitz et al. (2008)	South Africa	68	44.7	–	72.1	24.2 ± 11.2
Scassellati et al. (2007)	Italy	179	42.1	63.7	–	26.8 ± 12.6
Schaffer et al. (2006)	Canada	852	37.3	54.8	100	22.5 ± 12.0
Schoeyen et al. (2011)	Norway	482	39.3	55.6	65.4	21.2 ± 10.7
Schroeter et al. (2002)	Germany	11	44.2	36.4	100	34.5 ± 8.6
Seidman et al. (2003)	USA	14	39.1	50.0	100	28.1 ± 10.3
Serretti et al. (2002)	Italy	1004	46.5	60.3	86.0	30.9 ± 11.5
Serretti et al. (2004)	Greece	83	45.5	66.3	77.1	19.9 ± 9.7
Serretti et al. (2013)	Cross-national	686	–	–	–	28.1 ± 13.0
Sethi and Khanna (1993)	India	100	27.7	20.0	100	23.1 ± 6.7
Shabani et al. (2013)	Iran	100	35.8	33.0	100	26.6 ± 9.2
Shah et al. (2006)	USA	32	38.7	75.0	78.0	32.0 ± 11.0
Sierra et al. (2005)	Spain	50	45.1	60.0	90.0	29.4 ± 11.1
Skjelstad et al. (2011)	Norway	15	26.7	74.0	0	15.9 ± 3.6
Slama et al. (2004)	France	303	–	–	–	26.7 ± 11.2
Sonne et al. (1994)	USA	44	40.9	56.8	–	22.2 ± 10.7
Souery et al. (1999)	Cross-national	401	47.1	55.9	–	28.5 ± 9.6
Souery et al. (2012)	Belgium	168	44.7	62.5	61.9	21.6 ± 12.0
Spijker et al. (2011)	Netherlands	326	48.0	60.1	75.5	25.6 ± 11.7
Squassina et al. (2011)	Italy	300	42.9	63.3	–	25.8 ± 10.2
Strakowski et al. (1998)	USA	83	25.0	44.6	–	22.0 ± 7.0
Strakowski et al. (2005)	USA	144	21.7	47.9	100	18.7 ± 7.6
Suominen et al. (2007)	Finland	191	37.7	52.9	47.1	23.7 ± 9.8
Swann et al. (2013)	USA	55	37.3	47.3	7.3	17.3 ± 9.4
Sylvia et al. (2014)	USA	283	39.1	57.0	76.0	15.4 ± 7.6

(continued)

Table 5.6 (continued)

Authors (year)	Country	Subjects (*n*)	Mean age	% Females	% Bipolar I	Onset age ±SD
Szadoczky et al. (1998)	Hungary	149	–	–	31.5	19.9 ± 13.1
Szczepankiewicz et al. (2009)	Poland	101	52.4	57.4	–	29.6 ± 9.3
Takei et al. (2014)	Japan	31	34.9	54.8	3.2	26.0 ± 6.4
Tamam et al. (2006)	Turkey	44	33.7	56.8	100	22.7 ± 6.6
Tamam et al. (2008)	Turkey	159	33.8	49.7	91.8	23.7 ± 8.0
Taylor Tavares et al. (2007)	UK	17	32.6	70.6	0	17.0 ± 1.7
Thomé et al. (2012)	Brazil	60	47.6	73.3	96.7	26.2 ± 12.1
Tohen et al. (2007)	USA	833	41.7	63.0	100	24.0 ± 11.4
Tondo et al. (2014)	Italy	642	42.9	60.9	–	29.8 ± 13.3
Toniolo et al. (2009)	Brazil	95	40.5	61.1	100	20.2 ± 11.6
Torrent et al. (2006)	Spain	71	41.5	57.7	53.5	26.9 ± 9.4
Torrent et al. (2013)	Spain	239	40.1	–	–	25.6 ± 8.3
Torres et al. (2010)	USA	45	22.2	49.0	100	19.3 ± 4.4
Tozzi et al. (2011)	Cross-national	964	47.2	64.0	91.4	21.4 ± 9.5
Tundo et al. (2013)	Italy	140	39.2	58.0	55.0	27.6 ± 10.5
Turecki et al. (2001)	Canada	31	45.1	41.9	–	23.8 ± 7.2
Van den Bossche et al. (2012)	Cross-national	709	50.1	60.1	–	28.3 ± 13.5
Verdolini et al. (2014)	UK	65	35.0	–	–	15.7 ± 6.3
Verdoux et al. (1996)	France	40	33.4	62.5	–	22.5 ± 6.7
Versace et al. (2008)	USA	31	35.9	64.5	100	23.4 ± 8.9
Vieta et al. (1997)	Spain	60	37.1	63.3	63.3	25.3 ± 8.7
Vieta et al. (2008)	Spain	118	42.0	61.9	52.5	26.6 ± 8.8
Wang et al. (2012)	China	342	36.9	55.5	83.6	26.0 ± 9.8
Washizuka et al. (2003)	Japan	54	46.3	68.5	63.0	33.2 ± 12.8
Wehr et al. (1988)	USA	70	–	94.3	57.1	29.2 ± 11.6
Welge et al. (2004)	USA	357	39.4	47.0	100	24.6 ± 10.5
Wilson and Sponheim (2014)	USA	31	47.6	29	–	21.7 ± 7.2
Wu et al. (2009)	USA	49	39.4	40.8	–	19.0 ± 9.4
Xiang et al. (2013)	China	309	35.5	52.1	38.2	28.5 ± 10.8
Yildiz and Sachs (2003)	USA	328	–	56.7	81.1	21.3 ± 9.8
Zander et al. (1998)	France	119	46.1	54.6	71.4	28.1 ± 12.5
Zeschel et al. (2013)	Germany	42	35.1	59.5	64.3	30.5 ± 9.5
Zhang et al. (1997)	Japan	31	–	42.0	55.0	27.4 ± 11.9
Zhang et al. (2013)	China	286	32.7	59.4	–	25.5 ± 4.5
Zuncheddu and Carpiniello (2006)	Italy	51	33.1	52.9	–	30.9 ± 9.4
Zutshi et al. (2006)	India	80	30.1	28.8	81.3	21.5 ± 5.9

References

Aghanwa HS. Recurrent unipolar mania in a psychiatric hospital setting in the Fiji Islands. Psychopathology. 2001;34:312–7.

Akdeniz F, Vahip S, Pirildar S, et al. Risk factors associated with childbearing-related episodes in women with bipolar disorder. Psychopathology. 2003;36:234–8.

Akiskal HS, Walker P, Puzantian VR, et al. Bipolar outcome in the course of depressive illness. Phenomenologic, familial, and pharmacologic predictors. J Affect Disord. 1983;5:115–28.

Aldana LL, Miguel PS, Lopez MR, et al. Bipolar patients in community mental health centers and specialized units. Could they be pooled? Rev Psiquiatr Salud Ment. 2009;2:128–32.

Altamura AC, Dell'Osso B, Berlin HA, et al. Duration of untreated illness and suicide in bipolar disorder: a naturalistic study. Eur Arch Psychiatry Clin Neurosci. 2010;260:385–91.

Altindag A, Yanik M, Nebioglu M. Comorbid personality disorders in subjects with bipolar I disorder. Int J Psychiatry Clin Pract. 2006;10:33–7.

Altshuler LL, Curran JG, Hauser P, et al. T2 hyperintensities in bipolar disorder: magnetic resonance imaging comparison and literature meta-analysis. Am J Psychiatry. 1995;152:1139–44.

Ancın I, Santos JL, Teijeira C, et al. Sustained attention as a potential endophenotype for bipolar disorder. Acta Psychiatr Scand. 2010;122:235–45.

Andersson S, Barder HE, Hellvin T, et al. Neuropsychological and electrophysiological indices of neurocognitive dysfunction in bipolar II disorder. Bipolar Disord. 2008;10:888–99.

Andreazza AC, Kapczinski F, Kauer-Sant'Anna M, et al. 3-Nitrotyrosine and glutathione antioxidant system in patients in the early and late stages of bipolar disorder. J Psychiatry Neurosci. 2009;34:263–71.

Arai M, Obata N, Kockelkorn TT, et al. Lack of association between polymorphisms in the 5' upstream region of the DISC1 gene and mood disorders. Psychiatr Genet. 2007;17:357.

Arnold LM. Gender differences in bipolar disorder. Psychiatr Clin North Am. 2003;26:595–620.

Atkinson M, Zibin S, Chuang H. Characterizing quality of life among patients with chronic mental illness: a critical examination of the self-report methodology. Am J Psychiatry. 1997;154:99–105.

Atmaca M, Yildirim H, Ozdemir H, et al. Hippocampal 1H MRS in first-episode bipolar I patients. Prog Neuropsychopharmacol Biol Psychiatry. 2006;30:1235–9.

Azorin JM, Kaladjian A, Adida M, et al. Factors associated with rapid cycling in bipolar I manic patients: findings from a French national study. CNS Spectr. 2008;13:780–7.

Baethge C, Smolka MN, Gruschka P, et al. Does prophylaxis-delay in bipolar disorder influence outcome? Results from a long-term study of 147 patients. Acta Psychiatr Scand. 2003a;107:260–7.

Baethge C, Tondo L, Bratti IM, et al. Prophylaxis latency and outcome in bipolar disorders. Can J Psychiatry. 2003b;48:449–57.

Baethge C, Tondo L, Baldessarini RJ. Methodological considerations in a review of effects of earlier treatment of bipolar disorder. Int J Bipolar Disord. 2017;5:12–4.

Baldessarini RJ. Chemotherapy in Psychiatry. 3rd ed. New York: Springer Press; 2013.

Baldessarini RJ, Tondo L, Hennen J, et al. Latency and episodes before treatment: response to lithium maintenance in bipolar I and II disorders. Bipolar Disord. 1999;1:91–7.

Baldessarini RJ, Bolzani L, Cruz N, et al. Onset-age of bipolar disorders at six international sites. J Affect Disord. 2010;121:143–6.

Baldessarini RJ, Salvatore P, Khalsa HK, et al. Episode cycles with increasing recurrences in first-episode bipolar-I disorder patients. J Affect Disord. 2012a;136:149–54.

Baldessarini RJ, Tondo L, Vazquez GH, et al. Age at onset versus family history and clinical outcomes in 1,665 international bipolar-I disorder patients. World Psychiatry. 2012b;11:40–6.

Baldessarini RJ, Tondo L, Visioli C. First-episode types in bipolar disorder: predictive associations with later illness. Acta Psychiatr Scand. 2014;129:383–92.

Baron M, Risch N, Mendlewicz J. Age at onset in bipolar-related major affective illness: clinical and genetic implications. J Psychiatr Res. 1982;17:5–18.

Basso MR, Lowery N, Neel J, et al. Neuropsychological impairment among manic, depressed, and mixed-episode inpatients with bipolar disorder. Neuropsychology. 2002;16:84–91.
Bauer MS, Whybrow PC, Gyulai L, et al. Testing definitions of dysphoric mania and hypomania: prevalence, clinical characteristics and inter-episode stability. J Affect Disord. 1994;32:201–11.
Bauer M, Glenn T, Rasgon N, et al. Association between age of onset and mood in bipolar disorder: comparison of subgroups identified by cluster analysis and clinical observation. J Psychiatr Res. 2010;44:1170–5.
Bauer M, Glenn T, Alda M, et al. Relationship between sunlight and the age of onset of bipolar disorder: an international multisite study. J Affect Disord. 2014;167:104–11.
Beckmann H, Goodwin FK. Urinary MHPG in subgroups of depressed patients and normal controls. Neuropsychobiology. 1980;6:91–100.
Bellantuono C, Barraco A, Rossi A, et al. The management of bipolar mania: a national survey of baseline data from the EMBLEM study in Italy. BMC Psychiatry. 2007;7:33.
Bellivier F, Golmard JL, Rietschel M, et al. Age at onset in bipolar I affective disorder: further evidence for three subgroups. Am J Psychiatry. 2003;160:999–1001.
Bellivier F, Etain B, Malafosse A, et al. Age at onset in bipolar I affective disorder in the USA and Europe. World J Biol Psychiatry. 2014;15:369–76.
Benazzi F. Gender differences in bipolar II and unipolar depressed outpatients: a 557-case study. Ann Clin Psychiatry. 1999;11:55–9.
Benazzi F. A tetrachoric factor analysis validation of mixed depression. Prog Neuropsychopharmacol Biol Psychiatry. 2008;32:186–92.
Benedetti A, Scarpellini P, Casamassima F, et al. Bipolar disorder in late life: clinical characteristics in a sample of older adults admitted for manic episode. Clin Pract Epidemiol Ment Health. 2008;4:22. https://doi.org/10.1186/1745-0179-4-22.
Benedetti F, Dallaspezia S, Lorenzi C, et al. Gene-gene interaction of glycogen synthase kinase 3-beta and serotonin transporter on human antidepressant response to sleep deprivation. J Affect Disord. 2012;136:514–9.
Benedetti F, Riccaboni R, Poletti S, et al. The serotonin transporter genotype modulates the relationship between early stress and adult suicidality in bipolar disorder. Bipolar Disord. 2014;16:857–66.
Berk M, Hallam K, Lucas N, et al. Early intervention in bipolar disorders: opportunities and pitfalls. Med J Aust. 2007;187:S11–4.
Beyer JL, Kuchibhatla M, Cassidy F, et al. Stressful life events in older bipolar patients. Int J Geriatr Psychiatry. 2008;23:1271–5.
Biffin F, Tahtalian S, Filia K, et al. The impact of age at onset of bipolar I disorder on functioning and clinical presentation. Acta Neuropsychiatr. 2009;21:191–6.
Birmaher B, Axelson D, Goldstein B, et al. Psychiatric disorders in preschool offspring of parents with bipolar disorder: the Pittsburgh Bipolar Offspring Study (BIOS). Am J Psychiatry. 2010;167:321–30.
Blumberg HP, Kaufman J, Martin A, et al. Amygdala and hippocampal volumes in adolescents and adults with bipolar disorder. Arch Gen Psychiatry. 2003;60:1201–8.
Bora E, Vahip S, Akdeniz F, et al. The effect of previous psychotic mood episodes on cognitive impairment in euthymic bipolar patients. Bipolar Disord. 2007;9:468–77.
Bozikas VP, Tonia T, Fokas K, et al. Impaired emotion processing in remitted patients with bipolar disorder. J Affect Disord. 2006;91:53–6.
Brambilla P, Harenski K, Nicoletti M, et al. Differential effects of age on brain gray matter in bipolar patients and healthy individuals. Neuropsychobiology. 2001;43:242–7.
Bratti IM, Baldessarini RJ, Baethge C, et al. Pretreatment episode count and response to lithium treatment in manic-depressive illness. Harv Rev Psychiatry. 2003;11:245–56.
Braunig P, Sarkar R, Effenberger S, et al. Gender differences in psychotic bipolar mania. Gend Med. 2009;6:356–61.
Brugue E, Colom F, Sanchez-Moreno J, et al. Depression subtypes in bipolar I and II disorders. Psychopathology. 2008;41:111–4.

Carballo JJ, Harkavy-Friedman J, Burke AK, et al. Family history of suicidal behavior and early traumatic experiences: additive effect on suicidality and course of bipolar illness? J Affect Disord. 2008;109:57–63.

Cardoso BM, Kauer Sant'Anna M, Dias VV, et al. The impact of co-morbid alcohol use disorder in bipolar patients. Alcohol. 2008;42:451–7.

Carlson GA, Pataki C. Understanding early age of onset: a review of the last 5 years. Curr Psychiatry Rep. 2016;18:114.

Carlson GA, Kotov R, Chang SW, et al. Early determinants of four-year clinical outcomes in bipolar disorder with psychosis. Bipolar Disord. 2012;14:19–30.

Casas-Barquero N, Garcia-Lopez O, Fernandez-Arguelles P, et al. Clinical variables and implications of the personality on the outcome of bipolar illness: a pilot study. Neuropsychiatr Dis Treat. 2007;3:269–75.

Cervantes P, Gelber S, Kin FN, et al. Circadian secretion of cortisol in bipolar disorder. J Psychiatry Neurosci. 2001;26:411–6.

Cha B, Kim JH, Ha TH, et al. Polarity of the first episode and time to diagnosis of bipolar I disorder. Psychiatry Investig. 2009;6:96–101.

Chen YW, Dilsaver SC. Comorbidity of panic disorder in bipolar illness: evidence from the Epidemiologic Catchment Area Survey. Am J Psychiatry. 1995;152:280–2.

Cichon S, Nothen MM, Catalano M, et al. Identification of two novel polymorphisms and a rare deletion variant in the human dopamine D4 receptor gene. Psychiatr Genet. 1995;5:97–103.

Col SE, Caykoylu A, Karakas Ugurlu G, et al. Factors affecting treatment compliance in patients with bipolar I disorder during prophylaxis: a study from Turkey. Gen Hosp Psychiatry. 2014;36:208–13.

Colom F, Vieta E, Daban C, et al. Clinical and therapeutic implications of predominant polarity in bipolar disorder. J Affect Disord. 2006;93:13–7.

Colom F, Reinares M, Pacchiarotti I, et al. Has number of previous episodes any effect on response to group psychoeducation in bipolar patients? A 5-year follow-up post hoc analysis. Acta Neuropsychiatrica. 2010;22:50–3.

Conus P, Abdel-Baki A, Harrigan S, et al. Pre-morbid and outcome correlates of first episode mania with psychosis: is a distinction between schizoaffective and bipolar I disorder valid in the early phase of psychotic disorders? J Affect Disord. 2010;126:88–95.

Conus P, Macneil C, McGorry PD. Public health significance of bipolar disorder: implications for early intervention and prevention. Bipolar Disord. 2014;16:548–56.

Dagani J, Signorini G, Nielssen O, et al. Meta-analysis of the interval between the onset and management of bipolar disorder. Can J Psychiatry. 2017;62:247–58.

Dawson EL, Shear PK, Howe SR, et al. Impulsivity predicts time to reach euthymia in adults with bipolar disorder. Bipolar Disord. 2014;16:846–56.

Deeks JJ, Dinnes J, D'Amico R, et al. Evaluating non-randomised intervention studies. Health Technol Assess. 2003;7:iii–x, 1–173.

Del Grande C, Muti M, Musetti L, et al. Long-term treatment of bipolar disorder: how should we use lithium salts? Riv Psichiatr. 2012;47:515–26.

Dell'Osso B, Grancini B, Vismara M, et al. Age at onset in patients with bipolar I and II disorder: a comparison of large sample studies. J Affect Disord. 2016;201:57–63.

Demirel H, Yesilbas D, Ozver I, et al. Psychopathy and facial emotion recognition ability in patients with bipolar affective disorder with or without delinquent behaviors. Compr Psychiatry. 2014;55:542–6.

Derntl B, Seidel EM, Kryspin-Exner I, et al. Facial emotion recognition in patients with bipolar I and bipolar II disorder. Br J Clin Psychol. 2009;48:363–75.

DeRosse P, Burdick KE, Lencz T, et al. Empirical support for DSM-IV schizoaffective disorder: clinical and cognitive validators from a large patient sample. PLoS One. 2013;8(5):e63734. https://doi.org/10.1371/journal.pone.0063734.

Dervic K, Garcia-Amador M, Sudol K, et al. Bipolar I and II versus unipolar depression: clinical differences and impulsivity/aggression traits. Eur Psychiatry. 2015;30:106–13.

Di Florio A, Jones L, Forty L, et al. Mood disorders and parity—a clue to the aetiology of the postpartum trigger. J Affect Disord. 2014;152–154:334–9.
Dias VV, Brissos S, Cardoso C, et al. Serum homocysteine levels and cognitive functioning in euthymic bipolar patients. J Affect Disord. 2009;113:285–90.
Diflorio A, Jones I. Is sex important? Gender differences in bipolar disorder. Int Rev Psychiatry. 2010;22:437–52.
Ehnvall A, Agren H. Patterns of sensitisation in the course of affective illness. A life-charting study of treatment-refractory depressed patients. J Affect Disord. 2002;70:67–75.
El Kissi Y, Krir MW, Ben Nasr S, et al. Life events in bipolar patients: a comparative study with siblings and healthy controls. J Affect Disord. 2013;151:378–83.
El-Hadidy MA, Abdeen HM, Abd El-Aziz SM, et al. WITHDRAWN:C677T Methylenetetrahydrofolate reductase gene polymorphism in schizophrenia and bipolar disorder. Psychiatr Genet. 2013; https://doi.org/10.1097/YPG.0000000000000020.
Engström C, Brandstrom S, Sigvardsson S, et al. Bipolar disorder. II: personality and age of onset. Bipolar Disord. 2003;5:340–8.
Ernst CL, Goldberg JF. Clinical features related to age at onset in bipolar disorder. J Affect Disord. 2004;82:21–7.
Eryilmaz G, Hizli Sayar G, Ozten E, et al. Effect of valproate on the plasma concentrations of aripiprazole in bipolar patients. Int J Psychiatry Clin Pract. 2014;18:288–92.
Etain B, Roy I, Henry C, et al. No evidence for physical anhedonia as a candidate symptom or an endophenotype in bipolar affective disorder. Bipolar Disord. 2007;9:706–12.
Etain B, Aas M, Andreassen OA, et al. Childhood trauma is associated with severe clinical characteristics of bipolar disorders. J Clin Psychiatry. 2013;74:991–8.
Evans DL. Bipolar disorder: diagnostic challenges and treatment considerations. J Clin Psychiatry. 2000;61(Supp 13):26–31.
Faedda GL, Axelson DB, Baldessarini RJ, et al. International Society of Bipolar Disorders task force report: review of factors predicting bipolar disorder. Bipolar Disord. 2018 (in press).
Fagiolini A, Frank E, Rucci P, et al. Mood and anxiety spectrum as a means to identify clinically relevant subtypes of bipolar I disorder. Bipolar Disord. 2007;9:462–7.
Feinman JA, Dunner DL. The effect of alcohol and substance abuse on the course of bipolar affective disorder. J Affect Disord. 1996;37:43–9.
Ferrari AJ, Stockings E, Khoo JP, et al. The prevalence and burden of bipolar disorder: findings from the Global Burden of Disease Study 2013. Bipolar Disord. 2016;18:440–50.
Forbes EE, Miller A, Cohn JF, et al. Affect-modulated startle in adults with childhood-onset depression: relations to bipolar course and number of lifetime depressive episodes. Psychiatry Res. 2005;134:11–25.
Fornaro M, Perugi G, Gabrielli F, et al. Lifetime co-morbidity with different subtypes of eating disorders in 148 females with bipolar disorders. J Affect Disord. 2010;121:147–51.
Franchini L, Zanardi R, Smeraldi E, et al. Early onset of lithium prophylaxis as a predictor of good long-term outcome. Eur Arch Psychiatry Clin Neurosci. 1999;249:227–30.
Francis A, Gasparo P. Interval between symptom onset and hospitalization in mania. J Affect Disord. 1994;31:179–85.
Frangou S. Predictors of outcome in a representative population of bipolar disorder. Bipolar Disord. 2002;4(Suppl 1):41–2.
Frey BN, Zunta-Soares GB, Caetano SC, et al. Illness duration and total brain gray matter in bipolar disorder: evidence for neurodegeneration? Eur Neuropsychopharmacol. 2008;18:717–22.
Gan Z, Diao F, Wei Q, et al. A predictive model for diagnosing bipolar disorder based on the clinical characteristics of major depressive episodes in Chinese population. J Affect Disord. 2011;134:119–25.
Gao K, Kemp DE, Ganocy SJ, et al. Treatment-emergent mania/hypomania during antidepressant monotherapy in patients with rapid cycling bipolar disorder. Bipolar Disord. 2008;10:907–15.
Garcia-Amador M, Colom F, Valenti M, et al. Suicide risk in rapid cycling bipolar patients. J Affect Disord. 2009;117:74–8.

Gasperini M, Scherillo P, Manfredonia MG, et al. A study of relapses in subjects with mood disorder on lithium treatment. Eur Neuropsychopharmacol. 1993;3:103–10.

Gassab L, Mechri A, Gaha L, et al. Bipolarity correlated factors in major depression: about 155 Tunisian inpatients. Encephale. 2002;28:283–9.

Ghaemi SN, Hsu DJ, Ko JY, et al. Bipolar spectrum disorder: a pilot study. Psychopathology. 2004;37:222–6.

Glenn T, Whybrow PC, Rasgon N, et al. Approximate entropy of self-reported mood prior to episodes in bipolar disorder. Bipolar Disord. 2006;8:424–9.

Goghari VM, Sponheim SR. Differential association of the COMT Val158Met polymorphism with clinical phenotypes in schizophrenia and bipolar disorder. Schizophr Res. 2008;103:186–91.

Gogos A, Joshua N, Rossell SL. Use of the Repeatable Battery for the Assessment of Neuropsychological Status (RBANS) to investigate group and gender differences in schizophrenia and bipolar disorder. Aust N Z J Psychiatry. 2010;44:220–9.

Goldberg JF, Garno JL. Age at onset of bipolar disorder and risk for comorbid borderline personality disorder. Bipolar Disord. 2009;11:205–8.

Goldberg JF, Garno JL, Leon AC, et al. Association of recurrent suicidal ideation with nonremission from acute mixed mania. Am J Psychiatry. 1998;155:1753–5.

Goldstein BI, Levitt AJ. Further evidence for a developmental subtype of bipolar disorder defined by age at onset: results from the national epidemiologic survey on alcohol and related conditions. Am J Psychiatry. 2006;163:1633–6.

Grande I, Magalhaes PV, Chendo I, et al. Staging bipolar disorder: clinical, biochemical, and functional correlates. Acta Psychiatr Scand. 2014;129:437–44.

Grigoroiu-Serbanescu M, Nöthen MM, Ohlraun S, et al. Family history influences age of onset in bipolar I disorder in females but not in males. Am J Med Genet B Neuropsychiatr Genet. 2005;133B:6–11.

Grigoroiu-Serbanescu M, Rietschel M, Hauser J, et al. Commingling analysis of age-of-onset in bipolar I disorder and the morbid risk for major psychoses in first degree relatives of bipolar I probands. J Affect Disord. 2014;168:197–204.

Gruber SA, Rosso IM, Yurgelun-Todd D. Neuropsychological performance predicts clinical recovery in bipolar patients. J Affect Disord. 2008;105:253–60.

Gulseren S, Gurcan M, Gulseren L, et al. T2 hyperintensities in bipolar patients and their healthy siblings. Arch Med Res. 2006;37:79–85.

Gutiérrez-Rojas L, Gurpegui M, Ayuso-Mateos JL, et al. Quality of life in bipolar disorder patients: a comparison with a general population sample. Bipolar Disord. 2008;10:625–34.

Harnic D, Pompili M, Mazza M, et al. Affective temperaments and psychopathological dimensions of personality in bipolar and cyclothymic patients. Behav Med. 2013;39:17–23.

Haro JM, van Os J, Vieta E, et al. Evidence for three distinct classes of 'typical', 'psychotic' and 'dual' mania: results from the EMBLEM study. Acta Psychiatr Scand. 2006;113:112–20.

Hauser P, Matochik J, Altshuler LL, et al. MRI-based measurements of temporal lobe and ventricular structures in patients with bipolar I and bipolar II disorders. J Affect Disord. 2000;60:25–32.

Hays JC, Krishnan KR, George LK, et al. Age of first onset of bipolar disorder: demographic, family history, and psychosocial correlates. Depress Anxiety. 1998;7:76–82.

Hendrick V, Altshuler LL, Gitlin MJ, et al. Gender and bipolar illness. J Clin Psychiatry. 2000;61:393–6; quiz 397.

Henry C, Van den Bulke D, Bellivier F, et al. Affective lability and affect intensity as core dimensions of bipolar disorders during euthymic period. Psychiatry Res. 2008;159:1–6.

Herrman H. Early intervention as a priority for world psychiatry. Early Interv Psychiatry. 2014;8:305–6.

Holtzman JN, Miller S, Hooshmand F, et al. Gender by onset age interaction may characterize distinct phenotypic subgroups in bipolar patients. J Psychiatr Res. 2016;76:128–35.

Horesh N, Apter A, Zalsman G. Timing, quantity and quality of stressful life events in childhood and preceding the first episode of bipolar disorder. J Affect Disord. 2011;134:434–7.

Hosang GM, Korszun A, Jones L, et al. Life-event specificity: bipolar disorder compared with unipolar depression. Br J Psychiatry. 2012a;201:458–65.

Hosang GM, Uher R, Maughan B, et al. The role of loss and danger events in symptom exacerbation in bipolar disorder. J Psychiatr Res. 2012b;46:1584–9.
Johnson L, Andersson-Lundman G, Aberg-Wistedt A, et al. Age of onset in affective disorder: its correlation with hereditary and psychosocial factors. J Affect Disord. 2000;59:139–48.
Joslyn C, Hawes DJ, Hunt C, et al. Is age of onset associated with severity, prognosis, and clinical features in bipolar disorder? A meta-analytic review. Bipolar Disord. 2016;18:389–403.
Joyce K, Thompson A, Marwaha S. Is treatment for bipolar disorder more effective earlier in illness course? A comprehensive literature review. Int J Bipolar Disord. 2016;4:19. https://doi.org/10.1186/s40345-016-0060-6. Epub 2016 Sep 9.
Kanske P, Heissler J, Schonfelder S, et al. Neural correlates of emotional distractibility in bipolar disorder patients, unaffected relatives, and individuals with hypomanic personality. Am J Psychiatry. 2013;170:1487–96.
Kato T, Winokur G, Coryell W, et al. Failure to demonstrate parent-of-origin effect in transmission of bipolar II disorder. J Affect Disord. 1998;50:135–41.
Kato T, Kunugi H, Nanko S, et al. Association of bipolar disorder with the 5178 polymorphism in mitochondrial DNA. Am J Med Genet. 2000;96:182–6.
Kauer-Sant'Anna M, Tramontina J, Andreazza AC, et al. Traumatic life events in bipolar disorder: impact on BDNF levels and psychopathology. Bipolar Disord. 2007;9(Suppl 1):128–35.
Kawa I, Carter JD, Joyce PR, et al. Gender differences in bipolar disorder: age of onset, course, comorbidity, and symptom presentation. Bipolar Disord. 2005;7:119–25.
Keck PE Jr, McElroy SL, Strakowski SM, et al. Outcome and comorbidity in first- compared with multiple-episode mania. J Nerv Ment Dis. 1995;183:320–4.
Kennedy N, Boydell J, Kalidindi S, et al. Gender differences in incidence and age at onset of mania and bipolar disorder over a 35-year period in Camberwell, England. Am J Psychiatry. 2005;162:257–62.
Kesebir S, Isitmez S, Gundogar D. Compulsive buying in bipolar disorder: is it a comorbidity or a complication? J Affect Disord. 2012;136:797–802.
Khess CR, Das J, Akhtar S. Four year follow-up of first episode manic patients. Indian J Psychiatry. 1997;39:160–5.
Kim MJ, Lyoo IK, Dager SR, et al. The occurrence of cavum septi pellucidi enlargement is increased in bipolar disorder patients. Bipolar Disord. 2007;9:274–80.
Kim B, Kim SJ, Son JI, et al. Weight change in the acute treatment of bipolar I disorder: a naturalistic observational study of psychiatric inpatients. J Affect Disord. 2008;105:45–52.
Kim YK, Hwang JA, Lee HJ, et al. There is no association between the serotonin receptor gene and bipolar I disorder in the Korean population. Nord J Psychiatry. 2014;68:488–93.
Koc I, Kesebir S. The subgroup effect of adult attention deficit hyperactivity on disability and quality of life among bipolar patients. Bull Clin Psychopharmacol. 2014;24:49–54.
Kucukali CI, Aydin M, Ozkok E, et al. Angiotensin-converting enzyme polymorphism in schizophrenia, bipolar disorders, and their first-degree relatives. Psychiatr Genet. 2010;20:14–9.
Kudo T, Ishida S, Kubota H, et al. Manic episode in epilepsy and bipolar I disorder: a comparative analysis of 13 patients. Epilepsia. 2001;42:1036–42.
Kumar CT, Christodoulou T, Vyas NS, et al. Deficits in visual sustained attention differentiate genetic liability and disease expression for schizophrenia from Bipolar Disorder. Schizophr Res. 2010;124:152–60.
Kunugi H, Iijima Y, Tatsumi M, et al. No association between the Val66Met polymorphism of the brain-derived neurotrophic factor gene and bipolar disorder in a Japanese population: a multicenter study. Biol Psychiatry. 2004;56:376–8.
Kurumaji A, Narushima K, Ooshima K, et al. Clinical course of the bipolar II disorder in a Japanese sample. J Affect Disord. 2014;168:363–6.
Lagerberg TV, Kvitland LR, Aminoff SR, et al. Indications of a dose-response relationship between cannabis use and age at onset in bipolar disorder. Psychiatry Res. 2014;215:101–4.
Lambert M, Niehaus V, Correll C. Pharmacotherapy in children and adolescents at clinical-high risk for psychosis and bipolar disorder. Pharmacopsychiatry. 2016;49:229–44.

Large M, Nielssen O, Slade T, et al. Measurement and reporting of the duration of untreated psychosis. Early Interv Psychiatry. 2008;2:201–11.
Latalova K, Prasko J, Pastucha P, et al. Bipolar affective disorder and dissociation—comparison with healthy controls. Biomed Pap Med Fac Univ Palacky Olomouc Czech Repub. 2011;155:181–6.
Lee JH, Dunner DL. The effect of anxiety disorder comorbidity on treatment resistant bipolar disorders. Depress Anxiety. 2008;25:91–7.
Lee KY, Song JY, Kim SH, et al. Association between CLOCK 3111T/C and preferred circadian phase in Korean patients with bipolar disorder. Prog Neuropsychopharmacol Biol Psychiatry. 2010;34:1196–201.
Lev-Ran S, Le Foll B, McKenzie K, et al. Bipolar disorder and co-occurring cannabis use disorders: characteristics, co-morbidities and clinical correlates. Psychiatry Res. 2013;209:459–65.
Levin JB, Seifi N, Cassidy KA, et al. Comparing medication attitudes and reasons for medication nonadherence among three disparate groups of individuals with serious mental illness. J Nerv Ment Dis. 2014;202:769–73.
Levy B, Medina AM, Manove E, et al. The characteristics of a discrete mood episode, neuro-cognitive impairment and re-hospitalization in bipolar disorder. J Psychiatr Res. 2011;45:1048–54.
Lex C, Hautzinger M, Meyer TD. Cognitive styles in hypomanic episodes of bipolar I disorder. Bipolar Disord. 2011;13:355–64.
Li M, Cui L, Deng W, et al. Voxel-based morphometric analysis on the volume of gray matter in bipolar I disorder. Psychiatry Res. 2011;191:92–7.
Li J, Kale Edmiston E, Chen K, et al. A comparative diffusion tensor imaging study of corpus callosum subregion integrity in bipolar disorder and schizophrenia. Psychiatry Res. 2014;221:58–62.
Li Z, Deng W, Liu X, et al. Contingent negative variation in patients with deficit schizophrenia or bipolar I disorder with psychotic features: measurement and correlation with clinical characteristics. Nord J Psychiatry. 2015;69:196–203.
Licht RW, Gouliaev G, Vestergaard P, et al. Treatment of manic episodes in Scandinavia: the use of neuroleptic drugs in a clinical routine setting. J Affect Disord. 1994;32:179–85.
Lopez P, Mosquera F, de Leon J, et al. Suicide attempts in bipolar patients. J Clin Psychiatry. 2001;62:963–6.
Lopez-Jaramillo C, Lopera-Vasquez J, Gallo A, et al. Effects of recurrence on the cognitive performance of patients with bipolar I disorder: implications for relapse prevention and treatment adherence. Bipolar Disord. 2010;12:557–67.
Loranger AW, Levine PM. Age at onset of bipolar affective illness. Arch Gen Psychiatry. 1978;35:1345–8.
Maina G, Albert U, Bellodi L, et al. Health-related quality of life in euthymic bipolar disorder patients: differences between bipolar I and II subtypes. J Clin Psychiatry. 2007;68:207–12.
Maina G, Bechon E, Rigardetto S, et al. General medical conditions are associated with delay to treatment in patients with bipolar disorder. Psychosomatics. 2013;54:437–42.
Malhi GS, Bargh DM, Coulston CM, et al. Predicting bipolar disorder on the basis of phenomenology: implications for prevention and early intervention. Bipolar Disord. 2014;16:455–70.
Marshall M, Lewis S, Lockwood A, et al. Association between duration of untreated psychosis and outcome in cohorts of first-episode patients: a systematic review. Arch Gen Psychiatry. 2005;62:975–83.
Martínez-Arán A, Vieta E, Reinares M, et al. Cognitive function across manic or hypomanic, depressed, and euthymic states in bipolar disorder. Am J Psychiatry. 2004;161:262–70.
Martínez-Arán A, Vieta E, Colom F, et al. Do cognitive complaints in euthymic bipolar patients reflect objective cognitive impairment? Psychother Psychosom. 2005;74:295–302.
Mathieu F, Etain B, Daban C, et al. Affect intensity measure in bipolar disorders: a multidimensional approach. J Affect Disord. 2014;157:8–13.
Matsuo K, Walss-Bass C, Nery FG, et al. Neuronal correlates of brain-derived neurotrophic factor Val66Met polymorphism and morphometric abnormalities in bipolar disorder. Neuropsychopharmacology. 2009;34:1904–13.

Mazza M, Mandelli L, Zaninotto L, et al. Bipolar disorder: "pure" versus mixed depression over a 1-year follow-up. Int J Psychiatry Clin Pract. 2012;16:113–20.
Mazzarini L, Colom F, Pacchiarotti I, et al. Psychotic versus non-psychotic bipolar II disorder. J Affect Disord. 2010;126:55–60.
McCraw S, Parker G, Graham R, et al. The duration of undiagnosed bipolar disorder: effect on outcomes and treatment response. J Affect Disord. 2014;168:422–9.
McElroy SL, Keck PE Jr, Pope HG Jr, et al. Correlates of antimanic response to valproate. Psychopharmacol Bull. 1991;27:127–33.
McElroy SL, Frye MA, Hellemann G, et al. Prevalence and correlates of eating disorders in 875 patients with bipolar disorder. J Affect Disord. 2011;128:191–8.
McGorry PD, Killackey E, Yung AR. Early intervention in psychotic disorders: detection and treatment of the first episode and the critical early stages. Med J Aust. 2007;187:S8–10.
McGorry P, Johanessen JO, Lewis S, et al. Early intervention in psychosis: keeping faith with evidence-based health care. Psychol Med. 2010;40:399–404.
McIntyre RS, Soczynska JK, Mancini D, et al. Comparing features of bipolar disorder to major depressive disorder in a tertiary mood disorders clinic. Ann Clin Psychiatry. 2007;19:313–7.
McIntyre RS, Kennedy SH, Soczynska JK, et al. Attention-deficit/hyperactivity disorder in adults with bipolar disorder or major depressive disorder: results from the international mood disorders collaborative project. Prim Care Companion J Clin Psychiatry. 2010;12. https://doi.org/10.4088/PCC.09m00861gry.
Medda P, Perugi G, Zanello S, et al. Comparative response to electroconvulsive therapy in medication-resistant bipolar I patients with depression and mixed state. J ECT. 2010;26:82–6.
Miklowitz DJ, George EL, Richards JA, et al. A randomized study of family-focused psychoeducation and pharmacotherapy in the outpatient management of bipolar disorder. Arch Gen Psychiatry. 2003;60:904–12.
Miller S, Hallmayer J, Wang PW, et al. Brain-derived neurotrophic factor val66met genotype and early life stress effects upon bipolar course. J Psychiatr Res. 2013;47:252–8.
Min HJ, Cho HS, Kim SJ, et al. Association of the brain-derived neurotrophic factor gene and clinical features of bipolar disorder in Korea. Clin Psychopharmacol Neurosci. 2012;10:163–7.
Mitchell PB, Johnston AK, Corry J, et al. Characteristics of bipolar disorder in an Australian specialist outpatient clinic: comparison across large datasets. Aust N Z J Psychiatry. 2009;43:109–17.
Moher D, Liberati A, Tetzlaff J, et al. Preferred reporting items for systematic reviews and meta-analyses: the PRISMA statement. Int J Surg. 2010;8:336–41.
Montlahuc C, Curis E, Jonas SF, et al. Age-at-onset subsets of bipolar I disorders: a critical insight into admixture analyses. Int J Methods Psychiatr Res. 2016;26(3). https://doi.org/10.1002/mpr.1536.
Morselli PL, Elgie R, GAMIAN-Europe. GAMIAN-Europe/BEAM survey I—global analysis of a patient questionnaire circulated to 3450 members of 12 European advocacy groups operating in the field of mood disorders. Bipolar Disord. 2003;5:265–78.
Mosolov S, Ushkalova A, Kostukova E, et al. Bipolar II disorder in patients with a current diagnosis of recurrent depression. Bipolar Disord. 2014;16:389–99.
Mrad A, Mechri A, Rouissi K, et al. Clinical characteristics of bipolar I patients according to their family history of affective disorders. Encephale. 2007;33:762–7.
Mula M, Pini S, Monteleone P, et al. Different temperament and character dimensions correlate with panic disorder comorbidity in bipolar disorder and unipolar depression. J Anxiety Disord. 2008;22:1421–6.
Mula M, Pini S, Calugi S, et al. Distinguishing affective depersonalization from anhedonia in major depression and bipolar disorder. Compr Psychiatry. 2010;51:187–92.
Nardi AE, Nascimento I, Freire RC, et al. Demographic and clinical features of schizoaffective (schizobipolar) disorder—a 5-year retrospective study. Support for a bipolar spectrum disorder. J Affect Disord. 2005;89:201–6.
Negash A, Alem A, Kebede D, et al. Prevalence and clinical characteristics of bipolar I disorder in Butajira, Ethiopia: a community-based study. J Affect Disord. 2005;87:193–201.

Nehra R, Chakrabarti S, Pradhan BK, et al. Comparison of cognitive functions between first- and multi-episode bipolar affective disorders. J Affect Disord. 2006;93:185–92.

Nery FG, Miranda-Scippa A, Nery-Fernandes F, et al. Prevalence and clinical correlates of alcohol use disorders among bipolar disorder patients: results from the Brazilian Bipolar Research Network. Compr Psychiatry. 2014;55:1116–21.

Neves FS, Malloy-Diniz LF, Barbosa IG, et al. Bipolar disorder first episode and suicidal behavior: are there differences according to type of suicide attempt? Rev Bras Psiquiatr. 2009;31:114–8.

Neves FS, Malloy-Diniz LF, Romano-Silva MA, et al. Is the serotonin transporter polymorphism (5-HTTLPR) a potential marker for suicidal behavior in bipolar disorder patients? J Affect Disord. 2010;125:98–102.

Nguyen TV, Low NC. Comorbidity of migraine and mood episodes in a nationally representative population-based sample. Headache. 2013;53:498–506.

Nivoli AM, Murru A, Pacchiarotti I, et al. Bipolar disorder in the elderly: a cohort study comparing older and younger patients. Acta Psychiatr Scand. 2014;130:364–73.

Oepen G, Baldessarini RJ, Salvatore P, et al. On the periodicity of manic-depressive insanity, by Eliot Slater (1938): translated excerpts and commentary. J Affect Disord. 2004;78:1–9.

Ohara K, Nagai M, Suzuki Y, et al. Low activity allele of catechol-o-methyltransferase gene and Japanese unipolar depression. Neuroreport. 1998;9:1305–8.

Okan Ibiloglu A, Caykoylu A. The comorbidity of anxiety disorders in bipolar I and bipolar II patients among Turkish population. J Anxiety Disord. 2011;25:661–7.

Onyeama M, Agomoh A, Jombo E. Bipolar disorder in Enugu, South East Nigeria: demographic and diagnostic characteristics of patients. Psychiatr Danub. 2010;22(Suppl 1):S152–7.

Oquendo MA, Waternaux C, Brodsky B, et al. Suicidal behavior in bipolar mood disorder: clinical characteristics of attempters and nonattempters. J Affect Disord. 2000;59:107–17.

Ortiz A, Bradler K, Slaney C, et al. An admixture analysis of the age at index episodes in bipolar disorder. Psychiatry Res. 2011;188:34–9.

Ostacher MJ, Perlis RH, Nierenberg AA, et al. Impact of substance use disorders on recovery from episodes of depression in bipolar disorder patients: prospective data from the Systematic Treatment Enhancement Program for Bipolar Disorder (STEP-BD). Am J Psychiatry. 2010;167:289–97.

Oswald P, Souery D, Kasper S, et al. Current issues in bipolar disorder: a critical review. Eur Neuropsychopharmacol. 2007;17:687–95.

Ozerdem A, Tunca Z, Kaya N. The relatively good prognosis of bipolar disorders in a Turkish bipolar clinic. J Affect Disord. 2001;64:27–34.

Ozgürdal S, van Haren E, Hauser M, et al. Early mood swings as symptoms of the bipolar prodrome: preliminary results of a retrospective analysis. Psychopathology. 2009;42:337–42.

Ozyildirim I, Cakir S, Yazici O. Impact of psychotic features on morbidity and course of illness in patients with bipolar disorder. Eur Psychiatry. 2010;25:47–51.

Pacheco A, Barguil M, Contreras J, et al. Social and clinical comparison between schizophrenia and bipolar disorder type I with psychosis in Costa Rica. Soc Psychiatry Psychiatr Epidemiol. 2010;45:675–80.

Pae CU, Serretti A, Mandelli L, et al. Effect of 5-haplotype of dysbindin gene (DTNBP1) polymorphisms for the susceptibility to bipolar I disorder. Am J Med Genet B Neuropsychiatr Genet. 2007;144B:701–3.

Paholpak S, Kongsakon R, Pattanakumjorn W, et al. Risk factors for an anxiety disorder comorbidity among Thai patients with bipolar disorder: results from the Thai Bipolar Disorder Registry. Neuropsychiatr Dis Treat. 2014;10:803–10.

Papadimitriou GN, Dikeos DG, Karadima G, et al. Association between the GABA(A) receptor alpha5 subunit gene locus (GABRA5) and bipolar affective disorder. Am J Med Genet. 1998;81:73–80.

Pardoen D, Bauwens F, Dramaix M, et al. Life events and primary affective disorders. A one year prospective study. Br J Psychiatry. 1996;169:160–6.

Parmentier C, Etain B, Yon L, et al. Clinical and dimensional characteristics of euthymic bipolar patients with or without suicidal behavior. Eur Psychiatry. 2012;27:570–6.

Patrick V, Dunner DL, Fieve RR. Life events and primary affective illness. Acta Psychiatr Scand. 1978;58:48–55.

Patton GC, Hetrick SE, McGorry P. Service responses for youth onset mental disorders. Curr Opin Psychiatry. 2007;20:319–24.

Pavlickova H, Turnbull O, Bentall RP. Cognitive vulnerability to bipolar disorder in offspring of parents with bipolar disorder. Br J Clin Psychol. 2014;53:386–401.

Perich T, Mitchell PB, Loo C, et al. Cognitive styles and clinical correlates of childhood abuse in bipolar disorder. Bipolar Disord. 2014;16:600–7.

Perron H, Hamdani N, Faucard R, et al. Molecular characteristics of Human Endogenous Retrovirus type-W in schizophrenia and bipolar disorder. Transl Psychiatry. 2012;2:e201. https://doi.org/10.1038/tp.2012.125.

Perroud N, Cordera P, Zimmermann J, et al. Comorbidity between attention deficit hyperactivity disorder (ADHD) and bipolar disorder in a specialized mood disorders outpatient clinic. J Affect Disord. 2014;168:161–6.

Perugi G, Akiskal HS, Micheli C, et al. Clinical subtypes of bipolar mixed states: validating a broader European definition in 143 cases. J Affect Disord. 1997;43:169–80.

Perugi G, Micheli C, Akiskal HS, et al. Polarity of the first episode, clinical characteristics, and course of manic depressive illness: a systematic retrospective investigation of 320 bipolar I patients. Compr Psychiatry. 2000;41:13–8.

Piccardi MP, Ardau R, Chillotti C, et al. Manic-depressive illness: an association study with the inositol polyphosphate 1-phosphatase and serotonin transporter genes. Psychiatr Genet. 2002;12:23–7.

Pinto C, Souza RP, Lioult D, et al. Parent of origin effect and allelic expression imbalance of the serotonin transporter in bipolar disorder and suicidal behaviour. Eur Arch Psychiatry Clin Neurosci. 2011;261:533–8.

Pope M, Dudley R, Scott J. Determinants of social functioning in bipolar disorder. Bipolar Disord. 2007;9:38–44.

Popescu C, Ionescu R, Jipescu I, et al. Psychomotor functioning in unipolar and bipolar affective disorders. Rom J Neurol Psychiatry. 1991;29:17–33.

Porcelli S, Balzarro B, de Ronchi D, et al. Quetiapine extended release: preliminary evidence of a rapid onset of the antidepressant effect in bipolar depression. J Clin Psychopharmacol. 2014;34:303–6.

Post RM, Leverich GS, Kupka RW, et al. Early-onset bipolar disorder and treatment delay are risk factors for poor outcome in adulthood. J Clin Psychiatry. 2010;71:864–72.

Primavera D, Carta R, Lepori T, et al. Duration of untreated psychosis and cognitive deficits in a cohort of chronic psychotic patients. Clin Ter. 2013;164(4):e263–71. https://doi.org/10.7417/CT.2013.1586.

Radonic E, Rados M, Kalember P, et al. Comparison of hippocampal volumes in schizophrenia, schizoaffective and bipolar disorder. Coll Antropol. 2011;35(Suppl 1):249–52.

Ram D, Ram D. Subsyndromal states in bipolar disorder. Indian J Psychiatry. 2010;52:367–70.

Ramacciotti CE, Paoli RA, Marcacci G, et al. Relationship between bipolar illness and binge-eating disorders. Psychiatry Res. 2005;135:165–70.

Ratheesh A, Davey C, Hetrick S, et al. A systematic review and meta-analysis of prospective transition from major depression to bipolar disorder. Acta Psychiatr Scand. 2017;135:273–84.

Ravizza L, Tiraferri R, Rebaudengo P, et al. Age of onset and familial occurrence of manic-depressive psychosis. Riv Patol Nerv Ment. 1982;103:97–104.

Reinares M, Papachristou E, Harvey P, et al. Towards a clinical staging for bipolar disorder: defining patient subtypes based on functional outcome. J Affect Disord. 2013;144:65–71.

Rinieris PM, Stefanis CN, Lykouras EP, et al. Affective disorders and ABO blood types. Acta Psychiatr Scand. 1979;60:272–8.

Robb JC, Young LT, Cooke RG, et al. Gender differences in patients with bipolar disorder influence outcome in the medical outcomes survey (SF-20) subscale scores. J Affect Disord. 1998;49:189–93.

Robertson A, de Moore G, Boyce P. Bipolar II disorder in rural New South Wales. Australas Psychiatry. 2012;20:203–7.

Roiser JP, Cannon DM, Gandhi SK, et al. Hot and cold cognition in unmedicated depressed subjects with bipolar disorder. Bipolar Disord. 2009;11:178–89.

Rosa AR, Andreazza AC, Kunz M, et al. Predominant polarity in bipolar disorder: diagnostic implications. J Affect Disord. 2008;107:45–51.

Rydén E, Thase ME, Straht D, et al. A history of childhood attention-deficit hyperactivity disorder (ADHD) impacts clinical outcome in adult bipolar patients regardless of current ADHD. Acta Psychiatr Scand. 2009;120:239–46.

Safari R, Tunca Z, Ozerdem A, et al. New alterations at potentially regulated regions of the glial derived neurotrophic factor gene in bipolar disorder. J Affect Disord. 2014;167:244–50.

Sassi RB, Nicoletti M, Brambilla P, et al. Increased gray matter volume in lithium-treated bipolar disorder patients. Neurosci Lett. 2002;329:243–5.

Sato T, Bottlender R, Kleindienst N, et al. Syndromes and phenomenological subtypes underlying acute mania: a factor analytic study of 576 manic patients. Am J Psychiatry. 2002;159:968–74.

Saus E, Soria V, Escaramis G, et al. A haplotype of glycogen synthase kinase 3beta is associated with early onset of unipolar major depression. Genes Brain Behav. 2010;9:799–807.

Savitz JB, van der Merwe L, Stein DJ, et al. Neuropsychological task performance in bipolar spectrum illness: genetics, alcohol abuse, medication and childhood trauma. Bipolar Disord. 2008;10:479–94.

Scassellati C, Rotondo A, Bonvicini C, et al. Further evidence on the lack of association between glycogen synthase kinase 3beta gene polymorphisms and bipolar disorder. Psychiatr Genet. 2007;17:249–50.

Schaffer A, Cairney J, Cheung A, et al. Community survey of bipolar disorder in Canada: lifetime prevalence and illness characteristics. Can J Psychiatry. 2006;51:9–16.

Schoeyen HK, Vaaler AE, Auestad BH, et al. Despite clinical differences, bipolar disorder patients from acute wards and outpatient clinics have similar educational and disability levels compared to the general population. J Affect Disord. 2011;132:209–15.

Schroeter ML, Abdul-Khaliq H, Diefenbacher A, et al. S100B is increased in mood disorders and may be reduced by antidepressive treatment. Neuroreport. 2002;13:1675–8.

Seidman LJ, Lanca M, Kremen WS, et al. Organizational and visual memory deficits in schizophrenia and bipolar psychoses using the Rey-Osterrieth complex figure: effects of duration of illness. J Clin Exp Neuropsychol. 2003;25:949–64.

Serretti A, Mandelli L, Lattuada E, et al. Clinical and demographic features of mood disorder subtypes. Psychiatry Res. 2002;112:195–210.

Serretti A, Malitas PN, Mandelli L, et al. Further evidence for a possible association between serotonin transporter gene and lithium prophylaxis in mood disorders. Pharmacogenomics J. 2004;4:267–73.

Serretti A, Chiesa A, Calati R, et al. Influence of family history of major depression, bipolar disorder, and suicide on clinical features in patients with major depression and bipolar disorder. Eur Arch Psychiatry Clin Neurosci. 2013;263:93–103.

Sethi S, Khanna R. Phenomenology of mania in eastern India. Psychopathology. 1993;26:274–8.

Shabani A, Teimurinejad S, Kokar S, et al. Suicide risk factors in iranian patients with bipolar disorder: a 21-month follow-up from BDPF study. Iran J Psychiatry Behav Sci. 2013;7:16–23.

Shah A, Shen N, El-Mallakh RS. Weight gain occurs after onset of bipolar illness in overweight bipolar patients. Ann Clin Psychiatry. 2006;18:239–41.

Sierra P, Livianos L, Rojo L. Quality of life for patients with bipolar disorder: relationship with clinical and demographic variables. Bipolar Disord. 2005;7:159–65.

Skjelstad DV, Malt UF, Holte A. Symptoms and behaviors prior to the first major affective episode of bipolar II disorder. An exploratory study. J Affect Disord. 2011;132:333–43.

Slama F, Bellivier F, Henry C, et al. Bipolar patients with suicidal behavior: toward the identification of a clinical subgroup. J Clin Psychiatry. 2004;65:1035–9.

Sonne SC, Brady KT, Morton WA. Substance abuse and bipolar affective disorder. J Nerv Ment Dis. 1994;182:349–52.

Souery D, Lipp O, Rivelli SK, et al. Tyrosine hydroxylase polymorphism and phenotypic heterogeneity in bipolar affective disorder: a multicenter association study. Am J Med Genet. 1999;88:527–32.

Souery D, Zaninotto L, Calati R, et al. Depression across mood disorders: review and analysis in a clinical sample. Compr Psychiatry. 2012;53:24–38.

Spijker AT, Giltay EJ, van Rossum EF, et al. Glucocorticoid and mineralocorticoid receptor polymorphisms and clinical characteristics in bipolar disorder patients. Psychoneuroendocrinology. 2011;36:1460–9.

Squassina A, Manchia M, Costa M, et al. Age at onset in bipolar disorder: Investigation of the role of TaqIA polymorphism of DRD2 gene in a Sardinian sample. Eur Psychiatry. 2011;26:141–3.

Strakowski SM, Keck PE Jr, McElroy SL, et al. Twelve-month outcome after a first hospitalization for affective psychosis. Arch Gen Psychiatry. 1998;55:49–55.

Strakowski SM, DelBello MP, Fleck DE, et al. Effects of co-occurring alcohol abuse on the course of bipolar disorder following a first hospitalization for mania. Arch Gen Psychiatry. 2005;62:851–8.

Suominen K, Mantere O, Valtonen H, et al. Early age at onset of bipolar disorder is associated with more severe clinical features but delayed treatment seeking. Bipolar Disord. 2007;9:698–705.

Swann AC, Lijffijt M, Lane SD, et al. Antisocial personality disorder and borderline symptoms are differentially related to impulsivity and course of illness in bipolar disorder. J Affect Disord. 2013;148:384–90.

Sylvia LG, Rabideau DJ, Nierenberg AA, et al. The effect of personalized guideline-concordant treatment on quality of life and functional impairment in bipolar disorder. J Affect Disord. 2014;169:144–8.

Szadoczky E, Papp Z, Vitrai J, et al. The prevalence of major depressive and bipolar disorders in Hungary. Results from a national epidemiologic survey. J Affect Disord. 1998;50:153–62.

Szczepankiewicz A, Skibinska M, Suwalska A, et al. The association study of three FYN polymorphisms with prophylactic lithium response in bipolar patients. Hum Psychopharmacol. 2009;24:287–91.

Takei Y, Suda M, Aoyama Y, et al. Near-infrared spectroscopic study of frontopolar activation during face-to-face conversation in major depressive disorder and bipolar disorder. J Psychiatr Res. 2014;57:74–83.

Tamam L, Tuglu C, Karatas G, et al. Adult attention-deficit hyperactivity disorder in patients with bipolar I disorder in remission: preliminary study. Psychiatry Clin Neurosci. 2006;60:480–5.

Tamam L, Karakus G, Ozpoyraz N. Comorbidity of adult attention-deficit hyperactivity disorder and bipolar disorder: prevalence and clinical correlates. Eur Arch Psychiatry Clin Neurosci. 2008;258:385–93.

Taylor Tavares JV, Clark L, Cannon DM, et al. Distinct profiles of neurocognitive function in unmedicated unipolar depression and bipolar II depression. Biol Psychiatry. 2007;62:917–24.

Thesing CS, Stek ML, van Grootheest DS, et al. Childhood abuse, family history and stressors in older patients with bipolar disorder in relation to age at onset. J Affect Disord. 2015;184:249–55.

Thomé ES, Dargel AA, Migliavacca FM, et al. Stigma experiences in bipolar patients: the impact upon functioning. J Psychiatr Ment Health Nurs. 2012;19:665–71.

Tohen M, Calabrese J, Vieta E, et al. Effect of comorbid anxiety on treatment response in bipolar depression. J Affect Disord. 2007;104:137–46.

Tondo L, Baldessarini RJ. Suicide in bipolar disorder. In: Yildiz A, Nemeroff C, Ruiz P, editors. The bipolar book: history, neurobiology, and treatment. New York: Oxford University Press; 2015. p. 509–28.

Tondo L, Lepri B, Cruz N, et al. Age at onset in 3014 Sardinian bipolar and major depressive disorder patients. Acta Psychiatr Scand. 2010;121:446–52.

Tondo L, Visioli C, Preti A, et al. Bipolar disorders following initial depression: modeling predictive clinical factors. J Affect Disord. 2014;167:44–9.

Tondo L, Pompili M, Forte A, et al. Suicide attempts in bipolar disorders: comprehensive review of 101 reports. Acta Psychiatr Scand. 2016;133:174–86.

Toniolo RA, Caetano SC, da Silva PV, et al. Clinical significance of lifetime panic disorder in the course of bipolar disorder type I. Compr Psychiatry. 2009;50:9–12.

Torrent C, Martínez-Arán A, Daban C, et al. Cognitive impairment in bipolar II disorder. Br J Psychiatry. 2006;189:254–9.

Torrent C, Bonnin Cdel M, Martínez-Arán A, et al. Efficacy of functional remediation in bipolar disorder: a multicenter randomized controlled study. Am J Psychiatry. 2013;170:852–9.

Torres IJ, DeFreitas VG, DeFreitas CM, et al. Neurocognitive functioning in patients with bipolar I disorder recently recovered from a first manic episode. J Clin Psychiatry. 2010;71:1234–42.

Tozzi F, Manchia M, Galwey NW, et al. Admixture analysis of age at onset in bipolar disorder. Psychiatry Res. 2011;185:27–32.

Tundo A, Calabrese JR, Marchetti F, et al. Continuous circular cycling in bipolar disorder as a predictor of poor outcome. J Affect Disord. 2013;150:823–8.

Turecki G, Grof P, Grof E, et al. Mapping susceptibility genes for bipolar disorder: a pharmacogenetic approach based on excellent response to lithium. Mol Psychiatry. 2001;6:570–8.

Van Den Bossche MJ, Strazisar M, De Bruyne S, et al. Identification of a CACNA2D4 deletion in late onset bipolar disorder patients and implications for the involvement of voltage-dependent calcium channels in psychiatric disorders. Am J Med Genet B Neuropsychiatr Genet. 2012;159B:465–75.

Verdolini N, Dean J, Elisei S, et al. Bipolar disorder: the importance of clinical assessment in identifying prognostic factors—an audit. Part 1: an analysis of potential prognostic factors. Psychiatr Danub. 2014;26(Suppl 1):289–300.

Verdoux H, Mury M, Besancon G, et al. Comparative study of substance dependence comorbidity in bipolar, schizophrenic and schizoaffective disorders. Encephale. 1996;22:95–101.

Versace A, Almeida JR, Hassel S, et al. Elevated left and reduced right orbitomedial prefrontal fractional anisotropy in adults with bipolar disorder revealed by tract-based spatial statistics. Arch Gen Psychiatry. 2008;65:1041–52.

Vieta E, Suppes T. Bipolar II disorder: arguments for and against a distinct diagnostic entity. Bipolar Disord. 2008;10:163–78.

Vieta E, Gasto C, Otero A, et al. Differential features between bipolar I and bipolar II disorder. Compr Psychiatry. 1997;38:98–101.

Vieta E, Sanchez-Moreno J, Lahuerta J, et al. Subsyndromal depressive symptoms in patients with bipolar and unipolar disorder during clinical remission. J Affect Disord. 2008;107:169–74.

Vinberg M, Mikkelsen RL, Kirkegaard T, et al. Differences in clinical presentation between bipolar I and II disorders in the early stages of bipolar disorder: a naturalistic study. J Affect Disord. 2017;208:521–7.

Wang Z, Li Z, Chen J, Huang J, et al. Association of BDNF gene polymorphism with bipolar disorders in Han Chinese population. Genes Brain Behav. 2012;11:524–8.

Washizuka S, Ikeda A, Kato N, et al. Possible relationship between mitochondrial DNA polymorphisms and lithium response in bipolar disorder. Int J Neuropsychopharmacol. 2003;6:421–4.

Wehr TA, Sack DA, Rosenthal NE, et al. Rapid cycling affective disorder: contributing factors and treatment responses in 51 patients. Am J Psychiatry. 1988;145:179–84.

Welge JA, Keck PE Jr, Meinhold JM. Predictors of response to treatment of acute bipolar manic episodes with divalproex sodium or placebo in 2 randomized, controlled, parallel-group trials. J Clin Psychopharmacol. 2004;24:607–12.

Wilson S, Sponheim SR. Dimensions underlying psychotic and manic symptomatology: extending normal-range personality traits to schizophrenia and bipolar spectra. Compr Psychiatry. 2014;55:1809–19.

Wu JC, Kelsoe JR, Schachat C, et al. Rapid and sustained antidepressant response with sleep deprivation and chronotherapy in bipolar disorder. Biol Psychiatry. 2009;66:298–301.

Xiang YT, Zhang L, Wang G, et al. Sociodemographic and clinical features of bipolar disorder patients misdiagnosed with major depressive disorder in China. Bipolar Disord. 2013;15:199–205.

Yildiz A, Sachs GS. Age onset of psychotic versus non-psychotic bipolar illness in men and in women. J Affect Disord. 2003;74:197–201.

Yildiz A, Nemeroff C, Ruiz P, editors. The bipolar book: history, neurobiology, and treatment. New York: Oxford University Press; 2015.
Zander C, Schurhoff F, Laurent C, et al. CAG repeat sequences in bipolar affective disorder: no evidence for association in a French population. Am J Med Genet. 1998;81:338–41.
Zeschel E, Correll CU, Haussleiter IS, et al. The bipolar disorder prodrome revisited: is there a symptomatic pattern? J Affect Disord. 2013;151:551–60.
Zhang HY, Ishigaki T, Tani K, et al. Serotonin2A receptor gene polymorphism in mood disorders. Biol Psychiatry. 1997;41:768–73.
Zhang X, Zhang C, Wu Z, et al. Association of genetic variation in CACNA1C with bipolar disorder in Han Chinese. J Affect Disord. 2013;150:261–5.
Zuncheddu C, Carpiniello B. Sexual dysfunctions and bipolar disorder: a study of patients submitted to a long-term lithium treatment. Clin Ter. 2006;157:419–24.
Zutshi A, Reddy YC, Thennarasu K, et al. Comorbidity of anxiety disorders in patients with remitted bipolar disorder. Eur Arch Psychiatry Clin Neurosci. 2006;256:428–36.

The Age of Onset of Unipolar Depression

6

Nefize Yalin and Allan H. Young

6.1 Age of Onset in the Scope of Major Depressive Disorder

Major depressive disorder (MDD) is a common and frequently recurrent mental illness that might occur at any time during the lifespan (American Psychiatric Association 2013). It is associated with increased morbidity and mortality worldwide and has been ranked as the third leading cause of all-cause disability in the Global Burden of Disease Study 2015 (GBD 2015 Disease and Injury Incidence and Prevalence Collaborators 2016). In a meta-analysis of 18 prevalence and 5 incidence studies, annual and lifetime prevalence and annual incidence for MDD were found as 4.1%, 6.7% and 2.9%, respectively (Waraich et al. 2004). A recent meta-analysis also revealed similar results with a point prevalence of 4.7% (4.4–5.0%) and annual incidence of 3.0% (2.4–3.8%) (Ferrari et al. 2013).

MDD is defined as a major depressive episode (MDE) in the absence of a history of manic or hypomanic episodes in both widely accepted classification systems for mental disorders, namely, the *Diagnostic and Statistical Manual of Mental Disorders*, fifth Edition (DSM-5) and the 10th Revision of the *International Classification of Diseases* (ICD-10) (American Psychiatric Association 2013; World Health Organization 1992). Considering MDE, both classification systems are again similar apart from the threshold for required symptoms and define MDE as 2 weeks or longer of depressed mood or anhedonia accompanied by psychomotor and weight changes, sleep disturbances, fatigue, feelings of worthlessness and guilt, difficulty in concentrating and suicidal ideation (American Psychiatric Association 2013; World Health Organization 1992). Diagnostic criteria for MDE are the same for all age groups with the exception of an additional DSM-5 criteria whereby depressed mood can be replaced by irritable mood and weight loss could manifest

N. Yalin · A. H. Young (✉)
Centre for Affective Disorders, Department of Psychological Medicine, Institute of Psychiatry, Psychology and Neuroscience, King's College of London, London, UK
e-mail: nefize.yalin@kcl.ac.uk; allan.young@kcl.ac.uk

G. de Girolamo et al. (eds.), *Age of Onset of Mental Disorders*,
https://doi.org/10.1007/978-3-319-72619-9_6

as a failure to make expected weight in children and adolescents (American Psychiatric Association 2013).

Age of onset (AOO) of mental health disorders is an important clinical measure to understand the potential causes and underlying mechanisms for each illness, calculate the lifetime risk and target the appropriate age range for prevention and early intervention (Kessler et al. 2007; Jones 2013). Although most of the mental health disorders begin in childhood, adolescence or early adulthood, effective treatment is typically not initiated until a number of years later. Increasing evidence suggests that intervention during the early stages of the disorder may help to reduce the severity and/or the persistence of the initial or primary disorder and prevent secondary disorders (Kessler et al. 2007; de Girolamo et al. 2012). Therefore, AOO is not only important to understand the illness better but also may be crucial for restructuring existing mental health prevention strategies and developing more appropriate service design (Jones 2013; McGorry et al. 2011).

In terms of MDD, AOO is a particular research area of interest. There is a significant heterogeneity in symptomatology, comorbidities, treatment response, prognosis and clinical outcomes among depressed individuals, and differentiating them into more homogenous subgroups using AOO as a clinical indicator might help us to better understand disease pathology (Zhu et al. 2012). Compared to many other mental disorders that have an onset during childhood or adolescence, MDD usually has a later average AOO circa mid-20s (Kessler and Bromet 2013). The peak risk period for the onset extends from mid- to late adolescence to early 40s across all countries (Kessler and Bromet 2013); however, the late-life onset is also not uncommon (American Psychiatric Association 2013). According to the World Mental Health Survey Initiative, the median AOO for MDD is 25.7 (17.3–37.2) in high-income and 24.0 (17.0–34.8) in middle- to low-income countries (Kessler and Bromet 2013). There are no significant mean AOO differences between females and males, but age-specific incidence rates are reported to vary according to gender (Bogren et al. 2018; Martin-Merino et al. 2010). One cohort study of a source population of 1,287,829 subjects found the highest incidence for MDD between the ages of 20 and 29 with a trend of decreasing rate in incidence from 30 to 69 years of age in both genders. The incidence rates were higher in females for all age groups, and the fall of the rates after the age of 30 was more marked in women than it is in men (Martin-Merino et al. 2010). Another prospective community study found a distinct preponderance of MDD incidence for females in the 40–49 age band. The female rates increase from the 15–29 to the 40–49 age bands and start to decrease in the 60–69 age band; on the contrary male rates are rather stable throughout the age bands with a decreasing tendency in the 60–69 and 70+ age bands (Bogren et al. 2018).

So far, aetiological factors and clinical outcomes in relation to AOO of MDD were subjected to several studies, but there is a considerable variability in how "early-onset" and "late-onset" MDD have been defined. Cut-off points distinguishing "early-onset" and "late-onset" ranges from onset in childhood or adolescence up to the age of 60. Moreover, different terms were used as "pre-adult onset" and "adult onset" instead of "early onset" and "late onset" in the studies that included childhood-, adolescent- and adult-onset patients with MDD. If we consider the studies that were comprised of both pre-adult and adult-onset MDD patients, although different cut-off points between 17 and 30 years of age were used, the most frequently used cut-off point was 18 years of age for distinguishing "early onset" (pre-adult onset, <18 years of age) and "late onset" (adult onset, ≥18 years of age) (Fernando et al. 2011; van Noorden et al. 2011; Korczak and Goldstein 2009; Zisook et al. 2007). In these studies, further differentiation has also been made in the "early-onset" group as childhood onset (<12 years of age) and adolescent onset (≥12 to <18 years of age) (Fernando et al. 2011; van Noorden et al. 2011; Korczak and Goldstein 2009; Zisook et al. 2007). In solely adult-onset MDD samples, although different cut-off points between 40 and 65 years of age were used, the majority of the studies defined the cut-off point as 60 years of age to differentiate "early-onset" (<60 years of age) and "late-onset" (≥60 years of age) MDD (Grayson and Thomas 2013). MDD in elderly adults could also be labelled as "late-life", "geriatric" or "old-age" MDD. It should be noted that these terms are broad and used to describe both the individuals whose first episode is later in life (late-onset MDD) and whose depression started earlier (early-onset MDD) but show recurring episodes later on (Vu and Aizenstein 2013). In terms of studies that included participants with MDD from the whole AOO spectrum, Sequenced Treatment Alternatives to Relieve Depression (STAR*D) is the best of its kind. In this study, over 4000 individuals with MDD were classified into five AOO groups as childhood onset (by age 12), adolescent onset (between ages 12 and 17), early adult onset (between ages 18 and 44), middle adult onset (between ages 45 and 59) and late adult onset (after age 60) (Zisook et al. 2007).

One method to compensate for the discrepancy in the definition of "early onset" and "late onset" and identify the most suitable cut-off ages for AOO subgroups in MDD is admixture analysis (Zhu et al. 2012). This analysis performs a decomposition of the AOO distribution into a mixture of normal components and estimates the number of components of such a mixture. The maximum likelihood estimation of the finite normal mixture was applied to determine a theoretical model that best fitted the observed distribution of AOO (Zhu et al. 2012). So far, there is only one study conducted in MDD that implemented admixture analysis using 531 patients with an AOO ranging from 6 to 61 years of age. This study identified three AOO subgroups as the early-onset group with mean AOO of 14.60 years, the intermediate-onset group with mean of 29.15 years and late-onset group with mean of 46.96 years and proposed 22 and 40 years of age as cut-off points to differentiate these three subgroups (Zhu et al. 2012).

6.2 Age of Onset-Specific Symptomatology and Clinical Outcomes in Major Depressive Disorder

To date, several studies with large sample sizes have been conducted to define specific characteristics of MDD in different AOO subgroups. In terms of studies that compared pre-adult to adult samples, a study by Fernando et al. that included approximately 400 participants with childhood-, adolescent- or adult-onset MDD showed that childhood- and adolescent-onset MDD groups were more likely to have attempted suicide and have increased rates of comorbid alcohol dependence, social phobia and avoidant personality disorder compared to the adult-onset group. In addition, participants with adolescent-onset depression were more likely to meet criteria for agoraphobia and any kind of personality disorder, while participants with childhood-onset depression were more likely to meet criteria for cannabis dependence, any substance dependence, obsessive-compulsive disorder and paranoid personality disorder compared to adult-onset participants. There were no differences among childhood-, adolescent- and adult-onset groups in terms of depression severity, depression subtype and childhood abuse or neglect (Fernando et al. 2011).

In another study conducted with 1552 MDD outpatients, pre-adult-onset MDD has been associated with more suicidal attempts and current suicidal thoughts and increased rates of comorbid social phobia and drug dependence or abuse than adult-onset MDD. No differences between the groups were found in Montgomery–Asberg Depression Rating Scale (MADRS) continuous scores or in MADRS categories (van Noorden et al. 2011). Another study, which enrolled a large sample of outpatients (N = 6778) diagnosed with childhood-, adolescent- or adult-onset MDD, reported that patients with adolescent- and childhood-onset MDD have greater mean number and length of episodes, increased number of attempted suicide, increased need for hospitalization and increased latency from MDD onset to treatment. This study also showed that both childhood- and adolescent-onset MDD patients have higher rates of comorbid dysthymic disorder, personality disorders and social phobia, and they are more likely to report parental history of MDD and familial history of substance use disorder, while only childhood-onset MDD was reported to have a greater prevalence of familial alcohol disorders compared to adult-onset MDD. The authors also noted that the results for adolescent-onset MDD were less pronounced than childhood-onset compared to adult-onset MDD, but this group also has the early-onset illness burden (Korczak and Goldstein 2009).

Another follow-up study reported that with the exception of more melancholic symptoms in the adolescent-onset group, patients with childhood- and adolescent-onset MDD have similar depressive symptomatology, duration and severity of the index depressive episode, rates of recovery and recurrence, comorbid disorders and parental history of psychiatric disorders (Birmaher et al. 2004).

Among studies which have included only adult-onset patients, a large investigation with 18,912 individuals suffering from MDD (early- and late-onset cut-off was set to 65 years old) reported that patients with late-onset MDD did not differ from their early-onset counterparts in terms of melancholic symptoms but were more often women, who presented with more severe depressive episodes and more often with psychotic features (Kessing 2006). With regard to psychotic features and AOO of MDD, a recent meta-analysis showed that psychotic symptoms are present to a greater extent in earlier AOO MDD in younger samples (<45 years old) and are also greater in later AOO MDD in older samples (>55 years old) (Jaaskelainen et al. 2017). In addition, a few small sample-sized studies have focused on delusional content in psychotic MDD considering AOO so far, and it seems that patients with later-onset MDD(>60 years old) show more somatic and impending disaster content on the contrary to the early-onset MDD patients (≤60 years old) who show more paranoid ideation (Gournellis et al. 2008, 2011).

Another study that included 6850 individuals with MDD defined three AOO groups as early onset (18–59 years old), late onset (60–74 years old) and later late onset (75 years of age and older). The authors showed that later late-onset MDD group were characterized by more frequent retardation/agitation and less frequent sleep disturbances compared to early- and late-onset MDD group. Furthermore, patients with both later late-onset and late-onset showed less frequent guilt feelings than patients with early-onset MDD. Although this study did not reveal any differences between three groups in the severity of MDD measured by MADRS, patients with later late-onset MDD showed more severe lassitude, apparent sadness and reduced appetite compared to early-onset MDD and less severe reduced sleep, pessimism and inner tension compared to both late- and early-onset MDD (Corruble et al. 2008).

Korten et al. (2012) recruited 1104 participants with a cut-off age of 40 years and found that late-onset MDD was associated with less years of education, being male, more decreased appetite/weight loss and less often feelings of sadness, worthlessness and guilt compared to early-onset MDD. In addition, late-onset MDD patients showed shorter duration of symptoms, less often recurrence and serious suicide attempt, decreased rates of family history of MDD and increased neuroticism and comorbidity with generalized anxiety disorder compared to early-onset MDD patients (Korten et al. 2012).

Apart from these three large sample-sized studies, one systematic review that critically analysed the literature was published in 2013. According to this review, several studies reported no statistically significant differences between the symptomatology of early- and late-onset MDD, and the most consistent findings were reduced family history of MDD and pessimistic/suicidal thinking in late-onset MDD compared to early-onset MDD (Grayson and Thomas 2013). In terms of response, remission and recurrence rates, most of the studies failed to show significant differences between early- and late-onset MDD (Grayson and Thomas 2013; Mitchell and Subramaniam 2005).

With regard to studies comparing the whole AOO spectrum, STAR*D study showed that no single AOO group stood out as distinct, but younger AOO was associated with a larger proportion of participants being employed, seeking care in a psychiatric care setting, having a family history of depression having alcohol or drug abuse, and a smaller proportion of participants being married. Younger AOO was also associated with longer duration of illness, greater number of lifetime episodes, higher levels of general medical comorbidity, greater depressive symptom severity, worse mental functioning, decreased quality of life, worse work and social adjustment, increased likelihood of past suicide attempts, greater present suicide risk, greater probability of comorbid anxiety disorder and social phobia and a greater number of concurrent anxiety disorders. Post-traumatic stress disorder (PTSD) was more frequent in the childhood-onset group than in the adolescent-onset group and more frequent in the early adult-onset group than in either the middle adult- or late adult-onset groups. Furthermore, bulimia was statistically more frequent in the childhood-onset and adolescent-onset group than in the early adult-onset group. In terms of depressive symptoms, negative view of self, negative view of future, suicidal ideation and interpersonal rejection sensitivity were significantly more prevalent in the youngest AOO groups (Zisook et al. 2007).

Another clinical outcome related to MDD is the impairment in cognitive functions, which has been shown to be different in different AOO groups. One meta-analysis of cognition studies in the adults with MDD reported that both early- and late-onset patients showed reduced function in all domains, but late-onset MDD patients showed greater reductions in processing speed and executive function compared to both early-onset MDD and healthy controls (Herrmann et al. 2007). Another meta-analysis revealed that the magnitude of cognitive impairment is larger in late-onset MDD than early-onset MDD compared to healthy controls in most of the cognitive domains. A direct comparison of cognitive functions between late- and early-onset MDD showed that late-onset MDD patients were significantly more impaired in processing speed and verbal memory compared to early-onset MDD patients. There were also trend level differences for more impairment in global cognition and executive function in late-onset group. The authors also noted that between-group differences in executive functions were driven by speed-dependent tasks (Bora et al. 2013).

About cognitive functions of pre-adult-onset samples, the literature is very limited. Although no AOO classification or comparison with an adult sample was made, it is worth to mention that one review in cognition of adolescents and younger adults (between 12 and 25 years of age) diagnosed with MDD suggested that this relatively young group already exhibits neurocognitive impairments very similar to that of adult patients, particularly in the areas of executive function, working memory and psychomotor and processing speed (Baune et al. 2014).

6.3 Age of Onset-Specific Aetiology of Major Depressive Disorder

Neurobiological findings on AOO-specific aetiology of MDD are limited, and most of the conducted studies investigated genetic underpinnings of AOO in MDD as one of the most consistent findings in clinical settings was increased rates of family history in early-onset MDD.

One twin study found that AOO of MDD between the ages of 15 and 35 is associated with increased MDD liability in family members (Kendler et al. 2005). In terms of molecular studies on familiality of AOO in MDD, one study found marginally significant single nucleotide polymorphism (SNP) heritability estimate of 0.17 for the AOO of MDD (Ferentinos et al. 2015). On the other hand, another study found that AOO is not significantly heritable, and polygenic risk derived from the aggregated effects of common genetic variants does not significantly predict AOO. This study also showed that AOO was modestly but significantly lower in cases with a first-degree family history of MDD (Docherty et al. 2017).

The largest study up to date on AOO and MDD was a discovery case-control genome-wide association study where cases were stratified using age-at-onset cut-offs and significant single nucleotide polymorphisms were studied with a total sample of 22,158 MDD cases and 133,749 control subjects. One replicated genome-wide significant locus (rs7647854) was identified as associated with adult-onset (>27 years) MDD, flanking with genes C3orf70, VPS8, EHHADH and MAP3K13. C3orf70, VPS8 and MAP3K13 all showed evidence of expression in the brain in several areas of potential interest for MDD including the hypothalamus, frontal cortex, pituitary and thyroid. Polygenic score analyses showed that earlier-onset MDD is genetically more similar to schizophrenia and bipolar disorder than adult-onset MDD, coronary artery diseases were weakly positively associated with MDD without any AOO difference and no association was seen for the scores generated for Alzheimer's disease (Power et al. 2017).

6.4 Age of Onset of Major Depressive Disorder and Brain Imaging

In terms of neuroimaging studies, mega-data analysis of ENIGMA consortium found that patients with an early age of onset (≤21 years) is associated with a smaller hippocampus and a trend towards smaller amygdala and larger lateral ventricles (Schmaal et al. 2016). Considering cortical abnormalities, no significant differences were detected in cortical thickness in patients with an adolescent age of onset (≤21 years,) compared to controls and when comparing adolescent-onset and adult-onset patients directly. Similarly, no surface area differences were detected in these subgroup analyses (Schmaal et al. 2017).

Looking at the neuroimaging findings in late-onset MDD, the most consistent finding is increased white matter hyperintensities in late-life depression and, to a greater extent, late-onset depression in late life. In particular, the odds of having white matter changes were over four for late- compared to early-onset depression (Herrmann et al. 2008). In terms of grey matter abnormalities in late-onset depression, a few studies have been conducted and have shown a significant decrease of grey matter volume (GMV) in amygdala, hippocampus, medial orbitofrontal cortex, insula, posterior anterior cingulate cortex, postcentral cortex, superior frontal cortex, and middle temporal cortex and an increase of GMV in cingulate cortex compared to controls (Egger et al. 2008; Hwang et al. 2010; Yuan et al. 2008).

6.5 Age of Onset of Major Depressive Disorder and Conversion to Bipolar Disorder

Conversion from MDD to another disorder is an important area that needs to be discussed as there is an established relationship between AOO of MDD and conversion to other neuropsychiatric disorders. One of the AOO-specific aetiologic factors that need to be considered in the children, adolescent and young adults with MDD is bipolarity. Several studies in the literature have identified a significant association between lower AOO of MDD and higher rates of transition to bipolar disorder (Ratheesh et al. 2017; Faedda et al. 2015). Some of these studies also specify cut-off ages for early-onset MDD as <17 and <25 years and found an increased risk of conversion to bipolarity in this particular AOO group (Tondo et al. 2014; Akiskal et al. 1983; Beesdo et al. 2009). In addition, one recent meta-analysis showed that AOO of MDD in cases that became bipolar disorder in the follow-up was approximately 5 years younger than the ones who didn't develop bipolar disorder (Ratheesh et al. 2017). All together, these results support that early-onset MDD could be a prodromal state of bipolar disorder and this specific AOO group should be assessed and monitored carefully for a possible bipolar disorder diagnosis with the evaluation of the presence of other established predictors for the transition to bipolar disorder such as family history of bipolar disorder and presence of psychotic and subsyndromal (hypo)manic symptoms (Ratheesh et al. 2017; Faedda et al. 2015).

6.6 Late-Onset Major Depressive Disorder and Cognitive Impairment

In terms of individuals with late-onset MDD, possible dementia and vascular depression diagnosis should be evaluated in every patient as AOO-specific aetiologic factors. Vascular depression was suggested as a subtype of late-life MDD by Alexopoulos et al. in 1997, who argued that cerebrovascular disease, including small-vessel ischemic changes, may predispose, precipitate or perpetuate some geriatric depressive symptoms as a consequence of structural damage of brain circuits (Alexopoulos et al. 1997; Aizenstein et al. 2016). From that day on, several studies were conducted, and in a consensus report published in 2016, vascular depression was characterized by the absence of family history of MDD, presence of executive dysfunctions, white matter hyperintensities, loss of energy, subjective feeling of sadness, anhedonia, psychomotor retardation, motivational problems, reduced processing speed and visuospatial skills, deficits in self-initiation and lack of insight, higher cardiac illness comorbidity and increased rates of vascular risk factors. It is also noted that depressive symptomatology of patients with this disease may not meet criteria for any mood disorder in DSM-5 and these patients may have higher risk for cognitive decline and progression to dementia, fluctuating course of cognitive impairment due to progression of white matter hyperintensities, greater treatment resistance and poorer outcome (Aizenstein et al. 2016). Late-onset MDD is particularly important and should be examined in this context as several studies showed that individuals with vascular depression tend to have a later age of onset of depression, specifically after 65 years of age or later (Aizenstein et al. 2016).

The relationship between dementia and MDD is complex, and several hypotheses have been suggested so far, including depression being a risk factor, a prodrome or a consequence of Alzheimer's disease (AD) and other dementia's as well as an independent comorbidity (Bennett and Thomas 2014). Only the prodromal hypotheses will be discussed here. The evidence supports that late-life depression could be a prodromal state for dementia (Bennett and Thomas 2014), and one recent cohort study revealed that very late-onset depression (>70 years of age) with ongoing depressive symptomatology of clinical relevance without remission predicts a subsequent dementia and might be a prodrome of particularly AD (Heser et al. 2013). The research highlights the need to carefully follow up individuals presenting with depression in old age for future cognitive decline, especially if the depression is late onset (Bennett and Thomas 2014).

6.7 Age-Specific Treatment Recommendations for Major Depressive Disorder

Although there are no AOO specific treatment guidelines, it is worth to consider the treatment recommendations for pre-adult and late-life MDD as these subgroups particularly include "early-onset" and "late-onset" patients and have distinct features compared to adult MDD treatment recommendations. Here we critically summarized recommendations of four different treatment guidelines published by British Association of Psychopharmacology, Canadian Network for Mood and Anxiety Treatments, Royal Australian and New Zealand College of Psychiatrists and World Federation of Societies of Biological Psychiatry for the treatment of pre-adult and late-life depression (Cleare et al. 2015; MacQueen et al. 2016; Malhi et al. 2015; Bauer et al. 2013, 2015). These four guidelines were chosen according to their novelty and inclusion of recommendations for these special subgroups of MDD population.

For the treatment of pre-adult MDD, first of all one should note that the drug-placebo difference for antidepressants are smaller for children and adolescents compared to adults and they are even smaller and not statistically significant under the age of 13. Furthermore, it should be taken into account that there is very limited evidence for psychological treatments for the children under the age of 13. Up to date, the evidence-based research for the acute treatment shows that there is no clear comparative advantage for pharmacotherapy or psychotherapy in treating childhood and adolescent MDD although cognitive behavioural therapy (CBT) and interpersonal therapy (IPT) are recommended as the first line of treatment in mild to moderate MDD. Pharmacotherapy could be considered as a first-line intervention in more severe cases of depression, if there is a history of moderate to severe recurrent depression or when psychotherapy is not accessible or effective. Fluoxetine is the first-choice antidepressant in pre-adult population, and if fluoxetine treatment is found ineffective, escitalopram, sertraline and, to a lesser extent, citalopram are generally considered as second-choice antidepressants. Paroxetine is not recommended. Tricyclic antidepressants (TCAs), monoamine oxidase inhibitors (MAOIs) and neurostimulation treatments are also not recommended and may only be considered for last option in nonresponsive or treatment-resistant situations due to very limited evidence for MDD treatment in this age group (Cleare et al. 2015; MacQueen et al. 2016; Malhi et al. 2015). Young people prescribed selective serotonin reuptake inhibitors (SSRIs) must be closely monitored for emergent suicidality as there is an increased risk for nonfatal suicidal thoughts and behaviours for those younger than 24, and FDA issued a black-box warning on SSRI use in this group of patients (Cleare et al. 2015; MacQueen et al. 2016; Malhi et al. 2015). For the maintenance-phase strategies in pre-adult populations, the literature is sparse, but there is an evidence for favouring medication over placebo in preventing new episodes (Bauer et al. 2015).

For the treatment of late-life MDD, there are particular challenges for the clinicians such as changes in drug metabolism and pharmacokinetics associated with advanced age and the greater chance of serious drug-drug interactions because of concurrent treatments for higher level of medical comorbidity. In addition, one should take into account that pathophysiology of depression in old age could be different (vascular depression, etc.) or depressive symptoms could be a prodrome for dementia. In terms of pharmacological treatments for late-life depression, the efficacy of different classes of antidepressants including selective noradrenalin reuptake inhibitors (SNRIs), SSRIs, TCAs and MAOs over placebo was shown in the adults 55+ years of age, but there is insufficient data for the patients aged 65 years or older. Nevertheless, the guidelines encourage the use of the whole spectrum of antidepressant options in old age despite the dearth of information of possible side effects such as falls, gastrointestinal bleeding, orthostatic hypotension, hyponatraemia and cardiovascular and anticholinergic effects. It should also be noted that higher plasma concentrations for a given dose are generally found in older adults and lower doses of antidepressants are recommended. Considering psychological treatments, problem-solving therapy has the strongest evidence for late-life depression (Cleare et al. 2015; MacQueen et al. 2016; Bauer et al. 2013, 2015). Although it is not discussed in detail within the mentioned guidelines, neuromodulation therapies could also be considered in late-life depression. Studies have proven that electroconvulsive therapy (ECT) is more effective and has a faster onset of action than antidepressants in the treatment of severe, geriatric depression and older age is a predictor of rapid ECT response and remission (Galvez et al. 2015). Findings in repetitive transcranial magnetic stimulation (rTMS) suggest that it is also a safe intervention (Galvez et al. 2015). For the maintenance phase, there is evidence for continuing antidepressant medication for 12 months, and nortriptyline, phenelzine and SSRIs including paroxetine, escitalopram and citalopram were shown to be efficacious compared to placebo in preventing recurrence (Cleare et al. 2015; MacQueen et al. 2016; Bauer et al. 2013, 2015).

Conclusions

In summary, compared to many other mental disorders that have an onset during childhood or adolescence, MDD usually has a later AOO circa mid-20s. There is a considerable variability in how "early-onset" and "late-onset" MDD have been defined in the literature with cut-off points distinguishing "early-onset" and "late-onset" ranges from onset in childhood or adolescence through the age of 60. In terms of compensating for this discrepancy and identifying the most suitable cut-off ages for AOO subgroups in MDD, more studies implementing admixture analysis to bigger MDD samples are needed.

AOO of MDD is associated with specific symptomatology and clinical outcomes. The most repeated findings in pre-adult MDD are the higher presence of family history, increased number of suicide attempts and suicidal thinking and higher rates of comorbid substance use and social phobia compared to adult-onset MDD. Regarding differences in adult-onset MDD groups, late-onset MDD seems to show decreased presence of feelings of sadness, pessimism, worthlessness and guilt, more impairment in cognition, more decreased appetite/weight loss, less disturbance in sleep and less suicidal thinking. The studies on neurobiological underpinnings of MDD with regard to AOO are limited, and the results are inconsistent. More studies in this area are warranted.

It must be always kept in mind that early-onset MDD could be a prodromal state of bipolar disorder and this specific AOO group should be assessed and monitored carefully for a possible bipolar disorder diagnosis. In terms of elderly individuals with late-onset MDD, possible dementia and vascular depression diagnosis should always be considered and evaluated. Although there are no AOO-specific treatment guidelines, the treatment recommendations for pre-adult and late-life MDD should be considered in the early- and late-onset MDD groups.

References

Aizenstein HJ, Baskys A, Boldrini M, Butters MA, Diniz BS, Jaiswal MK, Jellinger KA, Kruglov LS, Meshandin IA, Mijajlovic MD, Niklewski G, Pospos S, Raju K, Richter K, Steffens DC, Taylor WD, Tene O. Vascular depression consensus report—a critical update. BMC Med. 2016;14(1):161.

Akiskal HS, Walker P, Puzantian VR, King D, Rosenthal TL, Dranon M. Bipolar outcome in the course of depressive illness. Phenomenologic, familial, and pharmacologic predictors. J Affect Disord. 1983;5(2):115–28.

Alexopoulos GS, Meyers BS, Young RC, Campbell S, Silbersweig D, Charlson M. 'Vascular depression' hypothesis. Arch Gen Psychiatry. 1997;54(10):915–22.

American Psychiatric Association. Diagnostic and statistical manual of mental disorders. 5th ed. Washington, DC: American Psychiatric Press; 2013.

Bauer M, Pfennig A, Severus E, Whybrow PC, Angst J, Moller HJ, World Federation of Societies of Biological Psychiatry. Task Force on Unipolar Depressive Disorders. World Federation of Societies of Biological Psychiatry (WFSBP) guidelines for biological treatment of unipolar depressive disorders, part 1: update 2013 on the acute and continuation treatment of unipolar depressive disorders. World J Biol Psychiatry. 2013;14(5):334–85.

Bauer M, Severus E, Kohler S, Whybrow PC, Angst J, Moller HJ, Wfsbp Task Force on Treatment Guidelines for Unipolar Depressive Disorders. World Federation of Societies of Biological Psychiatry (WFSBP) guidelines for biological treatment of unipolar depressive disorders. part 2: maintenance treatment of major depressive disorder-update 2015. World J Biol Psychiatry. 2015;16(2):76–95.

Baune BT, Fuhr M, Air T, Hering C. Neuropsychological functioning in adolescents and young adults with major depressive disorder—a review. Psychiatry Res. 2014;218(3):261–71.

Beesdo K, Hofler M, Leibenluft E, Lieb R, Bauer M, Pfennig A. Mood episodes and mood disorders: patterns of incidence and conversion in the first three decades of life. Bipolar Disord. 2009;11(6):637–49.

Bennett S, Thomas AJ. Depression and dementia: cause, consequence or coincidence? Maturitas. 2014;79(2):184–90.

Birmaher B, Williamson DE, Dahl RE, Axelson DA, Kaufman J, Dorn LD, Ryan ND. Clinical presentation and course of depression in youth: does onset in childhood differ from onset in adolescence? J Am Acad Child Adolesc Psychiatry. 2004;43(1):63–70.

Bogren M, Bradvik L, Holmstrand C, Nobbelin L, Mattisson C. Gender differences in subtypes of depression by first incidence and age of onset: a follow-up of the Lundby population. Eur Arch Psychiatry Clin Neurosci. 2018;268:179–89. https://doi.org/10.1007/s00406-017-0778-x.

Bora E, Harrison BJ, Yucel M, Pantelis C. Cognitive impairment in euthymic major depressive disorder: a meta-analysis. Psychol Med. 2013;43(10):2017–26.

Cleare A, Pariante CM, Young AH, Anderson IM, Christmas D, Cowen PJ, Dickens C, Ferrier IN, Geddes J, Gilbody S, Haddad PM, Katona C, Lewis G, Malizia A, McAllister-Williams RH, Ramchandani P, Scott J, Taylor D, Uher R, Members of the Consensus Meeting. Evidence-based guidelines for treating depressive disorders with antidepressants: a revision of the 2008 British Association for Psychopharmacology guidelines. J Psychopharmacol. 2015;29(5):459–525.

Corruble E, Gorwood P, Falissard B. Association between age of onset and symptom profiles of late-life depression. Acta Psychiatr Scand. 2008;118(5):389–94.

de Girolamo G, Dagani J, Purcell R, Cocchi A, McGorry PD. Age of onset of mental disorders and use of mental health services: needs, opportunities and obstacles. Epidemiol Psychiatr Sci. 2012;21(1):47–57.

Docherty AR, Edwards AC, Yang F, Peterson RE, Sawyers C, Adkins DE, Moore AA, Webb BT, Bacanu SA, Flint J, Kendler KS. Age of onset and family history as indicators of polygenic risk for major depression. Depress Anxiety. 2017;34(5):446–52.

Egger K, Schocke M, Weiss E, Auffinger S, Esterhammer R, Goebel G, Walch T, Mechtcheriakov S, Marksteiner J. Pattern of brain atrophy in elderly patients with depression revealed by voxel-based morphometry. Psychiatry Res. 2008;164(3):237–44.

Faedda GL, Marangoni C, Serra G, Salvatore P, Sani G, Vazquez GH, Tondo L, Girardi P, Baldessarini RJ, Koukopoulos A. Precursors of bipolar disorders: a systematic literature review of prospective studies. J Clin Psychiatry. 2015;76(5):614–24.

Ferentinos P, Koukounari A, Power R, Rivera M, Uher R, Craddock N, Owen MJ, Korszun A, Jones L, Jones I, Gill M, Rice JP, Ising M, Maier W, Mors O, Rietschel M, Preisig M, Binder EB, Aitchison KJ, Mendlewicz J, Souery D, Hauser J, Henigsberg N, Breen G, Craig IW, Farmer AE, Muller-Myhsok B, McGuffin P, Lewis CM. Familiality and SNP heritability of age at onset and episodicity in major depressive disorder. Psychol Med. 2015;45(10):2215–25.

Fernando K, Carter JD, Frampton CM, Luty SE, McKenzie J, Mulder RT, Joyce PR. Childhood-, teenage-, and adult-onset depression: diagnostic and individual characteristics in a clinical sample. Compr Psychiatry. 2011;52(6):623–9.

Ferrari AJ, Somerville AJ, Baxter AJ, Norman R, Patten SB, Vos T, Whiteford HA. Global variation in the prevalence and incidence of major depressive disorder: a systematic review of the epidemiological literature. Psychol Med. 2013;43(3):471–81.

Galvez V, Ho KA, Alonzo A, Martin D, George D, Loo CK. Neuromodulation therapies for geriatric depression. Curr Psychiatry Rep. 2015;17(7):59.

GBD 2015 Disease and Injury Incidence and Prevalence Collaborators. Global, regional, and national incidence, prevalence, and years lived with disability for 310 diseases and injuries, 1990-2015: a systematic analysis for the Global Burden of Disease Study 2015. Lancet. 2016;388(10053):1545–602.

Gournellis R, Oulis P, Christodoulou C, Kaparoudaki A, Fortos A, Lykouras L. Delusional beliefs in psychotic depression vary according to age of onset. Int J Geriatr Psychiatry. 2008;23(10):1093–4.

Gournellis R, Oulis P, Rizos E, Chourdaki E, Gouzaris A, Lykouras L. Clinical correlates of age of onset in psychotic depression. Arch Gerontol Geriatr. 2011;52(1):94–8.

Grayson L, Thomas A. A systematic review comparing clinical features in early age at onset and late age at onset late-life depression. J Affect Disord. 2013;150(2):161–70.

Herrmann LL, Goodwin GM, Ebmeier KP. The cognitive neuropsychology of depression in the elderly. Psychol Med. 2007;37(12):1693–702.

Herrmann LL, Le Masurier M, Ebmeier KP. White matter hyperintensities in late life depression: a systematic review. J Neurol Neurosurg Psychiatry. 2008;79(6):619–24.
Heser K, Tebarth F, Wiese B, Eisele M, Bickel H, Kohler M, Mosch E, Weyerer S, Werle J, Konig HH, Leicht H, Pentzek M, Fuchs A, Riedel-Heller SG, Luppa M, Prokein J, Scherer M, Maier W, Wagner M, Age CoDe Study Group. Age of major depression onset, depressive symptoms, and risk for subsequent dementia: results of the German study on Ageing, Cognition, and Dementia in Primary Care Patients (AgeCoDe). Psychol Med. 2013;43(8):1597–610.
Hwang JP, Lee TW, Tsai SJ, Chen TJ, Yang CH, Lirng JF, Tsai CF. Cortical and subcortical abnormalities in late-onset depression with history of suicide attempts investigated with MRI and voxel-based morphometry. J Geriatr Psychiatry Neurol. 2010;23(3):171–84.
Jaaskelainen E, Juola T, Korpela H, Lehtiniemi H, Nietola M, Korkeila J, Miettunen J. Epidemiology of psychotic depression—systematic review and meta-analysis. Psychol Med. 2017;48:1–14. https://doi.org/10.1017/S0033291717002501.
Jones PB. Adult mental health disorders and their age at onset. Br J Psychiatry Suppl. 2013;54:s5–10.
Kendler KS, Gatz M, Gardner CO, Pedersen NL. Age at onset and familial risk for major depression in a Swedish national twin sample. Psychol Med. 2005;35(11):1573–9.
Kessing LV. Differences in diagnostic subtypes among patients with late and early onset of a single depressive episode. Int J Geriatr Psychiatry. 2006;21(12):1127–31.
Kessler RC, Bromet EJ. The epidemiology of depression across cultures. Annu Rev Public Health. 2013;34:119–38.
Kessler RC, Amminger GP, Aguilar-Gaxiola S, Alonso J, Lee S, Ustun TB. Age of onset of mental disorders: a review of recent literature. Curr Opin Psychiatry. 2007;20(4):359–64.
Korczak DJ, Goldstein BI. Childhood onset major depressive disorder: course of illness and psychiatric comorbidity in a community sample. J Pediatr. 2009;155(1):118–23.
Korten NC, Comijs HC, Lamers F, Penninx BW. Early and late onset depression in young and middle aged adults: differential symptomatology, characteristics and risk factors? J Affect Disord. 2012;138(3):259–67.
MacQueen GM, Frey BN, Ismail Z, Jaworska N, Steiner M, Lieshout RJ, Kennedy SH, Lam RW, Milev RV, Parikh SV, Ravindran AV, Group CDW. Canadian Network for Mood and Anxiety Treatments (CANMAT) 2016 clinical guidelines for the management of adults with major depressive disorder: section 6. Special populations: youth, women, and the elderly. Can J Psychiatr. 2016;61(9):588–603.
Malhi GS, Bassett D, Boyce P, Bryant R, Fitzgerald PB, Fritz K, Hopwood M, Lyndon B, Mulder R, Murray G, Porter R, Singh AB. Royal Australian and New Zealand College of Psychiatrists clinical practice guidelines for mood disorders. Aust N Z J Psychiatry. 2015;49(12):1087–206.
Martin-Merino E, Ruigomez A, Johansson S, Wallander MA, Garcia-Rodriguez LA. Study of a cohort of patients newly diagnosed with depression in general practice: prevalence, incidence, comorbidity, and treatment patterns. Prim Care Companion J Clin Psychiatry. 2010;12(1):PCC 08m00764.
McGorry PD, Purcell R, Goldstone S, Amminger GP. Age of onset and timing of treatment for mental and substance use disorders: implications for preventive intervention strategies and models of care. Curr Opin Psychiatry. 2011;24(4):301–6.
Mitchell AJ, Subramaniam H. Prognosis of depression in old age compared to middle age: a systematic review of comparative studies. Am J Psychiatry. 2005;162(9):1588–601.
Power RA, Tansey KE, Buttenschon HN, Cohen-Woods S, Bigdeli T, Hall LS, Kutalik Z, Lee SH, Ripke S, Steinberg S, Teumer A, Viktorin A, Wray NR, Arolt V, Baune BT, Boomsma DI, Borglum AD, Byrne EM, Castelao E, Craddock N, Craig IW, Dannlowski U, Deary IJ, Degenhardt F, Forstner AJ, Gordon SD, Grabe HJ, Grove J, Hamilton SP, Hayward C, Heath AC, Hocking LJ, Homuth G, Hottenga JJ, Kloiber S, Krogh J, Landen M, Lang M, Levinson DF, Lichtenstein P, Lucae S, MacIntyre DJ, Madden P, Magnusson PK, Martin NG, McIntosh AM, Middeldorp CM, Milaneschi Y, Montgomery GW, Mors O, Muller-Myhsok B, Nyholt DR, Oskarsson H, Owen MJ, Padmanabhan S, Penninx BW, Pergadia ML, Porteous DJ, Potash JB, Preisig M, Rivera M, Shi J, Shyn SI, Sigurdsson E, Smit JH, Smith BH, Stefansson H, Stefansson K, Strohmaier J, Sullivan PF, Thomson P, Thorgeirsson TE, Van der Auwera S,

Weissman MM, Converge Consortium CCGC, Breen G, Lewis CM. Genome-wide association for major depression through age at onset stratification: major depressive disorder working group of the Psychiatric Genomics Consortium. Biol Psychiatry. 2017;81(4):325–35.

Ratheesh A, Davey C, Hetrick S, Alvarez-Jimenez M, Voutier C, Bechdolf A, McGorry PD, Scott J, Berk M, Cotton SM. A systematic review and meta-analysis of prospective transition from major depression to bipolar disorder. Acta Psychiatr Scand. 2017;135(4):273–84.

Schmaal L, Veltman DJ, van Erp TG, Samann PG, Frodl T, Jahanshad N, Loehrer E, Tiemeier H, Hofman A, Niessen WJ, Vernooij MW, Ikram MA, Wittfeld K, Grabe HJ, Block A, Hegenscheid K, Volzke H, Hoehn D, Czisch M, Lagopoulos J, Hatton SN, Hickie IB, Goya-Maldonado R, Kramer B, Gruber O, Couvy-Duchesne B, Renteria ME, Strike LT, Mills NT, de Zubicaray GI, McMahon KL, Medland SE, Martin NG, Gillespie NA, Wright MJ, Hall GB, MacQueen GM, Frey EM, Carballedo A, van Velzen LS, van Tol MJ, van der Wee NJ, Veer IM, Walter H, Schnell K, Schramm E, Normann C, Schoepf D, Konrad C, Zurowski B, Nickson T, McIntosh AM, Papmeyer M, Whalley HC, Sussmann JE, Godlewska BR, Cowen PJ, Fischer FH, Rose M, Penninx BW, Thompson PM, Hibar DP. Subcortical brain alterations in major depressive disorder: findings from the ENIGMA Major Depressive Disorder working group. Mol Psychiatry. 2016;21(6):806–12.

Schmaal L, Hibar DP, Samann PG, Hall GB, Baune BT, Jahanshad N, Cheung JW, van Erp TGM, Bos D, Ikram MA, Vernooij MW, Niessen WJ, Tiemeier H, Hofman A, Wittfeld K, Grabe HJ, Janowitz D, Bulow R, Selonke M, Volzke H, Grotegerd D, Dannlowski U, Arolt V, Opel N, Heindel W, Kugel H, Hoehn D, Czisch M, Couvy-Duchesne B, Renteria ME, Strike LT, Wright MJ, Mills NT, de Zubicaray GI, McMahon KL, Medland SE, Martin NG, Gillespie NA, Goya-Maldonado R, Gruber O, Kramer B, Hatton SN, Lagopoulos J, Hickie IB, Frodl T, Carballedo A, Frey EM, van Velzen LS, Penninx B, van Tol MJ, van der Wee NJ, Davey CG, Harrison BJ, Mwangi B, Cao B, Soares JC, Veer IM, Walter H, Schoepf D, Zurowski B, Konrad C, Schramm E, Normann C, Schnell K, Sacchet MD, Gotlib IH, MacQueen GM, Godlewska BR, Nickson T, McIntosh AM, Papmeyer M, Whalley HC, Hall J, Sussmann JE, Li M, Walter M, Aftanas L, Brack I, Bokhan NA, Thompson PM, Veltman DJ. Cortical abnormalities in adults and adolescents with major depression based on brain scans from 20 cohorts worldwide in the ENIGMA Major Depressive Disorder Working Group. Mol Psychiatry. 2017;22(6):900–9.

Tondo L, Visioli C, Preti A, Baldessarini RJ. Bipolar disorders following initial depression: modeling predictive clinical factors. J Affect Disord. 2014;167:44–9.

van Noorden MS, Minkenberg SE, Giltay EJ, den Hollander-Gijsman ME, van Rood YR, van der Wee NJ, Zitman FG. Pre-adult versus adult onset major depressive disorder in a naturalistic patient sample: the Leiden Routine Outcome Monitoring Study. Psychol Med. 2011;41(7):1407–17.

Vu NQ, Aizenstein HJ. Depression in the elderly: brain correlates, neuropsychological findings, and role of vascular lesion load. Curr Opin Neurol. 2013;26(6):656–61.

Waraich P, Goldner EM, Somers JM, et al. Prevalence and incidence studies of mood disorders: a systematic review of the literature. Can J Psychiatry. 2004;49:124–38.

World Health Organization. The ICD-10 classification of mental and behavioural disorders-clinical descriptions and diagnostic guidelines. Geneva: World Health Organization; 1992.

Yuan Y, Zhu W, Zhang Z, Bai F, Yu H, Shi Y, Qian Y, Liu W, Jiang T, You J, Liu Z. Regional gray matter changes are associated with cognitive deficits in remitted geriatric depression: an optimized voxel-based morphometry study. Biol Psychiatry. 2008;64(6):541–4.

Zhu T, De Luca V, Gallaugher LA, Woldeyohannes HO, Soczynska JK, Szymkowicz S, Muzina DJ, Kennedy SH, McIntyre RS. Admixture analysis of age at onset in major depressive disorder. Gen Hosp Psychiatry. 2012;34(6):686–91.

Zisook S, Lesser I, Stewart JW, Wisniewski SR, Balasubramani GK, Fava M, Gilmer WS, Dresselhaus TR, Thase ME, Nierenberg AA, Trivedi MH, Rush AJ. Effect of age at onset on the course of major depressive disorder. Am J Psychiatry. 2007;164(10):1539–46.

The Age of Onset of Anxiety Disorders

7

Jeroen S. Legerstee, Bram Dierckx, Elisabeth M. W. J. Utens, Frank C. Verhulst, Carola Zieldorff, Gwen C. Dieleman, and Jasmijn M. de Lijster

7.1 Introduction

Anxiety disorders are a highly prevalent and debilitating group of psychiatric disorders that often follow a chronic and recurrent course. The point prevalence of anxiety disorders across numerous studies is estimated at 4% (Remes et al. 2016), and women are almost two times more likely to develop an anxiety disorder than men (McLean et al. 2011). There is substantial co-morbidity among anxiety disorder subtypes and between anxiety disorders and other psychiatric disorders, especially

J. S. Legerstee (✉) · B. Dierckx · C. Zieldorff · G. C. Dieleman · J. M. de Lijster
Department of Child and Adolescent Psychiatry/Psychology, Erasmus MC—Sophia Children's Hospital, Rotterdam, The Netherlands
e-mail: j.s.legerstee@erasmusmc.nl; b.dierckx@erasmusmc.nl; c.zieldorff@erasmusmc.nl; g.dieleman@erasmusmc.nl; j.delijster@erasmusmc.nl

Elisabeth M. W. J. Utens
Department of Child and Adolescent Psychiatry/Psychology, Erasmus MC—Sophia Children's Hospital, Rotterdam, The Netherlands

Research Institute of Child Development and Education, University of Amsterdam, Amsterdam, The Netherlands

Academic Center for Child Psychiatry the Bascule/Department Child and Adolescent Psychiatry, Academic Medical Center, Amsterdam, The Netherlands
e-mail: e.utens@erasmusmc.nl

F. C. Verhulst
Department of Child and Adolescent Psychiatry/Psychology, Erasmus MC—Sophia Children's Hospital, Rotterdam, The Netherlands

Child and Adolescent Mental Health Center, Mental Health Services, Capital Region of Denmark/Department of Clinical Medicine, Faculty of Health and Medical Sciences, Copenhagen University Hospital/University of Copenhagen, Copenhagen, Denmark
e-mail: f.verhulst@erasmusmc.nl

G. de Girolamo et al. (eds.), *Age of Onset of Mental Disorders*,
https://doi.org/10.1007/978-3-319-72619-9_7

with depressive disorders and substance dependence and abuse (Conway et al. 2006; Swendsen et al. 2010). People with an anxiety disorder also more often have suicidal ideations and attempt suicide (Sareen et al. 2005).

Worldwide, anxiety disorders were the sixth leading cause of disability in 2010 (Baxter et al. 2014) and they impose a large economic burden on patients and society (Wittchen 2002). In addition, they are related to a range of personal, academic and social problems. In a recent systematic review, we found that anxiety-disordered adolescents experience more negativity in interpersonal relationships, have a lower social competence, feel lonelier and have been victimised more often than healthy peers (de Lijster et al. 2018). Although their school grades are comparable to their healthy peers, they feel more impaired at school and might have a lower chance of entering university. Comparable psychosocial problems and poor overall quality of life have been reported for anxiety-disordered children and adults (Essau et al. 2014; Olatunji et al. 2007).

Despite the availability of evidence-based psychological and pharmacological treatments, anxiety disorders often remain unrecognised and untreated. For instance, Zarger and Rich documented that 85% of adolescents with social phobia have never received treatment (Zarger and Rich 2016). Likewise, in a large general population study of adults with an anxiety disorder, 66.5% reported that they had never used mental health services (Sihvo et al. 2006).

Given the high prevalence, chronicity, burden and under-treatment of anxiety disorders, there is a clear need for early detection and intervention. There is accumulative evidence that such approaches, especially targeted prevention programmes, could prevent or delay the onset of anxiety disorders (Dadds et al. 1997; Rapee et al. 2005; Werner-Seidler et al. 2017). To target prevention strategies in an efficient, timely and cost-effective manner, information about the age of onset (AOO) is essential (Kessler et al. 2007).

Some anxiety disorder subtypes typically emerge in childhood, whereas others have their onset in adolescence and early adulthood (Kessler et al. 2005, 2009). Findings suggest that the outcome severity of anxiety disorders differs between childhood and adulthood onset. Early (childhood) onset has been associated with more severe psychopathology and co-morbidity, more behavioural inhibition, and even with higher rates of suicide (Lim et al. 2013; Ramsawh et al. 2011; Rosellini et al. 2013; Tibi et al. 2015). Hoehnsaric and colleagues (1993) documented that early onset of generalized anxiety disorders, in contrast to late onset, is related to increased domestic disturbances and social maladjustment in childhood, more sensitivity in interpersonal relationships and more marital difficulties in adulthood. Another more recent study also documented that an early onset of generalized anxiety disorder is significantly associated with childhood physical abuse and worse clinical outcomes (Goncalves et al. 2011).

Studies vary greatly in the reported AOO of anxiety disorders. This is mainly due to differences in methodology and age range between study samples. Two previous reviews have estimated the AOO of anxiety disorders (Kessler et al. 2007; McGorry et al. 2011). Kessler and colleagues reviewed epidemiological research on AOO from World Mental Health (WMH) surveys. They found that phobias and separation anxiety disorders have a median AOO between 7 and 14 years, and between 25 and 53 years for other anxiety disorders (Kessler et al. 2007). McGorry and colleagues reviewed three studies on the AOO of major mental illnesses in 2011. They concluded that certain anxiety disorders emerge during childhood, whilst other emerge during adolescence and early adulthood (McGorry et al. 2011). Both reviews did not examine the AOO for specific anxiety disorders but collapsed AOO information in clusters of different anxiety disorder subtypes.

We recently published the paper "The Age of Onset of Anxiety Disorders: A Meta-Analysis" in the *Canadian Journal of Psychiatry* (de Lijster et al. 2017), in which we reviewed studies on the AOO of anxiety disorders that were published before 17 October 2014. However, several studies have been published since 2014 and, therefore, the aim of this chapter is to extent and update our previous paper with studies published until 27 June 2017. We carried out a review and meta-analysis on the AOO of anxiety disorders in general and of its subtypes.

7.2 Methods

The search method, study selection and data extraction process are described briefly here. The reader is referred to de Lijster et al. (2017) for more in-depth information about the methods of the previous meta-analysis.

On 17 October 2014, the combination of following keywords were searched in several databases: "Anxiety disorder" (i.e. anxiety disorder, acute stress disorder, generalized anxiety disorder, agoraphobia, [specific/isolated] phobia, social phobia, obsessive–compulsive disorder, post-traumatic stress disorder, adjustment disorder, separation anxiety disorder, stress disorder, panic disorder), "AOO" (i.e. onset age, AOO, age at onset) and "Study design" (i.e. cohort, longitudinal, prospective, retrospective). This resulted in 1029 articles (after deletion of duplicates), which were reviewed independently by two authors (JdL and CZ) based on title and abstract. Inclusion criteria for title/abstract and full-text were a general population sample, data on AOO, prevalence, incidence, lifetime occurrence or epidemiology of anxiety, psychiatric or mental disorders, and published in a peer-reviewed, indexed scientific journal. Exclusion criteria were no representative sample of the general population, reviews and subclinical anxiety (i.e. no diagnosis).

Of the 1029 articles, 189 were selected based on title and abstract. Thirty of the 189 articles were selected for data extraction based on full-text. Six studies were subsequently excluded because they did not report sample sizes, prevalence rates or spread measures of AOO. This resulted in 24 studies that were included.

We extended the search method, study selection and data extraction process with studies on anxiety disorder AOO published until 27 June 2017. We repeated the previous search in EMBASE (Excerpta Medica dataBASE) and searched for studies that were published between 17 October 2014 and 27 June 2017. This resulted in 89 articles, of which 11 were selected by two authors (JdL and JL) based on title and abstract.

Subsequently, two (Ajdacic-Gross et al. 2016; de Jonge et al. 2016) of the 11 articles were selected based on full-text, which reported on the age of panic disorder, separation anxiety disorder, specific phobia and social phobia onset. These AOO data were combined with data from our search in October 2014.

The statistical program Comprehensive Meta-Analysis (Borenstein et al. 2005) was used to analyse the results. A random-effects model was used because of the high study heterogeneity. Medians of AOO were transformed to means and standard deviations. Median AOO, interquartile range (25th and 75th percentiles) and sample size were used to perform the median-to-mean transformation as described by Wan and colleagues (2014). Median AOO was also presented and a weighted mean was calculated for all anxiety disorders.

For anxiety disorders in general, analyses were performed to examine study heterogeneity and publication bias. Meta-regressions were performed to examine the effect of maximum age of the study sample, Human Developmental Index (HDI), study design and gender on the AOO of anxiety disorders in general.

7.3 Age of Onset of Anxiety Disorders

7.3.1 Anxiety Disorders in General

Based on 14 studies (Table 7.1), the median AOO of anxiety disorders in general is estimated at 22 years and 7 months, and the mean AOO at 21 years and 3 months. The 95% confidence interval of mean anxiety disorder onset is between 17.46 and 25.07 years. Hence, most people have the first onset of anxiety disorder symptoms between late adolescence and early adulthood.

7.3.1.1 Between-Study Heterogeneity and Publication Bias

Meta-analysis shows a high level of between-study heterogeneity ($I^2 = 99\%$) with regard to studies on AOO of anxiety disorders in general. Moreover, there is evidence of publication bias. The Eggers's regression coefficient was significant ($t = 3.37$, $p < 0.01$). Visual inspection of the funnel plot shows that studies reporting lower AOOs have slightly lower standard errors (Fig. 7.1).

However, we argue that it is unlikely that differences in AOO are related to publication bias, as lower or higher AOO is not likely to influence the chance of publication. Instead, we believe that study heterogeneity underlies the significant publication bias findings. For instance, studies with a low standard error were often conducted in populations with a low age: moreover, retrospective reports of AOO in young populations might suffer less from recall bias than older populations.

7.3.1.2 Meta-Regressions

Meta-regressions indicate that the maximum age of the study sample, HDI, study design and gender were significantly related to the AOO of anxiety disorders in general. More specifically, a higher age, lower stage of development of a country, retrospective study design and higher percentage of males were related to a higher AOO of anxiety disorders in general.

Likewise, the mean AOO of anxiety disorders in general reported by studies is also heavily dependent on the anxiety disorder subtypes included in a study. For instance, the study of Lewinsohn and colleagues reported the highest AOO of anxiety disorders. In this study, anxiety disorders in general only comprised subtypes with a high AOO, namely panic disorder, agoraphobia, generalized anxiety disorder and post-traumatic stress disorder (Lewinsohn et al. 1998).

Alhasnawi et al. found that the AOO of behaviour disorders is earlier than that of anxiety disorders (Alhasnawi et al. 2009). However, the study of Gau et al. (2007) illustrates that this earlier AOO could be explained by the early onset of attention-deficit hyperactivity disorder at 7.2 years (Gau et al. 2007). This is supported by the study of Lee and colleagues (2007), which did not find any differences in AOO between anxiety disorders and conduct disorder and intermittent explosive disorder. Across studies, it was consistently found that anxiety disorders, in general, have an earlier AOO than mood disorders and substance use disorders (Alhasnawi et al. 2009; Bonnewyn et al. 2007; Cho et al. 2012; Gau et al. 2007; Gureje et al. 2008; Lee et al. 2007; Levinson et al. 2007; Ritchie et al. 2004; Stein et al. 2008; Viana and Andrade 2012). In addition, most studies found that the interquartile range of AOO is higher for anxiety disorders than for mood and substance disorders. Thus, although anxiety disorders have an early mean AOO, they develop in a relatively broad age period. The question arises whether this period of anxiety disorder onset varies between anxiety disorder subtypes.

7.3.2 Separation Anxiety Disorder

Based on five studies (Table 7.2), the mean onset of separation anxiety disorder is estimated at 9 years and 6 months, with a 95% confidence interval between 6.34 and 12.59 years. No overall weighted median could be calculated because most studies on separation anxiety disorder did not report a median AOO. Hence, the onset of separation anxiety disorder is in childhood, and it typically develops during a small time period of 6 years. Moreover, it has the earliest AOO of all anxiety disorder subtypes.

Four studies showed that separation anxiety disorder has its onset between the age of 5 and 7 years (Ajdacic-Gross et al. 2016; Kessler et al. 2005; Knappe et al. 2011; Lewinsohn et al. 1998). Viana and Andrade (2012) found a considerably higher AOO for separation anxiety disorder, namely at 22 years and 4 months. The recent meta-analyses of our research group showed that the level of development of a country, reflected in the HDI, is related to the AOO of separation anxiety disorder. More specifically, an earlier AOO of separation anxiety disorders is often found in countries with a higher HDI. The São Paulo Megacity Mental Health Survey was carried out in Brazil, which has a lower HDI value (i.e. 0.75) than the countries of the four other studies (i.e. 0.92–0.94).

Table 7.1 Studies on the age of onset of anxiety disorders in general

Study	Survey	*n*	Age (years)	Design	AOO (years)		
					Median	Mean	95% CI
Alhasnawi et al. (2009)	World Mental Health survey	4332	18–65	Retrospective	25.00	29.00	26.86–31.14
Becker et al. (2007)	Dresden Study of Mental Health	5204	18–24	Prospective	NR	9.88	9.35–10.41
Bonnewyn et al. (2007)	European Study on the Epidemiology of Mental Disorders	2419	18–65	Retrospective	14.00	18.33	15.64–21.02
Cho et al. (2012)	Korean Epidemiologic Catchment and Area Study Replication	7972	18–64	Retrospective	29.00	29.00	26.51–31.49
Gau et al. (2007)	Randomly selected high school sample	428	12.5–15.5	Prospective	NR	9.50	8.71–10.29
Gureje et al. (2008)	Nigerian Survey of Mental Health and Wellbeing	6752	18–65	Retrospective	8.00	8.33	7.78–8.89
Kessler et al. (2005)	National Comorbidity Survey Replication	9282	18–60	Retrospective	NR	12.67	12.13–13.21
Lee et al. (2007)	World Mental Health household survey	5201	18–70	Retrospective	17.00	21.00	16.64–25.36
Levinson et al. (2007)	Israel National Health Survey	4589	21–65	Retrospective	43.00	43.00	40.05–45.95
Lewinsohn et al. (1998)	Oregon Adolescent Depression Project	816	16–17	Prospective	NR	15.44	14.32–16.56
Marquenie (2007)	The Netherlands Mental Health Survey and Incidence Study[a]	7076	18–64	Retrospective	NR	24.60	23.83–25.37
Ritchie et al. (2004)	Random selection of the 15 electoral rolls	1873	65–85	Retrospective	NR	28.15	26.37–29.93
Stein et al. (2008)	South African Stress and Health Study	4351	18–65	Retrospective	32.00	35.00	32.74–37.27
Viana and Andrade (2012)	The São Paulo Megacity Mental Health Survey	5037	18–65	Retrospective	13.00	15.33	14.37–16.29
Estimated AOO					*22.58*	*21.27*	*17.46–25.07*

AOO age of onset, *CI* confidence interval, *NR* not reported
[a] weighted median AOO

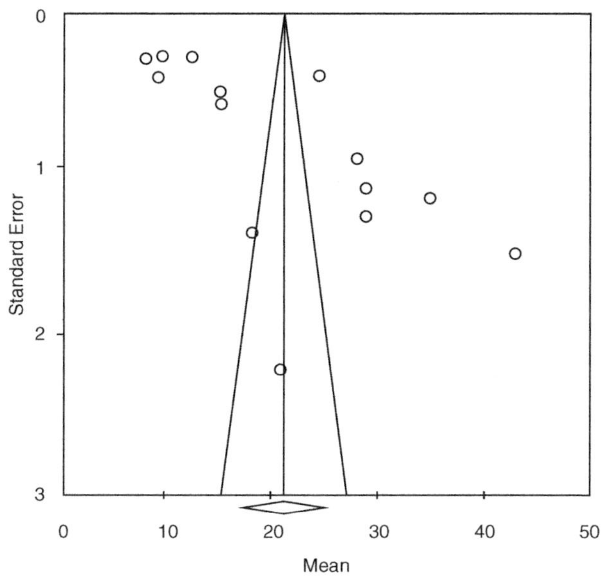

Fig. 7.1 Funnel plot of studies on the age of onset of anxiety disorders in general

7.3.3 Specific Phobia

Based on 12 studies (Table 7.3), the mean onset of specific phobia is estimated at 11 years and 1 month, with a 95% confidence interval between 8.52 and 13.57 years. The weighted median AOO of specific phobia is 10 years and 2 months. Hence, specific phobia has its onset in childhood, and it typically develops during a small time period of 5 years.

One study differentiated between specific phobia subtypes with regard to AOO. Becker and colleagues (2007) showed that animal, physical and environmental phobia typically have an early onset at age 6–7 years, whereas the mean onset of situational phobia is in mid-adolescence (i.e. 15.5 years).

7.3.4 Social Phobia

Based on 13 studies (Table 7.4), the mean onset of social phobia is estimated at 14 years and 1 month, with a 95% confidence interval between 12.99 and 15.02 years. The weighted median AOO was somewhat higher at 16 years and 9 months. Hence, the onset of separation anxiety disorder is in adolescence.

Of all anxiety disorder subtypes, social phobia has the lowest 95% confidence interval (i.e. 2 years), indicating that the 13 studies are quite homogenous in the reported AOO of social phobia. This also indicates that social phobia develops in a

Table 7.2 Studies on the age of onset of separation anxiety disorder

Study	Survey	*n*	Age (years)	Design	AOO (years)		
					Median	Mean	95% CI
Kessler et al. (2005)	National Comorbidity Survey Replication	9282	18–60	Retrospective	NR	7.67	7.22–8.13
Knappe et al. (2011)	Early Developmental Stages of Psychopathology Study	3021	14–34	Prospective	NR	5.31	4.00–6.63
Lewinsohn et al. (1998)	Oregon Adolescent Depression Project	816	16–17	Prospective	NR	7.53	6.64–8.43
Viana and Andrade (2012)	The São Paulo Megacity Mental Health Survey	5037	18–65	Retrospective	19.00	22.33	20.41–24.26
Ajdacic-Gross et al. (2016)	The Psychiatric arm of the Cohorte Lausannoise study (PsyCoLaus)	3720	35–66	Retrospective	NR	5.20	4.54–5.86
Estimated AOO					[a]	*9.47*	6.34–12.59

AOO age of onset, *CI* confidence interval, *NR* not reported
[a]Few data were available to calculate the estimated AOO

Table 7.3 Studies on the age of onset of specific phobia

Study	Survey	*n*	Age (years)	Design	AOO (years)		
					Median	Mean	95% CI
Alhasnawi et al. (2009)	World Mental Health survey	4332	18–65	Retrospective	7.00	8.33	7.46–9.20
Becker et al. (2007)	Dresden Study of Mental Health	5204	18–24	Prospective	7.90	7.20	6.44–7.96
Caraveo-Anduaga (2004)	Mexican household survey	1932	18–65	Retrospective	NR	16.95	13.91–20.00
Cho et al. (2012)	Korean Epidemiologic Catchment and Area Study Replication	7972	18–64	Retrospective	13.00	15.67	14.16–17.18
Falk et al. (2008)	National Epidemiologic Survey on Alcohol and Related Conditions	19,504	18–70	Retrospective	NR	14.60	14.59–14.61
Giaconia et al. (1994)	Follow-up of public kindergarten working community sample	386	18	Prospective	6.00	6.70	5.63–7.77
Kessler et al. (2005)	National Comorbidity Survey Replication	9282	18–60	Retrospective	NR	8.00	7.70–8.30
Knappe et al. (2011)	Early Developmental Stages of Psychopathology Study	3021	14–34	Prospective	NR	8.33	7.82–8.84
Lee et al. (2007)	World Mental Health household survey	5201	18–70	Retrospective	13.00	11.67	10.15–13.19
Lewinsohn et al. (1998)	Oregon Adolescent Depression Project	816	16–17	Prospective	NR	15.32	12.84–17.80
Viana and Andrade (2012)	The São Paulo Megacity Mental Health Survey	5037	18–65	Retrospective	8.00	8.67	8.20–9.14
Ajdacic-Gross et al. (2016)	The Psychiatric arm of the Cohorte Lausannoise study (PsyCoLaus)	3720	35–66	Retrospective	NR	12.10	11.26–12.94
Estimated AOO					*10.14*	*11.05*	*8.52–13.57*

AOO age of onset, *CI* confidence interval, *NR* not reported

Table 7.4 Studies on the age of onset of social phobia

Study	Survey	*n*	Age (years)	Design	AOO (years)		
					Median	Mean	95% CI
Alhasnawi et al. (2009)	World Mental Health survey	4332	18–65	Retrospective	14.00	15.00	13.72–16.28
Becker et al. (2007)	Dresden Study of Mental Health	5204	18–24	Prospective	NR	11.38	10.71–12.05
Caraveo-Anduaga (2004)	Mexican household survey	1932	18–65	Retrospective	NR	20.35	16.49–24.21
Chartier (2003)	Ontario Health Survey	8116	15–64	Retrospective	NR	13.00	12.19–13.81
Cho et al. (2012)	Korean Epidemiologic Catchment and Area Study Replication	7972	18–64	Retrospective	19.00	23.00	16.33–29.67
Giaconia et al. (1994)	Follow-up of public kindergarten working community sample	386	18	Prospective	12.00	10.83	9.70–11.96
Kessler et al. (2005)	National Comorbidity Survey Replication	9282	18–60	Retrospective	NR	12.00	11.70–12.30
Knappe et al. (2011)	Early Developmental Stages of Psychopathology Study	3021	14–34	Prospective	NR	13.05	12.32–13.79
Lewinsohn et al. (1998)	Oregon Adolescent Depression Project	816	16–17	Prospective	NR	15.54	13.05–18.03
Ritchie et al. (2004)	Random selection of the 15 electoral rolls	1873	65–85	Retrospective	NR	16.37	13.36–19.38
Stein et al. (2008)	South African Stress and Health Study	4351	18–65	Retrospective	19.00	21.33	19.01–23.65
Viana and Andrade (2012)	The São Paulo Megacity Mental Health Survey	5037	18–65	Retrospective	14.00	14.00	13.48–14.52
Ajdacic-Gross et al. (2016)	Psychiatric arm of the Cohorte Lausannoise study (PsyCoLaus)	3720	35–66	Retrospective	NR	10.90	10.01–11.79
Estimated AOO					*16.76*	*14.05*	*12.99–15.02*

AOO age of onset, *CI* confidence interval, *NR* not reported

very narrow and specific age period. The small difference in reported AOO between retrospective and prospective studies might suggest that the onset of social phobia is an event that individuals can recall quite accurately.

7.3.5 Agoraphobia Without Panic Disorder

Based on eight studies (Table 7.5), the mean onset of agoraphobia without panic disorder is estimated at 21 years and 2 months, with a 95% confidence interval between 17.02 and 25.23 years. The weighted median AOO was lower at 16 years and 6 months. Hence, the onset of agoraphobia without panic disorder is between late adolescence and early adulthood.

The prospective study of Bienvenu and colleagues (2006) is quite unique in that it has a long follow-up period. A sample of 1920 adults was assessed in 1981–1982 and 13 years later in 1993–1996. Agoraphobia was found to have its mean AOO at 21.2 years.

7.3.6 Obsessive–Compulsive Disorder

Based on 11 studies (Table 7.6), the mean onset of obsessive–compulsive disorder is estimated to lie in early adulthood, at 24 years, with a 95% confidence interval between 18.59 and 29.38 years. The weighted median AOO is higher, namely at 27 years and 6 months.

The estimate for AOO of obsessive–compulsive disorder had the largest 95% confidence interval of all anxiety disorder subtypes; the 11 studies vary in their reported AOO of obsessive–compulsive disorder. Recall bias might be a reason for this high 95% confidence interval. For obsessive–compulsive disorder, the discrepancy in findings between prospective and retrospective studies was especially pronounced. For prospective studies, AOO ranged between 11.33 and 19.10 years, whereas retrospective studies yielded significantly higher AOO estimates between 21.00 and 50.67 years. Another reason for the high 95% confidence interval is that the window in which obsessive–compulsive disorder develops is large. This is supported by the study of Vainganka r et al. (2013), which showed that obsessive–compulsive disorder onset is practically the same in various life stages up to 59 years. More specifically, they reported that 20% had their onset in childhood (< 12 years), 25% in adolescence (12–17 years), 32% in early adulthood (18–29 years), 21% in adulthood (30–59 years) and 2% in late adulthood (≥ 60 years). The large window of obsessive–compulsive disorder development implies that the reported AOO is dependent on the upper age limit of each study.

Table 7.5 Studies on the age of onset of agoraphobia without panic disorder

Study	Survey	*n*	Age (years)	Design	AOO (years)		
					Median	Mean	95% CI
Becker et al. (2007)	Dresden Study of Mental Health	5204	18–24	Prospective	13.00	14.67	12.99–16.36
Bienvenu et al. (2006)	Epidemiologic Catchment Area	816	18–86	Prospective	NR	21.20	16.06–26.34
Kessler et al. (2005)	National Comorbidity Survey Replication	9282	18–60	Retrospective	NR	22.00	19.42–24.58
Knappe et al. (2011)	Early Developmental Stages of Psychopathology Study	3021	14–34	Prospective	NR	15.41	14.01–16.81
Lewinsohn et al. (1998)	Oregon Adolescent Depression Project	816	16–17	Prospective	NR	17.30	9.56–25.04
Ritchie et al. (2004)	Random selection of the 15 electoral rolls	1873	65–85	Retrospective	NR	31.49	28.98–34.00
Stein et al. (2008)	South African Stress and Health Study	4351	18–65	Retrospective	18.00	22.00	20.46–23.54
Viana and Andrade (2012)	The São Paulo Megacity Mental Health Survey	5037	18–65	Retrospective	19.00	24.33	20.66–28.00
Estimated AOO					*16.56*	*21.12*	*17.02–25.23*

AOO age of onset, *CI* confidence interval, *NR* not reported

Table 7.6 Studies on the age of onset of obsessive–compulsive disorder

Study	Survey	*n*	Age (years)	Design	AOO (years)		
					Median	Mean	95% CI
Alhasnawi et al. (2009)	World Mental Health survey	4332	18–65	Retrospective	54.00	50.67	47.14–54.15
Angst (2004)	Zurich community	591	20–41	Prospective	18.00	19.10	17.06–21.14
Becker et al. (2007)	Dresden Study of Mental Health	5204	18–24	Prospective	NR	11.33	8.99–13.67
Caraveo-Anduaga (2004)	Mexican household survey	1932	18–65	Retrospective	NR	25.04	20.16–29.92
Cho et al. (2012)	Korean Epidemiologic Catchment and Area Study Replication	7972	18–64	Retrospective	25.00	26.00	23.19–28.81
Kessler et al. (2005)	National Comorbidity Survey Replication	9282	18–60	Retrospective	NR	21.00	16.46–25.54
Knappe et al. (2011)	Early Developmental Stages of Psychopathology Study	3021	14–34	Prospective	NR	14.37	12.94–15.80
Lewinsohn et al. (1998)	Oregon Adolescent Depression Project	816	16–17	Prospective	NR	18.32	13.58–23.06
Ritchie et al. (2004)	Random selection of the 15 electoral rolls	1873	65–85	Retrospective	NR	39.44	25.09–53.79
Vaingankar et al. (2013)	The Singapore mental health study	6616	18–65	Retrospective	19.00	21.10	19.36–22.85
Viana and Andrade (2012)	The São Paulo Megacity Mental Health Survey	5037	18–65	Retrospective	21.00	24.00	21.39–26.61
Estimated AOO					*27.51*	*23.99*	*18.59–29.38*

AOO age of onset, *CI* confidence interval, *NR* not reported

7.3.7 Post-Traumatic Stress Disorder

Based on 12 studies (Table 7.7), the mean onset of post-traumatic stress disorder is estimated to lie in early adulthood, at 26.50 years, with a 95% confidence interval between 22.38 and 30.73 years. The weighted median AOO was higher, namely at 32 years.

Estimates of onset of post-traumatic stress disorder are likely to be influenced by the occurrence of wars, systemic violence or high-impact events, such as in the study of Alhasnawi and colleagues (2009) in Iraq in 2009. These events can lead to an increase in the incidence of post-traumatic stress disorder and can bias AOO estimates in both prospective and retrospective designs if only participants of a certain age range are included. The age of the sample is related to the AOO of post-traumatic stress disorder. More specifically, studies with a higher maximum age had a higher AOO than those with a lower maximum age.

7.3.8 Panic Disorder

Based on 13 studies (Table 7.8), the mean onset of panic disorder is 26 years and 6 months, with a 95% confidence interval between 22.80 and 30.23 years. No weighted median AOO could be calculated because few of the included studies reported the median AOO of panic disorders. Hence, the average onset of panic disorder is in adulthood, and people typically develop a panic disorder in their twenties.

There is no clear difference in the AOO of panic disorder with (i.e. 22.26 years) or without (i.e. 24.59 years) agoraphobia. However, no definite conclusions regarding the effect of agoraphobia co-morbidity on panic disorder onset can be drawn because the AOO of panic disorder with agoraphobia has only been examined by a limited number of studies. Moreover, the AOO may be an underestimation because two of the three studies examined AOO in a relatively narrow age range. Indeed, the mean AOO of panic disorder with agoraphobia is almost two times higher in the study with a higher age upper limit (Falk et al. 2008). The same applies for studies on panic disorder where it is unspecified if there is any co-morbidity with agoraphobia. The upper age limit of these studies are higher and, as a consequence, the estimated AOO is also higher (37.21 years) than for panic disorder with (22.26 years) or without (26.52 years) agoraphobia.

7.3.9 Generalized Anxiety Disorder

Based on 15 studies (Table 7.9), the mean onset of generalized anxiety disorder is 34 years and 11 months, with a 95% confidence interval between 30.88 and 39.01 years. However, the weighted median AOO was higher, namely at 40 years and 7 months. Generalized anxiety disorder has the highest mean AOO of all anxiety disorder subtypes.

Table 7.7 Studies on the age of onset of post-traumatic stress disorder

Study	Survey	*n*	Age (years)	Design	AOO (years)		
					Median	Mean	95% CI
Alhasnawi et al. (2009)	World Mental Health survey	4332	18–65	Retrospective	16.00	18.00	16.30–19.70
Becker et al. (2007)	Dresden Study of Mental Health	5204	18–24	Prospective	NR	13.77	12.71–14.83
Chapman (2012)	Australian National Survey of Mental Health and Wellbeing	8841	16–85	Retrospective	26.00	27.67	25.66–29.69
Cho et al. (2012)	Korean Epidemiologic Catchment and Area Study Replication	7972	18–64	Retrospective	38.00	37.00	33.54–40.46
Giaconia et al. (1994)	Follow-up of public kindergarten working community sample	386	18	Prospective	16.00	14.79	13.63–15.95
Kessler et al. (2005)	National Comorbidity Survey Replication	9282	18–60	Retrospective	NR	25.67	23.89–27.45
Knappe et al. (2011)	Early Developmental Stages of Psychopathology Study	3021	14–34	Prospective	NR	18.27	16.90–19.64
Levinson et al. (2007)	Israel National Health Survey	4589	21–65	Retrospective	37.00	35.30	31.13–39.47
Lewinsohn et al. (1998)	Oregon Adolescent Depression Project	816	16–17	Prospective	NR	17.73	16.07–19.39
Ritchie et al. (2004)	Random selection of the 15 electoral rolls	1873	65–85	Retrospective	NR	40.47	31.87–49.07
Stein et al. (2008)	South African Stress and Health Study	4351	18–65	Retrospective	36.00	37.67	34.11–41.23
Viana and Andrade (2012)	The São Paulo Megacity Mental Health Survey	5037	18–65	Retrospective	40.00	37.67	33.87–41.48
Estimated AOO					*32.00*	*26.50*	*22.28–30.73*

AOO age of onset, *CI* confidence interval, *NR* not reported

Table 7.8 Studies on the age of onset of panic disorder

Study	Survey	*n*	Age (years)	Design	AOO (years)		
					Median	Mean	95% CI
PD (AGO unspecified)							
Alhasnawi et al. (2009)	World Mental Health survey	4332	18–65	Retrospective	35.00	32.33	27.38–37.28
Levinson et al. (2007)	Israel National Health Survey	4589	21–65	Retrospective	51.00	48.00	41.59–54.41
Lewinsohn et al. (1998)	Oregon Adolescent Depression Project	816	16–17	Prospective	NR	22.55	21.54–23.56
Ritchie et al. (2004)	Random selection of the 15 electoral rolls	1873	65–85	Retrospective	NR	44.22	38.01–50.43
Stein et al. (2008)	South African Stress and Health Study	4351	18–65	Retrospective	46.00	43.00	36.88–49.12
Viana and Andrade (2012)	The São Paulo Megacity Mental Health Survey	5037	18–65	Retrospective	37.00	34.67	31.64–37.70
Estimated AOO					*42.17*	*37.21*	*28.20–46.21*
PD with AGO							
Becker et al. (2007)	Dresden Study of Mental Health	5204	18–24	Prospective	NR	17.06	15.52–18.60
Falk et al. (2008)	National Epidemiologic Survey on Alcohol and Related Conditions	19,504	18–70	Retrospective	NR	32.30	32.28–32.32
Knappe et al. (2011)	Early Developmental Stages of Psychopathology Study	3021	14–34	Prospective	NR	17.35	15.73–18.97
Estimated AOO					[a]	*22.26*	*10.17–34.35*
PD without AGO							
Becker et al. (2007)	Dresden Study of Mental Health	5204	18–24	Prospective	NR	17.07	15.81–18.33
Caraveo-Anduaga (2004)	Mexican household survey	1932	18–65	Retrospective	NR	25.11	21.83–28.40
De Jonge et al. (2016)	World Mental Health surveys	142,949	18–65	Retrospective	32.00	33.00	32.20–33.80
Falk et al. (2008)	National Epidemiologic Survey on Alcohol and Related Conditions	19,504	18–70	Retrospective	NR	28.50	28.44–28.56
Kessler et al. (2005)	National Comorbidity Survey Replication	9282	18–60	Retrospective	NR	26.67	25.00–28.35
Knappe et al. (2011)	Early Developmental Stages of Psychopathology Study	3021	14–34	Prospective	NR	17.07	15.62–18.52
Estimated AOO					[a]	*24.59*	*20.25–28.92*
Overall estimated AOO						*26.52*	*22.80–30.23*

AGO agoraphobia, *AOO* age of onset, *CI* confidence interval, *NR* not reported, *PD* panic disorder
[a]Few data were available to calculate the estimated AOO

Table 7.9 Studies on the age of onset of generalized anxiety disorder

Study	Survey	*n*	Age (years)	Design	AOO (years)		
					Median	Mean	95% CI
Alhasnawi et al. (2009)	World Mental Health survey	4332	18–65	Retrospective	51.00	46.00	42.41–49.59
Becker et al. (2007)	Dresden Study of Mental Health	5204	18–24	Prospective	NR	17.91	16.85–18.97
Caraveo-Anduaga (2004)	Mexican household survey	1932	18–65	Retrospective	NR	33.92	30.96–36.88
Cho et al. (2012)	Korean Epidemiologic Catchment and Area Study Replication	7972	18–64	Retrospective	45.00	43.67	41.07–46.27
Falk et al. (2008)	National Epidemiologic Survey on Alcohol and Related Conditions	19,504	18–70	Retrospective	NR	33.30	33.28–33.32
Goncalves (2012)	Australian National Survey of Mental Health and Wellbeing	8841	16–85	Retrospective	26.00	27.00	25.87–28.13
Kessler et al. (2005)	National Comorbidity Survey Replication	9282	18–60	Retrospective	NR	32.67	30.96–34.38
Knappe et al. (2011)	Early Developmental Stages of Psychopathology Study	3021	14–34	Prospective	NR	17.01	15.78–18.24
Lee et al. (2007)	World Mental Health household survey	5201	18–70	Retrospective	44.00	44.00	39.36–48.64
Levinson et al. (2007)	Israel National Health Survey	4589	21–65	Retrospective	47.00	46.00	42.85–49.15
Lewinsohn et al. (1998)	Oregon Adolescent Depression Project	816	16–17	Prospective	NR	26.10	25.09–27.11
Ritchie et al. (2004)	Random selection of the 15 electoral rolls	1873	65–85	Retrospective	NR	32.99	30.20–35.78
Stein et al. (2008)	South African Stress and Health Study	4351	18–65	Retrospective	72.00	60.33	55.71–64.95
Vaingankar et al. (2013)	The Singapore mental health study	6616	18–65	Retrospective	20.00	24.40	21.89–26.91
Viana and Andrade (2012)	The São Paulo Megacity Mental Health Survey	5037	18–65	Retrospective	41.00	42.67	38.91–46.43
Estimated AOO					*40.61*	*34.94*	*30.88–39.01*

AOO age of onset, *CI* confidence interval, *NR* not reported

Vainganakar et al. (2013) reported the onset of generalized anxiety disorder during various life stages. Three percent had their onset in childhood (< 12 years), 21% in adolescence (12–17 years), 46% in early adulthood (18–29 years), 29% in adulthood (30–59 years) and 1% in late adulthood (≥ 60 years) (Vaingankar et al. 2013).

7.4 Discussion

Despite the fact that several studies have been published on the AOO of anxiety disorders since October 2014 (Albert et al. 2015; Rhebergen et al. 2017; Tibi et al. 2015), only two studies fulfilled our inclusion criteria. These two studies were combined with the studies included in our previous meta-analysis (de Lijster et al. 2017).

The mean onset of anxiety disorders in general was estimated at 21 years. Included studies consistently reported that anxiety disorders in general have an earlier AOO than mood disorders and substance use disorders, although anxiety disorders tend to develop over a larger age period. This finding is in line with previous studies that showed that anxiety disorders could be a pathway to later psychiatric disorders, also called heterotypic continuity. Indeed, many studies have shown that anxiety disorders precede the development of major depressive disorder (e.g. Bittner et al. 2004) and substance abuse (e.g. Goodwin and Stein 2013).

Substantial differences were found between anxiety disorder subtypes with regard to AOO. Separation anxiety disorder had the lowest estimated AOO, namely at 9 years. Overlapping confidence intervals were found for separation anxiety disorder, specific phobia and social phobia. The first onset of these anxiety disorder subtypes occurs in childhood and early adolescence. Overlapping confidence intervals were also found for agoraphobia, obsessive–compulsive disorder, post-traumatic stress disorder and panic disorder, all of which have their mean onset in early adulthood. Of all the anxiety disorder subtypes, generalized anxiety disorder had the latest mean onset at almost 35 years, and a median AOO of 40 years. The sequence of anxiety disorder subtypes validates the current taxonomy of anxiety disorders. Social and cognitive development has been shown to affect the timing of anxiety disorder subtypes (Broeren and Muris 2009). The later onset of agoraphobia, panic disorder and generalized anxiety disorders is in line with research that separates these disorders from specific phobia based on genetic predisposition (Hettema et al. 2005).

One reason for generalized anxiety disorder having the highest AOO might be that the percentage of studies with a maximum age above 60 years was highest for generalized anxiety disorder. Meta-regression for anxiety disorders in general has also shown that maximum age is positively related to the AOO reported. Another reason might be the diagnostic overlap between generalized anxiety disorder and major depressive disorder (Zbozinek et al. 2012). Because most studies relied on retrospective accounts, diagnostic overlap, in particular, can induce a reporting bias. Bonnewyn et al. (2007), for instance, found an AOO for mood disorders of 38 years, which more or less corresponds to the documented AOO of generalized anxiety disorder.

This meta-analysis indicated that social phobia develops in restricted age period within adolescence, which is valuable information for prevention strategies, particularly considering the fact that social phobia is prevalent, impairing and chronic (Wittchen et al. 1999). In contrast, obsessive–compulsive disorder develops in a broad age period, covering childhood, adolescence, and early and middle adulthood.

Meta-regressions indicated that the maximum age of the study sample, HDI, study design and gender were significantly related to the AOO of anxiety disorders in general. A higher maximum age of the study sample, lower stage of development of a country, retrospective study design and higher percentage of males were related to a higher AOO of anxiety disorders in general.

With regard to the effect of study design, the mean AOO of anxiety disorders was generally higher in retrospective studies. Recall bias of the exact onset of anxiety disorders might be an explanation for the later AOO in retrospective studies. Individuals might have a tendency to report the onset of anxiety disorders as being more recent, a phenomenon called forward telescoping (Simon and Vonkorff 1995). Another reason for the higher AOO in retrospective studies is the effect of age at interview, which was higher in retrospective than in prospective studies, and Vaingankar et al. (2013) showed that the age at interview and reported AOO are interrelated. In addition, the higher AOO in retrospective studies might be explained not only by forward telescoping, but also by the fact that patients that develop anxiety disorders at an older age are often outside the scope of prospective studies.

With regard to the developmental level of a country, anxiety disorders in general have an earlier onset in countries that provide better life expectancy, education and income. However, other factors can explain these findings as well. First, most studies had a retrospective design. As previously described, retrospective studies on AOOs rely heavily on the recall of the first onset of symptoms. More public awareness of and less prejudice against mental health problems in developed countries than in developing countries might result in the earlier recognition and recall of anxiety problems in people from developed countries (Lauber and Rössler 2007). Additionally, families in developing countries might have more pressing concerns, which could result in delayed recall of the onset of anxiety disorders when asked retrospectively. Second, most of the prospective studies were carried out in developed countries. Prospective studies are likely to achieve a more accurate AOO estimate than retrospective studies. This could be an explanation of why lower AOOs were found for developed countries.

Besides the clear female preponderance in the prevalence of anxiety disorders (McLean et al. 2011), the current findings on AOO of anxiety disorders in general also point to gender differences: the AOO of anxiety disorders in general was lower for females than for males. Multiple factors are likely to be involved in the earlier onset of anxiety disorders in females. However, the causes of gender differences in the prevalence and AOO of anxiety disorders are yet not fully understood (Riecher-Rössler 2017). Biological, personal and environmental factors have been associated with gender differences in anxiety. With regard to biological factors, sex hormones (Li and Graham 2017) and brain functioning have been shown to play a role in sex differences. Girls experience hormonal changes earlier in life than boys, which could result in an earlier onset of anxiety disorders. Also in girls an earlier pubertal timing is associated with higher levels of anxiety (Reardon et al. 2009). A paper by Oram et al. (2017) reported that women experience more violence than men, and that violence is related to an increased risk of mental disorders, including anxiety disorders. In addition, socialisation processes are hypothesised to contribute to gender differences in anxiety (McLean and Anderson 2009).

Conclusion

There is a wealth of studies on risk factors for anxiety disorder development (e.g. Hyland et al. 2016; Steinhausen et al. 2016; Zhang et al. 2015). The combination of the window of anxiety disorder development reported in this chapter and knowledge on risk factors for anxiety disorder onset could be highly informative for the timing of targeted prevention strategies. Primary prevention programmes have generally been provided at schools. However, the later onset of agoraphobia, obsessive–compulsive disorder, post-traumatic stress disorder, panic disorders and generalized anxiety disorder highlight the need for prevention beyond the education system.

References

Ajdacic-Gross V, Aleksandrowicz A, Rodgers S, Muller M, Kawohl W, Rossler W, et al. Social phobia is associated with delayed onset of chickenpox, measles, and mumps infections. Front Psychiatry. 2016;7:203.

Albert U, Manchia M, Tortorella A, Volpe U, Rosso G, Carpiniello B, et al. Admixture analysis of age at symptom onset and age at disorder onset in a large sample of patients with obsessive-compulsive disorder. J Affect Disord. 2015;187:188–96.

Alhasnawi S, Sadik S, Rasheed M, Baban A, Al-Alak MM, Othman AY, et al. The prevalence and correlates of DSM-IV disorders in the Iraq Mental Health Survey (IMHS). World Psychiatry. 2009;8(2):97–109.

Angst J, Gamma A, Endrass J, et al. Obsessive-compulsive severity spectrum in the community: prevalence, comorbidity, and course. Eur Arch Psychiatry Clin Neurosci. 2004;254(3):156–64.

Baxter AJ, Ferrari AJ, Erskine HE, Charlson FJ, Degenhardt L, Whiteford HA. The global burden of mental and substance use disorders: changes in estimating burden between GBD1990 and GBD2010. Epidemiol Psychiatr Sci. 2014;23(3):239–49.

Becker ES, Rinck M, Turke V, Kause P, Goodwin R, Neumer S, et al. Epidemiology of specific phobia subtypes: findings from the Dresden Mental Health Study. Eur Psychiatry. 2007;22(2):69–74.

Bienvenu OJ, Onyike CU, Stein MB, Chen LS, Samuels J, Nestadt G, et al. Agoraphobia in adults: incidence and longitudinal relationship with panic. Br J Psychiatry. 2006;188:432–8.

Bittner A, Goodwin RD, Wittchen HU, Beesdo K, Höfler M, Lieb R. What characteristics of primary anxiety disorders predict subsequent major depressive disorder. J Clin Psychiatry. 2004;65:618–26.

Bonnewyn A, Bruffaerts R, Vilagut G, Almansa J, Demyttenaere K. Lifetime risk and age-of-onset of mental disorders in the Belgian general population. Soc Psychiatry Psychiatr Epidemiol. 2007;42(7):522–9.

Borenstein M, Hedges L, Higgins J, Rothstein H. Comprehensive meta-analysis version 2. Engelwood: Biostat; 2005.

Broeren S, Muris P. The relation between cognitive development and anxiety phenomena in children. J Child Fam Stud. 2009;18:702–9.
Caraveo-Anduaga JJ, Colmenares Bermudez E. The epidemiology of obsessive-compulsive disorder in Mexico City. Salud Ment. 2004;27(2):1–6.
Chapman C, Mills K, Slade T, et al. Remission from posttraumatic stress disorder in the general population. Psychol Med. 2012;42(8):1695–703.
Chartier MJ, Walker JR, Stein MB. Considering comorbidity in social phobia. Soc Psychiatry Psychiatr Epidemiol. 2003;38(12):728–34.
Cho MJ, Chang SM, Hahm BJ, Chung IW, Bae A, Lee YM, et al. Lifetime risk and age of onset distributions of psychiatric disorders: analysis of national sample survey in South Korea. Soc Psychiatry Psychiatr Epidemiol. 2012;47(5):671–81.
Conway KP, Compton W, Stinson FS, Grant BF. Lifetime comorbidity of DSM-IV mood and anxiety disorders and specific drug use disorders: results from the national epidemiologic survey on alcohol and related conditions. J Clin Psychiatry. 2006;67(2):247–57.
Dadds MR, Spence SH, Holland DE, Barrett PM, Laurens KR. Prevention and early intervention for anxiety disorders: a controlled trial. J Consult Clin Psychol. 1997;65(4):627–35.
de Jonge P, Roest AM, Lim CCW, Florescu SE, Bromet EJ, Stein DJ, et al. Cross-national epidemiology of panic disorder and panic attacks in the World Mental Health surveys. Depress Anxiety. 2016;33(12):1155–77.
de Lijster JM, Dierckx B, Utens EM, Verhulst FC, Zieldorff C, Dieleman GC, et al. The age of onset of anxiety disorders: a meta-analysis. Can J Psychiatry. 2017;62(4):237–46.
de Lijster J, Dieleman GC, Utens EMWJ, Dierckx B, Wierenga M, Verhulst FC, et al. Social and academic functioning in adolescents with anxiety disorders: a systematic review. J Affect Disord. 2018;230:108–17.
Essau CA, Lewinsohn PM, Olaya B, Seeley JR. Anxiety disorders in adolescents and psychosocial outcomes at age 30. J Affect Disord. 2014;163:125–32.
Falk DE, Yi H-Y, Hilton ME. Age of onset and temporal sequencing of lifetime DSM-IV alcohol use disorders relative to comorbid mood and anxiety disorders. Drug Alcohol Depend. 2008;94(1–3):234–45.
Gau SSF, Chong MY, Yang PC, Yen CF, Liang KY, Cheng ATA. Psychiatric and psychosocial predictors of substance use disorders among adolescents—longitudinal study. Br J Psychiatry. 2007;190:42–8.
Giaconia RM, Reinherz HZ, Silverman AB, Pakiz B, Frost AK, Cohen E. Ages of onset of psychiatric-disorders in a community population of older adolescents. J Am Acad Child Adolesc Psychiatry. 1994;33(5):706–17.
Goncalves DC, Pachana NA, Byrne GJ. Prevalence and correlates of generalized anxiety disorder among older adults in the Australian National Survey of Mental Health and Well-Being. J Affect Disord. 2011;132(1–2):223–30.
Goncalves DC, Byrne GJ. Sooner or later: age at onset of generalized anxiety disorder in older adults. Depress Anxiety. 2012;29(1):39–46.
Goodwin RD, Stein DJ. Anxiety disorders and drug dependence: evidence on sequence and specificity among adults. Psychiatry Clin Neurosci. 2013;67(3):167–73.
Gureje O, Uwakwe R, Udofia O, Wakil A, Adeyemi O, Enyidah N. Common psychiatric disorders over a lifetime: age of onset, risk and treatment contact in the Nigerian survey of mental health and wellbeing. Afr J Med Med Sci. 2008;37(3):207–17.
Hettema JM, Prescott CA, Myers JM, Neale MC, Kendler KS. The structure of genetic and environmental risk factors for anxiety disorders in men and women. Arch Gen Psychiatry. 2005;62:182–9.
Hoehnsaric R, Hazlett RL, Mcleod DR. Generalized anxiety disorder with early and late-onset of anxiety symptoms. Compr Psychiatry. 1993;34(5):291–8.
Hyland P, Shevlin M, Elklit A, Christoffersen M, Murphy J. Social, familial and psychological risk factors for mood and anxiety disorders in childhood and early adulthood: a birth cohort study using the Danish Registry System. Soc Psychiatry Psychiatr Epidemiol. 2016;51(3):331–8.

Kessler RC, Berglund P, Demler O, Jin R, Merikangas KR, Walters EE. Lifetime prevalence and age-of-onset distributions of DSM-IV disorders in the National Comorbidity Survey Replication. Arch Gen Psychiatry. 2005;62(6):593–602.
Kessler RC, Amminger GP, Aguilar-Gaxiola S, Alonso J, Lee S, Ustun TB. Age of onset of mental disorders: a review of recent literature. Curr Opin Psychiatry. 2007;20(4):359–64.
Kessler RC, Aguilar-Gaxiola S, Alonso J, Chatterji S, Lee S, Ormel J, et al. The global burden of mental disorders: an update from the WHO World Mental Health (WMH) surveys. Epidemiol Psichiatr Soc. 2009;18(1):23–33.
Knappe S, Beesdo-Baum K, Lieb R, Wittchen HU. Specificity of family risk-factors for the onset and course of social phobia. Eur Neuropsychopharmacol. 2011;21:S532–3.
Lauber C, Rössler W. Stigma towards people with mental illness in developing countries in Asia. Int Rev Psychiatry. 2007;19:157–78.
Lee S, Tsang A, Zhang MY, Huang YQ, He YL, Liu ZR, et al. Lifetime prevalence and inter-cohort variation in DSM-IV disorders in metropolitan China. Psychol Med. 2007;37(1):61–71.
Levinson D, Zilber N, Lerner Y, Grinshpoon A, Levav I. Prevalence of mood and anxiety disorders in the community: results from the Israel National Health Survey. Isr J Psychiatry Relat Sci. 2007;44(2):94–103.
Lewinsohn PM, Gotlib IH, Lewinsohn M, Seeley JR, Allen NB. Gender differences in anxiety disorders and anxiety symptoms in adolescents. J Abnorm Psychol. 1998;107(1):109–17.
Li SH, Graham BM. Why are women so vulnerable to anxiety, trauma-related and stress-related disorders? The potential role of sex hormones. Lancet Psychiatry. 2017;4:73–82.
Lim SW, Ha J, Shin YC, Shin DW, Bae SM, Oh KS. Clinical differences between early- and late-onset social anxiety disorders. Early Interv Psychiatry. 2013;7(1):44–50.
Marquenie LA, Schade A, van Balkom AJLM, et al. Origin of the comorbidity of anxiety disorders and alcohol dependence: findings of a general population study. Eur Addict Res. 2007;13(1):39–49.
McGorry PD, Purcell R, Goldstone S, Amminger GP. Age of onset and timing of treatment for mental and substance use disorders: implications for preventive intervention strategies and models of care. Curr Opin Psychiatry. 2011;24(4):301–6.
McLean CP, Anderson ER. Brave men and timid women? A review of the gender differences in fear and anxiety. Clin Psychol Rev. 2009;29:496–505.
McLean CP, Asnaani A, Litz BT, Hofmann SG. Gender differences in anxiety disorders: prevalence, course of illness, comorbidity and burden of illness. J Psychiatr Res. 2011;45(8):1027–35.
Olatunji BO, Cisler JM, Tolin DF. Quality of life in the anxiety disorders: a meta-analytic review. Clin Psychol Rev. 2007;27(5):572–81.
Oram S, Khalifeh H, Howard LM. Violence against women and mental health. Lancet Psychiatry. 2017;4:159–70.
Ramsawh HJ, Weisberg RB, Dyck I, Stout R, Keller MB. Age of onset, clinical characteristics, and 15-year course of anxiety disorders in a prospective, longitudinal, observational study. J Affect Disord. 2011;132(1–2):260–4.
Rapee RM, Kennedy S, Ingram M, Edwards S, Sweeney L. Prevention and early intervention of anxiety disorders in inhibited preschool children. J Consult Clin Psychol. 2005;73(3):488–97.
Reardon LE, Leen-Feldner EW, Hayward C. Clin Psychol Rev. 2009;29:1–23.
Remes O, Brayne C, van der Linde R, Lafortune L. A systematic review of reviews on the prevalence of anxiety disorders in adult populations. Brain Behav. 2016;6:e00487.
Rhebergen D, Aderka IM, van der Steenstraten IM, van Balkom A, van Oppen P, Stek ML, et al. Admixture analysis of age of onset in generalized anxiety disorder. J Anxiety Disord. 2017;50:47–51.
Riecher-Rössler A. Sex and gender differences in mental disorders. Lancet Psychiatry. 2017;4:8–9.
Ritchie K, Artero S, Beluche I, Ancelin ML, Mann A, Dupuy AM, et al. Prevalence of DSM-IV psychiatric disorder in the French elderly population. Br J Psychiatry. 2004;184:147–52.
Rosellini AJ, Rutter LA, Bourgeois ML, Emmert-Aronson BO, Brown TA. The relevance of age of onset to the psychopathology of social phobia. J Psychopathol Behav Assess. 2013;35(3):356–65.

Sareen J, Cox BJ, Afifi TO, de Graaf R, Asmundson GJG, ten Have M, et al. Anxiety disorders and risk for suicidal ideation and suicide attempts—a population-based longitudinal study of adults. Arch Gen Psychiatry. 2005;62(11):1249–57.

Sihvo S, Hamalainen J, Kiviruusu O, Pirkola S, Isometsa E. Treatment of anxiety disorders in the Finnish general population. J Affect Disord. 2006;96(1–2):31–8.

Simon GE, Vonkorff M. Recall of psychiatric history in cross-sectional surveys—implications for epidemiologic research. Epidemiol Rev. 1995;17(1):221–7.

Stein DJ, Seedat S, Herman A, Moomal H, Heeringa SG, Kessler RC, et al. Lifetime prevalence of psychiatric disorders in South Africa. Br J Psychiatry. 2008;192(2):112–7.

Steinhausen HC, Jakobsen H, Meyer A, Jorgensen PM, Lieb R. Family aggregation and risk factors in phobic disorders over three-generations in a nation-wide study. PLoS One. 2016;11(1):e0146591.

Swendsen J, Conway KP, Degenhardt L, Glantz M, Jin R, Merikangas KR, et al. Mental disorders as risk factors for substance use, abuse and dependence: results from the 10-year follow-up of the National Comorbidity Survey. Addiction. 2010;105(6):1117–28.

Tibi L, van Oppen P, Aderka IM, van Balkom AJ, Batelaan NM, Spinhoven P, et al. An admixture analysis of age of onset in agoraphobia. J Affect Disord. 2015;180:112–5.

Vaingankar JA, Rekhi G, Subramaniam M, Abdin E, Chong SA. Age of onset of life-time mental disorders and treatment contact. Soc Psychiatry Psychiatr Epidemiol. 2013;48(5):835–43.

Viana MC, Andrade LH. Lifetime Prevalence, age and gender distribution and age-of-onset of psychiatric disorders in the Sao Paulo Metropolitan Area, Brazil: results from the Sao Paulo Megacity Mental Health Survey. Rev Bras Psiquiatr. 2012;34(3):249–60.

Wan X, Wang W, Liu J, et al. Estimating the sample mean and standard deviation from the sample size, median, range and/or interquartile range. BMC Med Res Methodol. 2014;14(1):135.

Werner-Seidler A, Perry Y, Calear AL, Newby JM, Christensen H. School-based depression and anxiety prevention programs for young people: a systematic review and meta-analysis. Clin Psychol Rev. 2017;51:30–47.

Wittchen HU. Generalized anxiety disorder: prevalence, burden, and cost to society. Depress Anxiety. 2002;16(4):162–71.

Wittchen HU, Stein MB, Kessler RC. Social fears and social phobia in a community sample of adolescents and young adults: prevalence, risk factors and co-morbidity. Psychol Med. 1999;29(2):309–23.

Zarger MM, Rich BA. Predictors of treatment utilization among adolescents with social anxiety disorder. Child Youth Serv Rev. 2016;71:191–8.

Zbozinek TD, Rose RD, Wollitzky-Taylor KB, Sherbourne C, Sullivan G, Stein MB, et al. Diagnostic overlap in generalized anxiety disorder and major depressive disorder on a primary care sample. Depress Anxiety. 2012;29:1065–71.

Zhang X, Norton J, Carriere I, Ritchie K, Chaudieu I, Ancelin ML. Risk factors for late-onset generalized anxiety disorder: results from a 12-year prospective cohort (the ESPRIT study). Transl Psychiatry. 2015;5:e536.

The Age of Onset of Substance Use Disorders

8

Adrian B. Kelly, Megan Weier, and Wayne D. Hall

8.1 Introduction

At a global level, the use of illicit drugs such as cannabis, opioids, amphetamines and cocaine is associated with substantial morbidity and mortality, particularly among young adults. Illicit drug use is estimated to account for 0.4% of all deaths worldwide and 0.8% of years of life lost due to disability (World Health Organization 2002). In 2012, an estimated 5.2% (range 3.5–7.0%) of the world

A. B. Kelly
School of Psychology and Counselling, Queensland University of Technology, Brisbane, QLD, Australia
e-mail: a.kelly@qut.edu.au

M. Weier
Centre for Youth Substance Abuse Research, Faculty of Health and Behavioural Sciences, The University of Queensland, St Lucia, QLD, Australia

National Drug and Alcohol Research Centre, The University of New South Wales, Sydney, NSW, Australia
e-mail: m.weier@unsw.edu.au

W. D. Hall (✉)
Centre for Youth Substance Abuse Research, Faculty of Health and Behavioural Sciences, The University of Queensland, St Lucia, QLD, Australia

Queensland Centre for Mental Health Research, School of Public Health, The University of Queensland, The Park Centre for Mental Health Treatment, Research and Education, Wacol, QLD, Australia

National Addiction Centre, Institute of Psychiatry, Psychology and Neuroscience, King's College London, London, UK
e-mail: w.hall@uq.edu.au

G. de Girolamo et al. (eds.), *Age of Onset of Mental Disorders*,
https://doi.org/10.1007/978-3-319-72619-9_8

population aged 15–64 years had used an illicit drug at least once in the previous year, from 162 to 324 million illicit drug users worldwide (United Nations Office on Drugs and Crime 2014).

Illicit drug use most commonly begins in the second and third decade of life, and ages of onset (AOO) are very consistent across developed countries. Degenhardt et al. (2008) compared World Health Organization (WHO) World Mental Health Survey data for cannabis and cocaine for the Americas, Europe, Asia, New Zealand, the Middle East and Africa. The median AOO for cannabis use in developed countries across these regions was 18–19 years (except for Nigeria, Israel and Lebanon where the AOO was 21–22 years). The most common age range for drug initiation (interquartile range, i.e. 25th–75th percentile) was 14–21 years. The median AOO for cocaine was 21–24 years for all countries meeting minimum data requirements (Degenhardt et al. 2008), and the age range for elevated risk of initiation was 19–28 years. These global data also show that the risk of starting cannabis use is higher for younger than older cohorts. This trend is consistent with other research (Colell et al. 2013).

The overall objective of this chapter is to review evidence on the links between AOO and long-term harm, outline contextual and developmental factors that may predict initial use and describe the implications of this research for policy and practice in preventing illicit drug use and its associated harms in young adults. Understanding why young people initiate illicit drug use has public health relevance, as early age of drug initiation is associated with an increased risk of long-term problems and premature death from drug-related causes. Knowledge of the factors associated with illicit drug use initiation can inform policy and practice to reduce their prevalence and associated harms. For the purposes of this review, we focus on cannabis, opioids, amphetamine-like stimulants and cocaine. In many American States (some 28 at the present point in time), and several other countries (e.g. Portugal, Uruguay, the Netherlands), the legal status of cannabis use is changing or has recently changed, in line with increased liberalisation of societal attitudes towards cannabis. We retain cannabis in our review compendium for several reasons, namely, because of its decades-long history as a restricted/illegal substance, because where cannabis laws have been liberalised age restrictions still apply that ban use during the critical age range for drug initiation (i.e. 21 years in American States) and because cannabis use commonly begins under legal ages of use. Also, we know much more about predictors and correlates of early cannabis use than we do for other drug use because cannabis is the most prevalent illicit drug and its early and regular use are strong predictors of the initiation and problem use of other illicit drugs (Degenhardt and Hall 2012). In terms of opioid use, we focus on nonmedical prescription drug use (NMPDU) because this is one of the most common forms of first opioid use; involvement in the illicit opioid market commonly follows NMPDU (Novak et al. 2016). We focus on routes of administration other than injecting, because these routes usually precede injection by several years (Rahimi-Movaghar et al. 2015).

8.2 The Effects and Prevalence of Illicit Drug Use in Young People

Cannabis. Cannabis (primary psychoactive constituent delta 9-tetrahydrocannabinol, or THC) is commonly viewed as a benign recreational drug. In recent years its medical use has been promoted in the United States, and its potentially harmful effects downplayed. Short- and long-term effects of cannabis are summarised in Table 8.1. About one in ten lifetime users develop cannabis dependence (Anthony et al. 1994), and the risk is one in six among those who initiate in their teens (Anthony 2006). Regular cannabis use is associated with an increased risk of psychosis in vulnerable individuals (most notably those with a family history of mental health problems) (Hall and Solowij 1998; Crean et al. 2011).

Cannabis remains by far the most commonly used illicit drug among adolescents and young people. In Central European countries, past year prevalence of cannabis use among young adults (aged 15–34 years) varies from 10% in Belgium and 11% in Germany to 22% in France (EMCDDA 2016a). Cannabis use in the United States is far higher than in other countries, including Europe, the Americas, Asia and the Middle East (Degenhardt et al. 2008). In the United States, about 10% of Grade 8 and 35% of Grade 12 students report cannabis use in the previous year (Johnston et al. 2016). Nationally representative surveys in Australia indicate that 12.1% of 14–17-year-olds have used cannabis in the previous year (Weier et al. 2016). These rates are higher than the global average estimated for the World Drug Report (United Nations Office on Drugs and Crime 2015) (1 year prevalence rate of 3.8% for 15–64-year-olds; see Table 8.1).

Opioids. Worldwide, the past year prevalence of opioid use among 15–64-year-olds is 0.7% (see Table 8.1), but as with other drug types, rates appear to be much higher for young people in Western countries. In the European Union, opioid use among adolescents (12–17 years of age) has a lifetime prevalence of 3.5%, and young adults aged 18–25 are most at risk for prescription drug abuse (13.1%; Novak et al. 2016). Around half of people who have misused prescription painkillers reported acquiring them from friends or relatives (Novak et al. 2016). In the United States, NMPDU is likely to be higher than in the European Union (Novak et al. 2016). In Australia, 3.4% of 18–24-year-olds in 2013 reported using painkillers for nonmedical reasons (AIHW 2014). Prescribed opioids (e.g. oxycodone, hydrocodone, codeine) and illegal opioids (e.g. heroin) have great propensity for abuse because of their powerful euphoric and analgesic properties, and they are associated with significant short- and long-term harm (see Table 8.1).

Amphetamine-like stimulants ('speed', 'ice', 'ecstasy') are typically used in party/club settings for their effects on energy, mood and sociability. The short- and long-term effects of speed and ice are well established (see Table 8.1). Global prevalence rates for amphetamine use (past year) are 0.8% (see Table 8.1), but rates in Western countries are probably much higher among young adults. In Australia (2013), 3% of Australians (aged 14+) reported ever using methamphetamines

Table 8.1 Summary data on the global prevalence of drug use, routes of administration and effects

Drug	Estimated past year prevalence % (lower and upper estimates)		Most common administration/forms	Short-term effects	Long-term effects
Cannabis (marijuana, pot, weed, ganja)	Africa	7.6 (3.4–9.7)	Smoked	Euphoria (or 'high'); dysphoria; changes to colour, spatial and time perception; impairs cognitive/psychomotor performance	Attention and memory impairment; inability to process complex information; possible dependence; risk of psychosis (Hall 2009)
	Americas	7.5 (7.4–7.7)			
	Asia	1.9 (1.0–3.1)			
	Europe	4.9 (4.8–5.1)			
	Oceania	10.2 (8.5–14.2)			
	Global	3.8 (2.7–4.9)			
Opioids (including heroin, oxycodone, codeine, morphine and opium)	Africa	0.33 (0.15–0.53)	Oral (capsule/liquid) Injection begins much later	Euphoria, analgesic properties, sedation	Accidental injury; cardiovascular pathology; liver disease; mental health problems; suicidality; fatal overdose (Degenhardt and Hall 2012)
	Americas	2.0 (2.0–2.1)			
	Asia	0.42 (0.32–0.54)			
	Europe	0.9 (0.8–0.9)			
	Oceania	3.0 (2.4–3.0)			
	Global	0.7 (0.6–0.8)			
Amphetamine-type stimulants (Meth, crystal, ice, MDMA, speed)	Africa	0.87 (0.23–1.50)	Snorting, oral Most prevalent—speed	Increased energy; positive mood; sociability; appetite suppression; drug-induced psychotic symptoms; myocardial infarction	Compulsivity; paranoid ideation; aggression/acute; depression and suicidality; cardiovascular disease (Degenhardt et al. 2007b)
	Americas	1.2 (1.1–1.2)			
	Asia	0.68 (0.15–1.21)			
	Europe	0.4 (0.4–0.5)			
	Oceania	1.9 (1.5–2.1)			
	Global	0.8 (0.3–1.2)			
Cocaine (coke, crack, powder, base)	Africa	0.4 (0.1–0.8)	Snorting	Mood, alertness and sexual arousal; anxiety; paranoia; hypertension; heart attack	Dependence; risk of overdose; cardiovascular pathology; mental health problems such as psychosis and depression (Degenhardt et al. 2007b)
	Americas	1.5 (1.4–1.5)			
	Asia	0.1 (0.0–0.1)			
	Europe	0.7 (0.7–0.8)			
	Oceania	1.5 (1.5–1.9)			
	Global	0.38 (0.31–0.46)			

Note: For greatest consistency in age and measures, prevalence estimates are based on the World Drug Report (United Nations Office on Drugs and Crime 2015)

(AIHW 2014). Crystal methamphetamine ('ice') more than doubled in prevalence between 2010 and 2013 based on Australian household surveys and wastewater analyses (now the standard for measuring population-scale use of various chemical compounds) (Hall et al. 2012) suggest that the rates of methamphetamine ('ice') use in Australia have increased more rapidly to far higher rates than surveys would suggest. Australia ranks second of 18 countries for consumption of methamphetamine (O'Brien et al. 2017). Among European young adults, 1.7% report using MDMA (ecstasy) in the past year. In the United Kingdom, 3.5% of young adults report using MDMA in the previous 12 months, and 3% of school students reported ever trying the substance (EMCDDA 2016b). In Australia, 3.9% of Australians aged 14–19 reported ever using MDMA (AIHW 2014).

Cocaine. Cocaine use typically begins around 20 years of age (Wagner and Anthony 2001) and is used for its powerful effects on mood and alertness. It has a number of adverse effects on mental and physical health (see Table 8.1). Global prevalence of past year cocaine use in adults ranges from 0.07 to 0.52% across Western Europe, southeast Asia and North America (Degenhardt and Hall 2012). Among young people in Europe and the United Kingdom, 1.9% and 4.2%, respectively, of young adults report using cocaine in the past year. Around 2% of school students in the United Kingdom report lifetime use of cocaine (EMCDDA 2016b), and around 2.1% of Australians aged 14–19 years old report lifetime use (AIHW 2014).

8.3 When Does Illicit Drug Use Typically Start?

For more than half of all new illicit drug users, cannabis is the first illicit drug used (NIDA 2015). Based on data on Americans aged 12–21 years from the 2013 National Survey on Drug Use and Health (NSDUH) ($n = 26{,}659$), the mean age of first use of cannabis was 16.5 years of age (Chen et al. 2017). In Australians aged under 20, the mean age for initiation of cannabis in 2007 was 15.2 years, and there is evidence that the age of initiation in Australia has increased since 1998 (when it was 14.6 years of age) (based on the National Drug Strategy Household Surveys; Lenton et al. 2012). The age at which amphetamine and cocaine use is often initiated is difficult to establish, as most studies are based on convenience samples. In one of the few nationally representative studies in Australia, past year prevalence rates were 12% among 24-year-olds, and almost half of those who reported amphetamine use at 24 years reported no amphetamine use at age 20 years (Degenhardt et al. 2007a; AIHW 2005). Among American adolescents seeking treatment for cocaine, the average age of first use was just over 15 years of age (Bracken et al. 2013). In Australia, the mean age of initiation among people brought to police stations on a wide variety of charges was 15 years for cannabis users, 18 for amphetamine and cocaine users and 19 for heroin users (Johnson 2001). Compared to the 1998 Australian National Drug Strategy Household Survey (NDSHS) (Adhikari and Summerill 2000), ages of initiation for Johnson's sample were lower (18 years for cannabis, 20 years for amphetamines and 22 years for cocaine and heroin). Among the general population and high-risk groups (including drug users, detainees and prisoners), the ages of initiation of cannabis were comparable, but the initiation of other illicit drugs followed soon after for those in high-risk groups, such as antisocial youth.

8.4 Age of Onset and Drug-Related Consequences

Findings on the consequences of drug use are typically derived from population-based longitudinal studies or clinically oriented samples with drug-related problems (e.g. young people seeking drug treatment). There are limitations to both methodologies. Community-based longitudinal studies often have insufficient numbers of people who develop drug dependence to study the risk factors for dependence, and the attrition of people with drug problems may be higher than for people who leave the study. For clinically oriented studies, methodologies are typically retrospective, and unknown pathways to sample inclusion make it impossible to draw firm conclusions about how AOO is related to drug problems. In this section we prioritise high-quality longitudinal studies that examine pathways into cannabis-related problems over studies based on clinically oriented samples and other drugs. We do this because the relatively high prevalence of cannabis use maximises statistical power to determine effects where they are present. Early initiation and the development of problematic cannabis use also predict an increased risk of using other illicit drugs.

When a young person begins cannabis use in their teen years, they have a greater risk of developing long-term problems than peers who begin to use at later ages or do not use at all. Research from the *Christchurch Health and Development Study* ($n = 1265$ followed from age 15 to adulthood) shows that early cannabis use is associated with increased risk of car accidents (Fergusson and Horwood 2001), arrests and convictions (Fergusson et al. 2003b), polydrug use (particularly hallucinogens and amphetamines) (Boden et al. 2006) and early school dropout (Lynskey and Hall 2000; Kelly et al. 2015). The Australian NDSHS (AIHW 2014) data indicate that among those adults who first tried marijuana at the age of 14 or younger, 13.2% were classified as having illicit drug dependence or abuse; this was six times higher than the risk for adults who first used marijuana at the age of 18 or older. For young people who develop cannabis dependence (nearly 10%), there is an increased risk of psychotic symptoms (Fergusson et al. 2003a). Cannabis use prior to the age of 15 years is associated with conduct disorders, offending, unexplained school absences, anxiety, depression and suicidality (Fergusson et al. 1996) with the increased odds of these outcomes ranging from 2.7 for anxiety disorders to 7.0 for conduct and oppositional problems and 9.3 for unexplained school absences. Fergusson et al. (1996) found that most of these risks were attributable to family disadvantage, early maladjustment and deviant peer group engagement, but early onset of cannabis use remained a significant predictor of these risks after accounting for all these other risk factors. Other nationally representative surveys in the United States show that early AOO is related to high chronicity and severity of illicit drug use. Based on the National Comorbidity Survey (adolescents, 13–18 years of age), the likelihood of drug abuse is tenfold among young drug users (13–14 years of age) compared to older adolescent drug users, where drug abuse was just over twice the sample base rates (Swendsen et al. 2012).

8.5 Why Do Young People Initiate Illicit Drug Use?

Contemporary aetiological frameworks for understanding the early phases of illicit drug use are complex and multidimensional (Dodge et al. 2009; Steinberg 2008). These include the *gateway hypothesis* (i.e. where an individual is thought to progress through a sequence from licit to illicit drugs), an *opportunistic* dimension (i.e. use begins because a drug is available), *person-centred vulnerabilities* to use (e.g. genetic vulnerabilities, personality traits, early puberty), a *social systems* approach (e.g. influence of families, peers) and *transactional approaches* (e.g. the cascading of multiple risks over time).

8.5.1 The Gateway Hypothesis

The gateway hypothesis (Kandel 1975) assumes a temporal sequence of drug initiation in which the effects of using one drug is thought to promote the initiation of the next drug in the sequence, with the use of later drugs usually attracting more severe social sanctions and/or illegal status than those earlier in the sequence (Kandel et al. 2006). From this perspective, the licit drugs alcohol and tobacco act as a gateway to cannabis use, and cannabis use, in turn, acts as a gateway to the use of other illicit drugs, such as cocaine and amphetamines. A large body of empirical literature reports patterns of initiation that are consistent with the gateway hypothesis. Early use of alcohol and tobacco predicts the early onset of cannabis and subsequent illicit drug use (Agrawal et al. 2006; Butterworth et al. 2014; Ellickson et al. 1992; Behrendt et al. 2012). In their cohort study of American twins ($n = 3729$), Agrawal et al. (2006) found that early onset of alcohol and tobacco use was a strong predictor of illicit drug use. Early intensive use (12 years or younger) of any substance (including alcohol/tobacco) predicted the later use of 'harder drugs' (most notably heroin, ketamine, gamma-hydroxybutyric acid (GHB)) (Baggio et al. 2013). In treatment samples, adolescents report that alcohol use usually precedes first use of cocaine (Apantaku-Olajide et al. 2013).

Some research findings are inconsistent with the gateway hypothesis. First, the association between early use of 'soft' drugs and subsequent use of 'hard' drugs has been found to be substantially weakened after accounting for childhood/familial vulnerabilities, suggesting that common vulnerabilities at least partially account for diversities in drug use and drug use trajectories (Tarter et al. 2006). Second, a large proportion (22.4%) of cannabis-using adolescents do not follow a gateway sequence to illicit drugs (Tarter et al. 2006), and some studies show reverse gateway effects in which cannabis use increases the risks of tobacco smoking (Becker et al. 2015; Bennett et al. 2000). In sum, there is little evidence that the use of one drug is aetiologically related to another or that there is a universal ordered sequence in the use of drugs that leads to dependence (Tarter et al. 2006).

8.5.2 Opportunity to Use Illicit Drugs

Adolescents vary in their perceived opportunities to use illicit drugs, and while these opportunities develop strongly during adolescence, not all adolescents who are exposed to opportunities to use a drug take up the opportunity. Opportunities to use illicit drugs rise dramatically from around 13 years of age (Swendsen et al. 2012). About 39% of 13–14-year-olds and 81% of 17–18-year-olds report opportunities to use illicit drugs, indicating a doubling of opportunities to use illicit drug use across the teen years (Swendsen et al. 2012). About 40.5% of adolescents who are exposed to illicit drugs actually report illicit drug use and 36.6% develop patterns of abuse (Swendsen et al. 2012). These results suggest that most adolescents who are exposed to illicit drugs do not use, but a substantial minority of those who do use go on to develop patterns of abuse. The research on exposure and uptake of illicit drug use has important implications for preventing the initiation of illicit drug use. It makes sense to investigate the reasons why the majority of adolescents resist opportunities to use illicit drugs. Factors that are associated with such resilience would be a useful focus for prevention programmes. It would also make sense to restrict opportunities to use illicit drugs by restricting supply routes and/or exposure to high-risk networks.

8.5.3 Person-Centred Vulnerabilities

An alternative account of the gateway pattern of drug use is that some individuals have a *common liability to addiction* (CLA) such as a genetic vulnerability to develop addiction or display socially deviant behaviour (Vanyukov et al. 2012; Mayet et al. 2016). Illicit drug use is more likely to begin in persons with a genetic or familial predisposition towards drug use or misuse. Sibling/twin/adoption studies are a powerful way of testing the contribution of genetic mechanisms to the initiation of substance use. Available evidence suggests that the genetic contribution to AOO of illicit drug use is significant but moderate in size. For example, Rhee et al. (2003) found evidence of moderate to substantial genetic influences on cannabis initiation during adolescence, but the heritability of substance initiation was lower than the heritability of problem drug use. Rhee et al. also found that there were significant environmental influences shared only by twin pairs on drug use, pointing to the importance of sibling and shared peer and drug accessibility influences (Rhee et al. 2003). Reviews of the empirical literature also indicate that heritability across all stages of cannabis use (use, abuse, dependence) is significant, but initiation of cannabis use is more strongly related to environmental factors than are cannabis abuse and dependence (Agrawal and Lynskey 2006; Lynskey et al. 2003). Agrawal and Lynskey (2006) also found that the links between early cannabis use and later use/abuse/dependence were not solely explained by common genetic/shared environmental factors; they proposed that peer contexts contributed significantly to the development of cannabis use and abuse. The heritability of early-onset drug use fits with established findings on early childhood traits and behaviours. Early childhood vulnerabilities include childhood conduct disorder, high novelty seeking, low harm avoidance and hyperactivity/attention deficit disorder, all of which are related to the onset of cannabis use in late adolescence (Cerda et al. 2013; Masse and Tremblay 1997; Galera et al. 2010; Charach et al. 2011).

In their longitudinal study of 10–12-year-olds followed to age 22, Kirisci et al. (2013) measured transmissible liability for addiction (including early impulsivity and antisocial behaviour), AOO of alcohol and cannabis and alcohol/cannabis use disorder. They found that transmissible liability negatively predicted AOO and that it mediated the association between AOO and alcohol/cannabis use disorder. Also consistent with the CLA model is the fact that problems cluster at the individual level (White et al. 2013; Quek et al. 2013) with troubled adolescents more likely to have multiple problems (e.g. polydrug problems, sexual risk-taking and depression) than one problem. For example, in the United Kingdom, 22% of 15-year-olds report 0–1 risk behaviours, 42% report 2–3 risk behaviours and 34% report four or more risk behaviours (Kipping et al. 2015). Onset of cannabis use in young adult males has been associated with depression, parental divorce and low parental monitoring, peer pressure and sensation-seeking traits (Haug et al. 2014). Early onset of 'hard drugs' in high-risk adolescents is associated with depression and suicidality (Cho et al. 2007).

The CLA model also better accounts for the fact that some young people skip some intermediary drug types (moving straight to using illicit drugs) and accounts for both early initiation of drug use and rapid progression to addiction (Kirisci et al. 2013). Research points to the likelihood that the gateway pattern probably reflects common causes rather than the causal effects of specific drugs on the subsequent use of other drugs (Degenhardt et al. 2010). In a study of early cannabis users and their co-twin controls, individuals who used cannabis by age 17 had increased odds of other drug use, and drug abuse/dependence was 2.1–5.2 times higher among these young people than their co-twins who did not use by age 17. These effects remain significant after controlling for a range of adverse psychosocial experiences (Lynskey et al. 2003).

8.5.4 Developmental Vulnerabilities

Social neuroscientists argue that neurological development processes make young people inherently vulnerable to the initiation of drug use (Steinberg 2008). Risky behaviours, including drug use, are a function of the development of socio-emotional brain systems around the time of puberty, which contributes to increases in risky behaviour that are especially likely to be expressed in socially permissive social contexts (e.g. drug-using peer groups) (Steinberg 2008). There is good evidence that key changes occur in brain structure from adolescence to the mid-20s, namely, synaptic pruning (key to information processing and logical reasoning), myelination (key to executive functioning) and projections of white matter across brain regions (key to improved emotional regulation) (Steinberg 2008; Gogtay et al. 2004). Social neuroscience predicts that illicit drug initiation will most likely begin during adolescence because this is when susceptibility to peer influence is highest. Vulnerability to early initiation will be elevated when puberty comes early. Consistent with these predictions, peer influences are closely associated with adolescent drug-taking (Monahan et al. 2009; Steinberg and Monahan 2007; Chan et al. 2013; Kelly et al. 2012; Clinton-Sherrod et al. 2005), and early onset of puberty is closely linked to risk-taking behaviour, including alcohol use and sexual risk-taking (Downing and Bellis 2009; Li et al. 2014) and early onset of illicit drug use (Dudovitz et al. 2015; Lanza and Collins 2002). A key implication of a social neuroscience perspective is that prevention programmes that build resistance to acting on drug-taking opportunities will be less effective in preventing illicit drug use than reducing drug supply.

8.5.5 Social Systems Models

The *social development model* (SDM) (Catalano et al. 1996) has been widely applied to substance use and misuse in young people. SDM integrates models that emphasise modelling and vicarious reinforcement (*social learning theory;* SLT) (Bandura 1969); bonding to prosocial institutions such as families, schools and the community (*social control theory;* SCT) (Hirschi 1971); and the role of potentially modifiable and often-nested social systems of influence (*ecology of human development theory*; EHDT) (Bronfenbrenner 1989; Ennett et al. 2008). From an SDM perspective, illicit drug experimentation is a consequence of individual differences (e.g. antisocial behaviour, genetic proneness), family environments (parental drug use, supervision, monitoring), peer networks (drug use, anti-establishment values) and broader macrosystems in which these proximal networks are located, such as schools (e.g. school engagement and support) (Kelly et al. 2015) and communities (e.g. clubs, sport infrastructure, law and order, drug sales networks) (Smith et al. 2014).

Studies based on SDM principles are consistent with the impact of social systems on drug use among young people. Drug use is significantly correlated with engagement and socialisation with drug using peers (Abar and Turrisi 2008; Martino et al. 2009; Bahr et al. 2005; Capaldi et al. 2009). Drug using peer groups promote anticonventional norms that isolate group members from prosocial influences (Donovan and Jessor 1985; Jessor 1991). Parental drug use (Tildesley and Andrews 2008; Simons-Morton 2004) and sibling alcohol and other drug use (Fagan and Najman 2005; Rajan et al. 2003; Kelly et al. 2011a) are also related to adolescent drug use. Perhaps the single strongest family-oriented predictor of adolescent drug initiation and use is parental monitoring and supervision (Haug et al. 2014). Emotionally close parent-child relationships predict less alcohol and other drug misuse in young cohorts (Brook et al. 2000; Choquet et al. 2008; Wills and Cleary 1996; Barnes et al. 2006; Barnes et al. 2000), and parent-child closeness predicts positive outcomes in adolescents receiving treatment for drug problems (Kelly 2008). Families characterised by low levels of emotional closeness and high conflict may indirectly contribute to the development of substance use by increasing the likelihood that young people form connections with deviant peer groups (Kelly in press; Kelly et al. 2011b, c) and neighbourhood disadvantage longitudinally predicts substance use (alcohol/tobacco/cannabis) initiation in at-risk children (Fite et al. 2009).

8.5.6 Transactional Models

A widely accepted example of transactional approaches to drug use is *dynamic cascade theory* (Dodge et al. 2009). DCT incorporates biological and social perspectives and emphasises the unfolding and expanding nature of adjustment problems in adolescence. From this perspective, early-onset illicit drug use is a temporal marker of an unfolding progression from early problems (e.g. difficult temperament, family history of substance use, social disadvantage) to progressively deepening problems (substance use, social isolation, school dropout) that may develop into severe drug problems (dependence, depression, crime). Consistent with DCT, young people who use illicit drugs usually report other problems, including heavy alcohol use, tobacco smoking, risky sexual behaviour, unexplained absences from school and other deviant behaviours (Kipping et al. 2015). Early onset of substance use is associated with a range of other risky/antisocial behaviours, lower academic performance and family instability (DuRant et al. 1999). In a longitudinal study of 585 boys from kindergarten to Grade 12, linkages between biological and social ecological variables with drug onset across time were assessed (Dodge et al. 2009). The key findings were that early influences on drug use initiation were significant, that problems were interrelated in a web of correlations that expanded over time and that problems at earlier periods incremented with subsequent problems. Other longitudinal research shows that the cascade model fits data on adolescent violence (Dodge et al. 2008).

8.5.7 Summary and Integration

Illicit drug use is a global problem that has wide-ranging effects on individuals, families and communities. It commonly begins in the mid to late teens through to the early 20s and initiation can be explained or understood by a range of conceptual models. These models vary in their unit of analysis (neuroscience through to macrosocial systems) and the extent to which they focus on the dynamics of change. Most of these conceptual models share some features, such as an acknowledgement of individual vulnerabilities, social processes and the worsening of problems over time in vulnerable young people.

Many studies provide data consistent with the *gateway hypothesis*, which emphasises sequential transitions to drugs with progressively greater social sanctions. However, trajectories of drug use are heterogeneous, and the gateway model does not clearly explain why a young person would initiate illicit drug use at a particular time. A model that fits the empirical data better is the *common liability model*, which proposes that the pattern of drug involvement reflects a predisposition to addiction that may be genetic, personal and social. This model explains why there are correlations between problem behaviours and why genetic and early childhood factors account for diverse outcomes. The model also fits with *social neuroscience* models of addiction, which emphasise the role of pubertal development and immaturity in executive functioning as important in the initiation and early development of adolescent drug use. There is also considerable evidence that potentially modifiable *social systems* around the adolescent predict early substance use, with the strongest effects attributable to peer networks and parental monitoring, supervision and substance use. Finally, *transactional models* emphasise that problems snowball over time and fit well with findings that adolescents with one type of problem usually have others and that webs of problems in young adulthood commonly develop from simpler problem profiles in adolescence.

8.6 Implications for Prevention of Illicit Drug Use

The evidence-based models reviewed above have a number of implications for prevention. Social neuroscience models emphasise traits and developmental stages that may be difficult to suppress. Initiation of drug use during adolescence and young adulthood is a high probability event, if drugs are available. From this perspective, policies and programmes that seek to reduce supply (e.g. minimising exposure to drugs and drug using networks) are likely to be more effective than demand reduction programmes (e.g. programmes that seek to teach adolescents how to avoid drug use opportunities or 'just say no' to peers' offers of drugs). School-based prevention programmes are oriented towards teaching adolescents to manage high-risk situations, through psychoeducation, training in resisting peer influences, promotion of norms that are negative towards drug use, problem-solving training and interpersonal skills training (Botvin 1986). Overall, primary prevention programmes have small effect sizes at best (Masterman and Kelly 2003). The most extensively evaluated primary prevention programme, DARE, shows few if any effects on drug use and may in fact stimulate drug experimentation (Masterman and Kelly 2003). Consistent with the possibility that supply reduction approaches are effective, parental supervision and monitoring of contacts with peer networks are among the strongest predictors of reduced drug involvement, and parent-oriented interventions show significant though modest effects (Kelly and Connor 2012).

Social developmental models that focus on multilevel social ecologies of substance use point to the utility of targeting school, family and community risks. Community-based prevention programmes like the *Communities That Care* (CTC) approach are good examples of social systemic approaches to prevention (Salom et al. 2012; Rowland et al. 2013). CTC initially identifies and quantifies community-level risk and protective profiles related to adolescent delinquency, including licit and illicit drug use and misuse. In the United States, randomised control trials of CTC (24 communities) that have followed students from 10 to 13 years of age show reductions in the initiation of delinquency and alcohol use (past 30 days) over 2 years (Greenberg et al. 2005; Hawkins et al. 2008, 2009). Reductions in cannabis use were not found, but this may have been because the sample was younger than the age at which cannabis use typically escalates in the United States (16–17 years).

A second example of a social systems approach to prevention is PROSPER (PROmoting School-community-university Partnerships to Enhance Resilience) (Spoth et al. 2004). PROSPER involves community-university partnerships to implement evidence-based programmes to prevent adolescent substance use and related problems. At 6.5-year follow-up (year 12 end), community-wide reductions of 10–35% in illicit drug use initiation were found for students who were nonusers prior to the programme (Redmond et al. 2009; Spoth et al. 2009).

The common liability to addiction (CLA) model points to the potential value of addressing core vulnerabilities such as conduct disorders rather than specifically focusing on preventing alcohol/drug use. The *Fast Track* programme (Conduct Problems Prevention Research Group 2002) is a good example of a multicomponent, intensive intervention for children with early-onset conduct problems. The programme includes a mix of school- and home-based strategic interventions from Grade 1 through high school. Fast Track has been shown to produce sustained reductions in conduct problems and involvement with deviant peer groups—two of the leading predictors of illicit drug use (Conduct Problems Prevention Research Group 2002).

A second evidence-based programme targeting core vulnerabilities is the *Life Skills Program* (Botvin et al. 1995, 2000). It seeks to improve health and well-being through a mix of school- and family-based sessions that target self-esteem, self-confidence, knowledge and cognitive and behavioural skills (Botvin et al. 2000). LSP has been shown to reduce alcohol, tobacco and cannabis during high school (Botvin et al. 1995) and to reduce the lifetime prevalence of illicit drug use (other than cannabis) by 25% (Botvin et al. 2000). These results suggest that enhancing social resistance skills and building a broad set of general life skills can prevent or at least delay the initiation of illicit drug use.

Conclusions

Adolescence and young adulthood is a developmental period of heightened vulnerability to the initiation of illicit drug use. Most young people who are exposed to illicit drugs do not initiate use, but a significant proportion of young people who do go on to develop drug-related problems and dependence. Evidence favours common liability models of illicit drug use over the gateway hypothesis and the impact of diverse and often-nested social systems on drug use. Consistent with the common liability and multilevel systems models, evidence-based prevention programmes include a mix of drug-focused and generic skills training and partnership approaches that build coalitions or partnerships between families, schools and communities.

Acknowledgements The first author was supported by the Australian National Health and Medical Research Council (Project APP1087781) and the Australian Research Council (Discovery Project DP100102015).

References

Abar C, Turrisi R. How important are parents during the college years? A longitudinal perspective of indirect influences parents yield on their college teens' alcohol use. Addict Behav. 2008;33:1360–8.

Adhikari P, Summerill A. 1998 National Drug Strategy Household Survey: detailed findings. Canberra: Australian Institute of Health and Welfare; 2000.

Agrawal A, Grant JD, Waldron M, Duncan AE, Scherrer JF, Lynskey MT, et al. Risk for initiation of substance use as a function of age of onset of cigarette, alcohol and cannabis use: findings in a Midwestern female twin cohort. Prev Med. 2006;43:125–8.

Agrawal A, Lynskey MT. The genetic epidemiology of cannabis use, abuse and dependence. Addiction. 2006;101:801–12.

AIHW. 2004 National Drug Strategy Household Survey: detailed findings. Canberra: Australian Institute of Health and Welfare; 2005.

AIHW. National Drug Strategy Household Survey detailed report 2013. Canberra: Australian Institute of Health and Welfare; 2014.

Anthony JC, Warner LA, Kessler RC. Comparative epidemiology of dependence on tobacco, alcohol, controlled substances, and inhalants: basic findings from the National Comorbidity Survey. Exp Clin Psychopharmacol. 1994;2:244–68.

Anthony JC. The epidemiology of cannabis dependence. In: Roffman RA, Stephens RS, editors. Cannabis dependence: its nature, consequences and treatment. Cambridge: Cambridge University Press; 2006. p. 58–105.

Apantaku-Olajide T, Darker CD, Smyth BP. Onset of cocaine use: associated alcohol intoxication and psychosocial characteristics among adolescents in substance abuse treatment. J Addict Med. 2013;7:183–8.

Baggio S, Studer J, Mohler-Kuo M, Daeppen JB, Gmel G. Profiles of drug users in Switzerland and effects of early-onset intensive use of alcohol, tobacco and cannabis on other illicit drug use. Swiss Med Wkly. 2013;143:w13805.

Bahr SJ, Hoffman JP, Yang X. Parental and peer influences on the risk of adolescent drug use. J Prim Prev. 2005;26:529–51.

Bandura A. Social-learning theory of identificatory processes. In: Goslin DA, editor. Handbook of socialization theory and research. Chicago: Rand McNally; 1969. p. 213–62.

Barnes GM, Reifman AS, Farrell MP, Dintcheff BA. The effects of parenting on the development of adolescent alcohol misuse: a six-wave latent growth model. J Marriage Fam. 2000;62:175–86.

Barnes GM, Hoffman JH, Welte JW, Farrell MP, Dintcheff BA. Effects of parental monitoring and peer deviance on substance use and delinquency. J Marriage Fam. 2006;68:1084–104.

Becker J, Schaub MP, Gmel G, Haug S. Cannabis use and other predictors of the onset of daily cigarette use in young men: what matters most? Results from a longitudinal study. BMC Public Health. 2015;15:843.

Behrendt S, Beesdo-Baum K, Hofler M, Perkonigg A, Buhringer G, Lieb R, et al. The relevance of age at first alcohol and nicotine use for initiation of cannabis use and progression to cannabis use disorders. Drug Alcohol Depend. 2012;123:48–56.

Bennett ME, Walters ST, Miller JH, Woodall WG. Relationship of early inhalant use to substance use in college students. J Subst Abus. 2000;12:227–40.

Boden JM, Fergusson DM, Horwood LJ. Illicit drug use and dependence in a New Zealand birth cohort. Aust N Z J Psychiatry. 2006;40:156–63.

Botvin GJ. Substance abuse prevention research: recent developments and future directions. J Sch Health. 1986;56:369–74.

Botvin GJ, Baker E, Dusenbury L, Botvin EM, Diaz T. Long-term follow-up results of a randomized drug abuse prevention trial in a White middle-class population. JAMA. 1995;273: 1106–12.

Botvin GJ, Griffin KW, Diaz T, Scheier LM, Williams C, Epstein JA. Preventing illicit drug use in adolescents: long-term follow-up data from a randomized control trial of a school population. Addict Behav. 2000;25:769–74.

Bracken BK, Rodolico J, Hill KP. Sex, age, and progression of drug use in adolescents admitted for substance use disorder treatment in the northeastern United States: comparison with a national survey. Subst Abus. 2013;34:263–72.

Bronfenbrenner U. Ecological systems theory. In: Vasta R, editor. Annals of child development, Six theories of child development: revised formulations and current issues, vol. 6. London: JAI Press; 1989. p. 197–249.

Brook JS, Whiteman M, Finch S, Cohen P. Longitudinally foretelling drug use in the late twenties: adolescent personality and social-environmental antecedents. J Genet Psychol. 2000;161: 37–51.

Butterworth P, Slade T, Degenhardt L. Factors associated with the timing and onset of cannabis use and cannabis use disorder: results from the 2007 Australian National Survey of Mental Health and Well-Being. Drug Alcohol Rev. 2014;33:555–64.

Capaldi DM, Stoolmiller M, Kim HK, Yoerger K. Growth in alcohol use in at-risk adolescent boys: two-part random effects prediction models. Drug Alcohol Depend. 2009;105:109–17.

Catalano RF, Kosterman R, Hawkins JD, Newcomb MD. Modeling the etiology of adolescent substance use: a test of the social development model. J Drug Issues. 1996;26:429–55.

Cerda M, Bordelois PM, Keyes KM, Galea S, Koenen KC, Pardini D. Cumulative and recent psychiatric symptoms as predictors of substance use onset: does timing matter? Addiction. 2013;108:2119–28.

Chan GCK, Kelly AB, Toumbourou JW, Hemphill SA, Young RM, Haynes MA, et al. Predicting steep escalations in alcohol use over the teenage years: age-related variations in key social influences. Addiction. 2013;108:1924–32.

Charach A, Yeung E, Climans T, Lillie E. Childhood attention-deficit/hyperactivity disorder and future substance use disorders: comparative meta-analyses. J Am Acad Child Adolesc Psychiatry. 2011;50:9–21.

Chen X, Yu B, Lasopa SO, Cottler LB. Current patterns of marijuana use initiation by age among US adolescents and emerging adults: implications for intervention. Am J Drug Alcohol Abuse. 2017;43(3):261–70.

Cho H, Hallfors DD, Iritani BJ. Early initiation of substance use and subsequent risk factors related to suicide among urban high school students. Addict Behav. 2007;32:1628–39.

Choquet M, Hassler C, Morin D, Falissard B, Chau N. Perceived parenting styles and tobacco, alcohol and cannabis use among French adolescents: gender and family structure differentials. Alcohol Alcohol. 2008;43:73–80.

Clinton-Sherrod M, Sobeck J, Abbey A, Agius E, Terry K. The role of psychosocial factors in the transition to substance use: are they protective among urban minority adolescents? J Prim Prev. 2005;26:511–28.

Colell E, Sanchez-Niubo A, Domingo-Salvany A. Sex differences in the cumulative incidence of substance use by birth cohort. Int J Drug Policy. 2013;24:319–25.

Conduct Problems Prevention Research Group. The implementation of the Fast Track Program: an example of a large-scale prevention science efficacy trial. J Abnorm Child Psychol. 2002;30:1–17.

Crean RD, Crane NA, Mason BJ. An evidence based review of acute and long-term effects of cannabis use on executive cognitive functions. J Addict Med. 2011;5(1):1–8.

Degenhardt L, Coffey C, Carlin JB, Moran P, Patton GC. Who are the new amphetamine users? A 10-year prospective study of young Australians. Addiction. 2007a;102:1269–79.

Degenhardt L, Coffey C, Moran P, Carlin JB, Patton GC. The predictors and consequences of adolescent amphetamine use: findings from the Victoria Adolescent Health Cohort Study. Addiction. 2007b;102:1076–84.

Degenhardt L, Chiu WT, Sampson N, Kessler RC, Anthony JC, Angermeyer M, et al. Toward a global view of alcohol, tobacco, cannabis, and cocaine use: findings from the WHO World Mental Health Surveys. PLoS Med. 2008;5:e141.

Degenhardt L, Dierker L, Chiu WT, Medina-Mora ME, Neumark Y, Sampson N, et al. Evaluating the drug use "gateway" theory using cross-national data: consistency and associations of the order of initiation of drug use among participants in the WHO World Mental Health Surveys. Drug Alcohol Depend. 2010;108:84–97.

Degenhardt L, Hall W. Extent of illicit drug use and dependence and their contribution to the global burden of disease. Lancet. 2012;379:55–70.

Dodge KA, Greenberg MT, Malone PS. Testing an idealized dynamic cascade model of the development of serious violence in adolescence. Child Dev. 2008;79:1907–27.

Dodge KA, Malone PS, Lansford JE, Miller S, Pettit GS, Bates JE. A dynamic cascade model of the development of substance-use onset. Monogr Soc Res Child Dev. 2009;74:1–31.

Donovan JE, Jessor R. Structure of problem behavior in adolescence and young adulthood. J Consult Clin Psychol. 1985;53:890–904.

Downing J, Bellis MA. Early pubertal onset and its relationship with sexual risk taking, substance use and anti-social behaviour: a preliminary cross-sectional study. BMC Public Health. 2009;9:446.

Dudovitz RN, Chung PJ, Elliott MN, Davies SL, Tortolero S, Baumler E, et al. Relationship of age for grade and pubertal stage to early initiation of substance use. Prev Chronic Dis. 2015;12:E203.

DuRant RH, Smith JA, Kreiter SR, Krowchuk DP. The relationship between early age of onset of initial substance use and engaging in multiple health risk behaviors among young adolescents. Arch Pediatr Adolesc Med. 1999;153:286–91.

Ellickson PL, Hays RD, Bell RM. Stepping through the drug use sequence: longitudinal scalogram analysis of initiation and regular use. J Abnorm Psychol. 1992;101:441–51.

EMCDDA. Prevalence maps—prevalence of drug use in Europe. Publications Office of the European Union, Luxembourg. 2016a. http://www.emcdda.europa.eu/countries/prevalence-maps. Accessed 13 Jan 2018.

EMCDDA. European Drug Report 2016: trends and developments. Luxembourg: Publications Office of the European Union; 2016b.

Ennett ST, Foshee VA, Bauman KE, Hussong A, Cai L, Luz H, et al. The social ecology of adolescent alcohol misuse. Child Dev. 2008;79:1777–91.

Fagan AA, Najman JM. The relative contributions of parental and sibling substance use to adolescent tobacco, alcohol and other drug use. J Drug Issues. 2005;35:531–44.

Fergusson DM, Lynskey MT, Horwood LJ. The short-term consequences of early onset cannabis use. J Abnorm Child Psychol. 1996;24:499–512.

Fergusson DM, Horwood LJ. Cannabis use and traffic accidents in a birth cohort of young adults. Accid Anal Prev. 2001;33:703–11.

Fergusson DM, Horwood LJ, Swain-Campbell NR. Cannabis dependence and psychotic symptoms in young people. Psychol Med. 2003a;33:15–21.

Fergusson DM, Swain-Campbell NR, Horwood LJ. Arrests and convictions for cannabis related offences in a New Zealand birth cohort. Drug Alcohol Depend. 2003b;70:53–63.

Fite PJ, Wynn P, Lochman JE, Wells KC. The influence of neighborhood disadvantage and perceived disapproval on early substance use initiation. Addict Behav. 2009;34:769–71.

Galera C, Bouvard MP, Melchior M, Chastang JF, Lagarde E, Michel G, et al. Disruptive symptoms in childhood and adolescence and early initiation of tobacco and cannabis use: the Gazel Youth study. Eur Psychiatry. 2010;25:402–8.

Gogtay N, Giedd JN, Lusk L, Hayashi KM, Greenstein D, Vaituzis AC, et al. Dynamic mapping of human cortical development during childhood through early adulthood. Proc Natl Acad Sci U S A. 2004;101:8174–9.

Greenberg MT, Feinberg M, Gomez BJ, Osgood DW. Testing a community prevention focused model of coalition functioning and sustainability: a comprehensive study of Communities That

Care in Pennsylvania. In: Stockwell PJ, Toumbourou JW, Loxley W, editors. Preventing harmful substance use: the evidence base for policy and practice. London: Wiley; 2005. p. 129–42.
Hall W, Solowij N. Adverse effects of cannabis. Lancet. 1998;352:1611–6.
Hall W. The adverse health effects of cannabis use: what are they, and what are their implications for policy? Int J Drug Policy. 2009;20:458–66.
Hall W, Prichard J, Kirkbride P, Bruno R, Thai P, Gartner C, et al. An analysis of ethical issues in using wastewater analysis to monitor illicit drug use. Addiction. 2012;107(10):1767–73.
Haug S, Nunez CL, Becker J, Gmel G, Schaub MP. Predictors of onset of cannabis and other drug use in male young adults: results from a longitudinal study. BMC Public Health. 2014;14:1202.
Hawkins JD, Brown EC, Oesterle S, Arthur MW, Abbott RD, Catalano P. Early effects of communities that care on targeted risks and intiation of delinquent behavior and substance use. J Adolesc Health. 2008;43:15–22.
Hawkins JD, Oesterle S, Brown EC, Arthur MW, Abbott RD, Fagan AA, et al. Results of a Type 2 translational research trial to prevent adolescent drug use and delinquency. Arch Pediatr Adolesc Med. 2009;163:789–98.
Hirschi T. Causes of delinquency. Berkeley: University of California Press; 1971.
Jessor R. Risk behavior in adolescence: a psychosocial framework for understanding and action. J Adolesc Health. 1991;12:597–605.
Johnson D. Age of illicit drug initiation. Canberra: Australian Institute of Criminology; 2001.
Johnston LD, Miech RA, O'Malley PM, Bachman JG, Schulenberg JE. University of Michigan News Service, December 13: Teen use of any illicit drug other than marijuana at new low, same true for alcohol. University of Michigan, Ann Arbor. 2016. http://ns.umich.edu/new/releases/24385-teen-use-of-any-illicit-drug-other-than-marijuana-at-new-low-same-true-for-alcohol. Accessed 13 Jan 2018.
Kandel D. Stages in adolescent involvement in drug use. Science. 1975;190:912–4.
Kandel DB, Yamaguchi K, Klein LC. Testing the gateway hypothesis. Addiction. 2006;101:470–2; discussion 4–6.
Kelly AB. Predictors of response to brief smoking cessation interventions for adolescents who have contravened school smoking policy. J Subst Use. 2008;13:219–24.
Kelly AB, O'Flaherty M, Connor JP, Homel R, Toumbourou JW, Patton GC, et al. The influence of parents, siblings, and peers on pre- and early-teen smoking: a multi-level model. Drug Alcohol Rev. 2011a;30:381–7.
Kelly AB, O'Flaherty M, Toumbourou JW, Connor JP, Hemphill S, Catalano RF. Gender differences in the impact of families on alcohol use: a lagged longitudinal study of pre-teens. Addiction. 2011b;106:1427–36.
Kelly AB, Toumbourou JW, O'Flaherty M, Patton GC, Homel R, Connor JP, et al. Family risks for early alcohol use: evidence for gender-specific risk processes. J Stud Alcohol Drugs. 2011c;72:399–407.
Kelly AB, Chan GCK, Toumbourou JW, O'Flaherty M, Homel R, Patton GC, et al. Very young adolescents and alcohol: evidence of a unique susceptibility to peer alcohol use. Addict Behav. 2012;37:414–9.
Kelly AB, Connor JP. Review: some universal family-based prevention programmes provide small reductions in alcohol use in youths in the short and long term. Evid Based Ment Health. 2012;15:16.
Kelly AB, Evans-Whipp TJ, Smith R, Chan GCK, Toumbourou JW, Patton GC, et al. A longitudinal study of the association of adolescent polydrug use, alcohol use and high school non-completion. Addiction. 2015;110:627–35.
Kelly AB. Perceived father's care: protects adolescents from transitions to tobacco use at a highly vulnerable age: a short-term longitudinal study. Ment Health Subst Use. 2012;5:173–81.
Kipping RR, Smith M, Heron J, Hickman M, Campbell R. Multiple risk behaviour in adolescence and socio-economic status: findings from a UK birth cohort. Eur J Pub Health. 2015;25:44–9.
Kirisci L, Tarter R, Ridenour T, Zhai ZW, Fishbein D, Reynolds M, et al. Age of alcohol and cannabis use onset mediates the association of transmissible risk in childhood and development

of alcohol and cannabis disorders: evidence for common liability. Exp Clin Psychopharmacol. 2013;21:38–45.
Lanza ST, Collins LM. Pubertal timing and the onset of substance use in females during early adolescence. Prev Sci. 2002;3:69–82.
Lenton S, Liang W, Chikritzhs T. Evidence of increasing age of onset of cannabis use among younger Australians. Addiction. 2012;107:650–7.
Li HK, Kelly AB, Chan GC, Toumbourou JW, Patton GC, Williams JW. The association of puberty and young adolescent alcohol use: do parents have a moderating role? Addict Behav. 2014;39:1389–93.
Lynskey M, Hall W. The effects of adolescent cannabis use on educational attainment: a review. Addiction. 2000;95:1621–30.
Lynskey MT, Heath AC, Bucholz KK, Slutske WS, Madden PA, Nelson EC, et al. Escalation of drug use in early-onset cannabis users vs co-twin controls. JAMA. 2003;289:427–33.
Martino SC, Ellickson PL, McCaffrey DF. Multiple trajectories of peer and parental influence and their association with the development of adolescent heavy drinking. Addict Behav. 2009;34:693–700.
Masse LC, Tremblay RE. Behavior of boys in kindergarten and the onset of substance use during adolescence. Arch Gen Psychiatry. 1997;54:62–8.
Masterman PW, Kelly AB. Reaching adolescents who drink harmfully: fitting intervention to developmental reality. J Subst Abus Treat. 2003;24:347–55.
Mayet A, Legleye S, Beck F, Falissard B, Chau N. The gateway hypothesis, common liability to addictions or the route of administration model: a modelling process linking the three theories. Eur Addict Res. 2016;22:107–17.
Monahan KC, Steinberg L, Cauffman E. Affiliation with antisocial peers, susceptability to peer influence, and antisocial behavior during the transition to adulthood. Dev Psychol. 2009;45:1520–30.
NIDA. Nationwide trends (National Survey on Drug Use and Health 2013). Bethesda, MD: National Institute on Drug Abuse, National Institutes of Health, U.S. Department of Health and Human Services; 2015.
Novak SP, Håkansson A, Martinez-Raga J, Reimer J, Krotki K, Varughese S. Nonmedical use of prescription drugs in the European Union. BMC Psychiatry. 2016;16:274.
O'Brien J, Grant S, Mueller J, Tscharke B, Gerber C, White J. National Wastewater Drug Monitoring Program Report 1, March 2017. The University of Queensland and The University of South Australia on behalf of the Australian Criminal Intelligence Commission. Canberra: Commonwealth of Australia; 2017.
Quek L-H, Chan GCK, White A, Connor JP, Baker P, Saunders JB, et al. Concurrent and simultaneous polydrug use: latent class analysis of an Australian nationally representative sample of young adults. Front Public Health. 2013;1:61. https://doi.org/10.3389/fpubh.2013.00061.
Rahimi-Movaghar A, Amin-Esmaeili M, Shadloo B, Noroozi A, Malekinejad M. Transition to injecting drug use in Iran: a systematic review of qualitative and quantitative evidence. Int J Drug Policy. 2015;26:808–19.
Rajan KB, Leroux BG, Peterson AV Jr, Bricker JB, Andersen MR, Kealey KA, et al. Nine-year prospective association between older siblings' smoking and children's daily smoking. J Adolesc Health. 2003;33:25–30.
Redmond C, Spoth R, Shin C, Schainker L, Greenberg M, Feinberg M. Long-term protective factor outcomes of evidence-based interventions implemented by community teams through a community–university partnership. J Prim Prev. 2009;30:513–30.
Rhee S, Hewitt JK, Young SE, Corley RP, Crowley TJ, Stallings MC. Genetic and environmental influences on substance initiation, use, and problem use in adolescents. Arch Gen Psychiatry. 2003;60:1256–64.
Rowland B, Toumbourou JW, Osborn A, Smith R, Hall JK, Kremer P, et al. A clustered randomised trial examining the effect of social marketing and community mobilisation on the age of uptake and levels of alcohol consumption by Australian adolescents. BMJ Open. 2013;3:e002423.

Salom C, Holman A, Connor JP, Toumbourou JW, Kelly AB. Evidence that community based prevention reduces adolescent alcohol use: a commentary on Gilligan et al. Drug Alcohol Rev. 2012;31:930–1.

Simons-Morton B. Prospective association of peer influence, school engagement, drinking expectancies, and parent expectations with drinking initiation among sixth graders. Addict Behav. 2004;29:299–309.

Smith D, Kelly AB, Chan GCK, Toumbourou JW, Patton GC, Williams J. Beyond the primary influences of parents and peers on very young adolescent alcohol use: evidence of independent neighbourhood effects. J Early Adolesc. 2014;34:568–83.

Spoth R, Greenberg M, Bierman K, Redmond C. PROSPER community-university partnership model for public education systems: capacity-building for evidence-based, competence-building prevention. Prev Sci. 2004;5:31–9.

Spoth R, Trudeau L, Guyll M, Shin C, Redmond C. Universal intervention effects on substance use among young adults mediated by delayed adolescent substance initiation. J Consult Clin Psychol. 2009;77:620–32.

Steinberg L, Monahan KC. Age differences in resistance to peer influence. Dev Psychol. 2007;43:1531–43.

Steinberg L. A social neuroscience perspective on adolescent risk-taking. Dev Rev. 2008;28:78–106.

Swendsen J, Burstein M, Case B, Conway KP, Dierker L, He J, et al. Use and abuse of alcohol and illicit drugs in US adolescents: results of the National Comorbidity Survey-Adolescent Supplement. Arch Gen Psychiatry. 2012;69:390–8.

Tarter RE, Vanyukov M, Kirisci L, Reynolds M, Clark DB. Predictors of marijuana use in adolescents before and after licit drug use: examination of the gateway hypothesis. Am J Psychiatry. 2006;163:2134–40.

Tildesley EA, Andrews JA. The development of children's intentions to use alcohol: direct and indirect effects of parent alcohol use and parenting behaviors. Psychol Addict Behav. 2008;22:326–39.

United Nations Office on Drugs and Crime. World drug report 2014. Vienna: UNODC; 2014.

United Nations Office on Drugs and Crime. World drug report 2015. Vienna: UNODC; 2015.

Vanyukov MM, Tarter RE, Kirillova GP, Kirisci L, Reynolds MD, Kreek MJ, et al. Common liability to addiction and "gateway hypothesis": theoretical, empirical and evolutionary perspective. Drug Alcohol Depend. 2012;123:S3–17.

Wagner FA, Anthony GC. From first drug use to drug dependence: developmental periods of risk for dependence upon marijuana, cocaine, and alcohol. Neuropsychopharmacology. 2001;26:479–88.

Weier M, Chan GCK, Quinn C, Hides L, Hall WD. Cannabis use in 14 to 25 year old Australians 1998–2013: Research Monograph 1. Brisbane: Centre for Youth Substance Abuse Research, The University of Queensland; 2016.

White A, Chan GCK, Quek LH, Connor JP, Baker P, Saunders JB, et al. The topography of multiple drug use among adolescent Australians: findings from the National Drug Strategy Household Survey. Addict Behav. 2013;38:2038–73.

Wills TA, Cleary SD. How are social support effects mediated? A test with parental support and adolescent substance use. J Pers Soc Psychol. 1996;71:937–52.

World Health Organization. World Health Report 2002: reducing risks, promoting healthy life. Geneva: WHO; 2002.

The Age of Onset of Alcohol Use Disorders

9

Jason P. Connor, Megan Weier, and Wayne D. Hall

9.1 Introduction

Alcohol remains the most widely used recreational drug among young adults despite an ever-increasing availability of novel psychoactive substances. Approximately 90% of adults in developed countries have consumed alcohol, and 17.6% of men and 10.4% of women in the USA met DSM-5 criteria for alcohol use disorder in the past year (Grant et al. 2015). Individuals with an alcohol use

J. P. Connor
Faculty of Medicine, The University of Queensland, Royal Brisbane and Women's Hospital, Herston, QLD, Australia

Centre for Youth Substance Abuse Research, Faculty of Health and Behavioural Sciences, The University of Queensland, St Lucia, QLD, Australia
e-mail: Jason.Connor@uq.edu.au

M. Weier
Centre for Youth Substance Abuse Research, Faculty of Health and Behavioural Sciences, The University of Queensland, St Lucia, QLD, Australia

National Drug and Alcohol Research Centre, The University of New South Wales, Sydney, NSW, Australia
e-mail: m.weier@unsw.edu.au

W. D. Hall (✉)
Centre for Youth Substance Abuse Research, Faculty of Health and Behavioural Sciences, The University of Queensland, St Lucia, QLD, Australia

Queensland Centre for Mental Health Research, School of Public Health, The University of Queensland, The Park Centre for Mental Health Treatment, Research and Education, Wacol, QLD, Australia

National Addiction Centre, Institute of Psychiatry, Psychology and Neuroscience, King's College London, London, UK
e-mail: w.hall@uq.edu.au

G. de Girolamo et al. (eds.), *Age of Onset of Mental Disorders*,
https://doi.org/10.1007/978-3-319-72619-9_9

disorder account for around half of all the alcohol-related harm in developed societies (Rehm et al. 2009) and contribute to an estimated 4% of the total global disease burden (Rehm et al. 2009).

There is accumulating evidence on the complex range of cultural, environmental and genetic factors associated with individual variations in age of alcohol onset patterns. This chapter summarizes what we know about age of onset of alcohol use and alcohol use disorders and identifies what remains to be understood. It examines factors associated with alcohol use initiation and the relationship between onset, severity of the disorder and individual functioning. It assesses patterns of early and late alcohol use as possible clinical markers for more effective treatment and prevention approaches. Evidence on the effectiveness of public policies to delay age of onset is reviewed. The existing evidence is considered in light of methodological challenges in age of onset research, particularly the more rigorous assessment of the possible causal role of early onset of drinking on risk of alcohol use disorders.

The absence of a standardized definition of age of onset of alcohol use is a major challenge in interpreting the impact on age of onset of alcohol use on psychological functioning, alcohol disorder severity, concurrent psychiatric comorbidity, potential diagnostic markers and prevention effectiveness. Age of onset (Sartor et al. 2016) is variously defined in the alcohol literature as:

- Age of onset of alcohol *initiation*
- Age of first alcohol *intoxication* or when *regularly* consumed
- Age of onset of an *alcohol use disorder*

There is strong cross-sectional evidence that the earlier the age of onset for each of these definitions, the more severe forms of the alcohol use disorder (Sartor et al. 2016). Measures used vary considerably between studies. Kuntsche et al. (2016), for example, cite over 20 examples of different questions used to assess age of onset of *initiation* in the literature. These items vary on the basis of how much was drunk, the definition of a 'sip' or 'taste', the use of dichotomous age thresholds, the presence or absence of adult supervision, the use of one's own drinking vessel (rather than someone else's glass), whether alcohol was used as part of a religious ceremony and the level of intoxication achieved. These variations in measurement are probably important. For example, Wadolowski et al. (2015) identified fundamental differences in risk between alcohol 'sippers' and those that had consumed a 'full' drink in a large sample of adolescent-parent dyads.

Age of onset of alcohol use typically commences in adolescence, and alcohol use disorders are most prevalent between 18 and 29 years of age (Grant et al. 2015). Research in this field therefore largely focuses on these age groups. Drinking pattern data are predominately drawn from high- and middle-income countries and so may not fully represent cultural, religious and economic diversity that may impact on the use and societal interpretation of alcohol onset (Alati 2016; Rehm and Room 2015). We know that age of alcohol initiation across western countries is very similar, with onset increasing from age 11 onwards and peaking in mid-adolescence, despite many cultural and legal differences (Vega et al. 2002).

9.2 Age of Onset of Alcohol Initiation

The most widely studied age of onset measure is the age of initiation. It is also the most controversial. Large-scale studies have consistently reported an association between initiation and subsequent alcohol–related problems (e.g. Hawkins et al. 1997; Rossow and Kuntsche 2013) and alcohol use disorders (e.g. Dawson et al. 2008; Grant and Dawson 1997; Hingson et al. 2006a; Sartor et al. 2016). International guidelines on safe levels of alcohol consumption (e.g. in Australia, the USA, the United Kingdom) that recommend delaying alcohol initiation for as long as possible (e.g. National Health and Medical Research Council 2009) underpin public prevention programmes for alcohol use among young people in many countries.

The body of research on age of first drink has predominately used cross-sectional or retrospective designs. An association is well documented between age of initiation of alcohol use and mood disorders (Birrell et al. 2016), psychosis and impaired interpersonal functioning (Compton et al. 2009), alcohol-related violence, drink driving, vocational absenteeism and the risk of using other drugs (Gruber et al. 1996; Pilatti et al. 2013; Sanchez et al. 2013). Studies that ask subjects to recall the age at which they had their first drink may introduce memory bias. For example, Sartor et al. (2011) asked over 1700 participants in a multi-wave prospective study to indicate the age they first consumed alcohol. Responding to the same question 4 years later, the majority reported an older age of onset than that originally provided, with one-third reporting an age of onset that differed by 2 years from their initial estimate.

A more fundamental challenge with cross-sectional or retrospective designs is demonstrating that age of initiation plays a causal role in the development of later alcohol use disorders and alcohol-related problems. This is because those who initiate alcohol use early are not a random sample of their birth cohort. It is well documented that they are more likely than their peers to have concurrent behavioural problems (Donovan 2004), to be impulsive (Mason and Spoth 2012) and to have heavier drinking parents and peers (Donovan 2004; Rothman et al. 2008), and they may have an increased genetic vulnerability to develop alcohol disorders and alcohol-related social problems (Schmid et al. 2010). Well-controlled cross-sectional studies that attempt to statistically account for these alterative explanations provide a stronger case for a causal effect of early alcohol initiation on future alcohol and non-alcohol-related problems, but possible causal mechanisms remain to be identified. Where prospective studies have been conducted, the evidence for causation still remains uncertain (see Maimaris and McCambridge 2014) because of a lack of replication due to measurement variation and inability to statistically control for important predictors of alcohol use disorders such as familial and genetic risk.

Even if studies used a reliable and valid approach to measure age of alcohol initiation, several key theoretical challenges remain in assessing the possible causal role of early initiation. Kuntsche et al. (2013, 2016) critique the theoretical behavioural, social and neurobiological early-onset mechanisms proposed to underpin subsequent heavy drinking. They challenge the notion that one sip or alcoholic drink early in a child or adolescent's life can fundamentally shift the trajectory of subsequent alcohol-related problems. Biological hypotheses that include neuroadaptation of the adolescent brain require repeated exposure to alcohol. Although no human thresholds of changes in brain architecture have been reliably established, it is unlikely that a single early exposure (either a sip or a full drink) would permanently affect neurological functioning in ways that make heavy drinking more likely in young adulthood. There is more compelling evidence that regular or 'intermittent' binge drinking in adolescent alcohol use can have a sustained impact on adult synaptic functioning and impair cognitive performance (Crews et al. 2016, p. 1100). Kuntsche et al. (2013, 2016) also identified poor coping strategies, social engagement and self-efficacy as key risk factors for both early initiation and the later development of alcohol problems.

Researchers agree that early initiation is reliably associated with an increased risk of a wide range of poor psychological, behavioural, social, academic, alcohol, and other substance use outcomes (Birrell et al. 2016; Crum et al. 2008; Guttmannova et al. 2011, 2012; Schmid et al. 2010; Warner et al. 2007). Satisfying the stringent methodological requirements to establish that early initiation plays a causal role in these outcomes may be less important if age of initiation is a robust risk marker that can inform the design of treatment and prevention approaches. In other words, are the underlying risk factors associated with early initiation the same ones that are associated with subsequent problem drinking? If so, establishing causation may not be necessary to use age of initiation to inform effective treatment and prevention programmes.

Guttmannova et al. (2011) tested the marker hypothesis by statistically controlling for mediating factors that were predictors of early onset of drinking and of developing alcohol problems in adulthood. In a two-decade-long prospective study (with 92% retention), they found that age of onset of drinking before 11 years of age was a predictor of increased chronicity of alcohol adult dependence, after controlling for potential mediating factors. Similar findings were observed in a 10-year prospective study by King and Chassin (2007) in which initiation before age 13 was a key predictor of the risk of adult substance dependence. Based on these findings, Guttmannova et al. (2011) and King and Chassin (2007) recommended delaying age of onset of initiation of drinking as a prevention strategy. Neither study measured genetic vulnerability to alcohol use disorder, which was a major limitation.

There is convincing evidence that age of drinking onset is related to familial risk factors for alcohol problems. The number of first-degree and second-degree relatives with alcohol dependence (familial density) is associated with a higher risk of early alcohol use onset in offspring. This probably reflects a combination of learned behaviour, other environmental characteristics and genetic risk. In a large-scale twin study, Prescott and Kendler (1999) found that the relationship between early age of initiation and alcohol dependence (DSM-IV) was explained by both shared environmental and genetic factors and the familial association was lower for alcohol abuse (DSM-IV). In a follow-up study that used newer diagnostic criteria (DSM-5) for alcohol use disorder which combine abuse and dependence into one diagnostic entity (Hasin et al. 2013), Ystrom et al. (2014) reported that the association between age of initiation and alcohol use disorders was primarily explained by a shared genetic vulnerability to initiate alcohol use early and later develop alcohol use disorders. Independent, non-genetic risk factors were estimated to contribute to only 1% of the risk of developing an alcohol use disorder. Both studies excluded a causal link and cautioned that prevention programmes that solely aim to delay the onset of alcohol use were unlikely to be successful.

9.3 Age of Onset of Alcohol Intoxication and Regular Drinking

Some have argued that age of first intoxication may be more important than age of alcohol initiation in predicting risk of future alcohol problems (Morean et al. 2014). These findings are consistent with the findings of Warner and White's (2003) 20-year prospective study which found that the best predictor of adult alcohol problems was feeling drunk at first use, after potential confounders were accounted for in the statistical analysis. These findings have been replicated in a large 'at-risk' sample study of European and African-Americans with a family history of alcohol problems (Sartor et al. 2016). Sartor et al. found that increasingly powerful predictors of risk of subsequent alcohol use disorder were age of onset of alcohol initiation, followed by age of onset of intoxication and age of onset of regular drinking (Sartor et al. 2016). These relationships persisted after accounting for a wide range of demographic, psychosocial and psychiatric factors. There is emerging evidence in some studies that a shorter latency between onset and first intoxication may be an additional clinical marker of increased risk (Morean et al. 2014). These findings suggest that the age of the first taste or sip of alcohol may not be the most robust indicator of the risk of future alcohol problems. Age of onset of more regular use and use to intoxication potentially may have more clinical and prevention utility.

The superior predictive power of early drunkenness over initiation was illustrated in a large-scale study of almost 45,000 students aged 15 years in North America and Europe (Kuntsche et al. 2013). All students, split relatively equally by gender, were recruited based on reported alcohol use. Age of first drink was not a direct risk factor for subsequent alcohol, other drug, violence and academic problems. Only after age of first episode of drunkenness was accounted for was there a strong association between age of onset and these problem behaviours. Consequently, Kuntsche et al. (2013) recommend a prevention focus that minimizes adolescent drunkenness, rather than on simply delaying first use of alcohol.

Prospective studies also point to age of regular drinking or drunkenness as a more robust indicator of the risk of later developing alcohol problems. In a three-decade follow-up study, Pitkanen et al. (2005) found early onset of regular drinking, measured as getting drunk or using regularly, was associated with all four CAGE screen items (Ewing 1984) and a modified Michigan Alcoholism Screening Test (MAST) (Seppa et al. 1990) in adulthood. These findings were replicated on the full MAST by Ohannessian et al. (2015). More severe alcohol problems were associated with higher morbidity (Connor et al. 2016), but few studies have examined the relationship between onset of drunkenness and premature death. A drunkenness-mortality association was found by Hu et al. (2017) who linked approximately 15,000 death records to survey data collected 27 years earlier. They found significantly higher mortality rates among those reporting their first episode of alcohol intoxication before 15 years of age. This finding remained after including those without an alcohol use disorder, indicating the direct and indirect effect of other concurrent risk factors in age of onset research. While recognizing methodological limitations in these studies, the body of current evidence suggests that the age of onset of regular alcohol consumption, and especially drunkenness, is more strongly associated with adult alcohol problems, mortality and psychiatric and physical morbidity than is the age at which a person has their first drink of alcohol.

9.4 Age of Onset of Alcohol Use Disorder

The earlier an individual has their first drink of alcohol, typically the shorter the time between their first use and the development of alcohol dependence (Sartor et al. 2009). The level of intoxication or drunkenness, as we have seen, may be a more nuanced indicator of later risk of alcohol use disorders. Age of onset of alcohol-related problems has been considered a key marker of alcohol use disorder severity and treatment outcome in common subtypes of drinking. For example, Cloninger's *Type II* (Cloninger 1987) and Babor's *Type B* (Babor et al. 1992) 'alcoholics' exhibit more severe alcohol problems at a much earlier age than Type 1 or Type A 'alcoholics', who have a later onset and develop less severe alcohol-related problems. The more severe subtypes of alcohol dependence are also more likely to include polysubstance use, chronic treatment history, the presence of other risky behaviour and a novelty-seeking personality. Early age of onset of alcohol dependence is also associated with a large maximum drinking quantity, rapid progression from regular drinking to dependence and greater psychiatric comorbidity (Chen et al. 2011). Although large-scale studies report early age of onset of alcohol problems as an important clinical marker of severity (Chen et al. 2011), this criterion is not reflected in any recognized international diagnostic system (i.e. DSM-5, ICD-10).

Those with early-onset alcohol dependence, often defined as before 22 years of age, have a strong family history of drinking problems (Chen et al. 2011; Chorlian et al. 2013; Le Strat et al. 2010), especially among females (Chen et al. 2011). These early typologies of alcohol dependence severity were proposed largely on the basis of statistical clusters in clinical observations, patient and family histories and theoretical assumptions. With the advent of more advanced approaches to genetic analysis, confirmation that there is a genetic liability for early onset of dependence is available from large genome-wide association studies (GWAS) (e.g. Kapoor et al. 2014). However recent GWAS with larger, more heterogeneous samples indicate that the association between specific genetic polymorphisms and age of onset may be more modest than originally thought (Kapoor et al. 2016). These findings are consistent with there being a general genetic risk factor for alcohol dependence in

GWAS in which individual risk alleles explain less than 1% of the overall association with dependence (Heath et al. 2011; Palmer et al. 2012). The risk alleles identified are implicated in neurotransmitter responses to alcohol (e.g. dopaminergic, GABAergic, serotonergic), impulsivity, psychiatric comorbidity and other drug use.

Few of the genes implicated in early age of onset of alcohol dependence have been replicated. Those identified in GWAS tend to be non-functional or lack a clear mechanism that would explain how they affect phenotypic variations in alcohol use. Among the potential candidate genes replicated in some, but not all, studies are those involved in dopaminergic function. One of the most widely studied age of dependence onset genetic markers is the *TaqI* A dopamine receptor (DRD2) polymorphism, which is strongly expressed in the brain, particularly in reward areas. Located on chromosome 11q22-23, the *A1* allele of the *TaqI* restriction fragment length DRD2 polymorphism is hypothesized to be associated with reduced dopamine function via lower neuronal expression of dopamine receptors. Carriers of the A1 risk allele are thought to require larger quantities of alcohol and other substances to produce the same dopamine response as their non-A1 counterparts (Noble 1998, 2000). This potentially places them at higher risk for early-onset alcohol dependence. Among treatment-seeking, alcohol-dependent inpatients, Connor et al. (2002, 2008) found that patients carrying the A1 risk allele were more likely to start problem drinking earlier and had a shorter latency between onset of drinking and development of dependence. These findings were not replicated in a later study (Pinto et al. 2009). While heritability estimates are high for age of onset of alcohol dependence, specific genetic markers for this risk are generally weak predictors, and their role is poorly understood. Future research is likely to employ higher-powered GWAS across large numbers of single-nucleotide polymorphisms (SNPS) in an attempt to identify remaining genetic risk factors.

Those with early-onset alcohol dependence have more impaired adult functioning than those with later onset. Many of the psychiatric and social correlates are similar to age of onset of initiation, reflecting challenges in identifying casual links between initiation and dependence. These risk factors can include more severe internalizing (Gorka et al. 2014; Le Strat et al. 2010; Meier et al. 2013; Menary et al. 2017) and externalizing (Meier et al. 2013) symptoms, more childhood developmental and behavioural problems (Charach et al. 2011; Le Strat et al. 2010) and other substance use disorders (Le Strat et al. 2010; Meier et al. 2013).

One risk domain that has received attention in age of onset of dependence research is cognitive functioning. Neuropsychological studies of early-onset dependence have confirmed hypotheses derived from clinical observation and alcohol assessment histories. Early onset of alcohol dependence is associated with higher impulsivity, antisocial traits and attention deficit hyperactivity (Joos et al. 2013). Imaging studies suggest that dependent early-onset drinkers are more likely to have brain structural abnormalities than their peers, predominately in the prefrontal cortex with smaller brain volume and reduced white matter volume (De Bellis et al. 2005).

9.5 Potential Clinical Utility

Can the association between age of onset of drinking and problem drinking be used to improve the effectiveness of alcohol dependence treatment? Despite the uncertainty about causal mechanisms, this chapter has highlighted that the risk of developing alcohol dependence is associated with a range of age markers, including age of onset of drinking. The research suggests that onset of regular drinking or intoxication may be a stronger clinical indicator of future problems than drinking initiation. In the three-decade long Dunedin birth cohort study, daily drinking before 18 years of age was the strongest predictor of alcohol dependence in adulthood (Meier et al. 2013). Based on these data, Meier et al. (2013) identified a number of fundamentally different developmental trajectories to persistent problem alcohol and other drug use in adulthood. In addition to early onset of drinking, individuals at greatest risk of persistent adult alcohol dependence had a history of early severe behavioural problems, a family history of psychiatric disorders and extreme levels of negative affect. For these reasons, they argued that age of onset should be incorporated into DSM-5 and ICD-10 diagnostic systems criteria for alcohol use disorders.

On the basis of existing knowledge, one may also anticipate that individuals with early-onset alcohol use and problems may benefit from more intensive treatment (behavioural and/or pharmacological) and may need clinical interventions tailored to their problem profile. Surprisingly there is a paucity of studies that have examined treatment response among persons with alcohol use disorders using age of onset of drinking or of problem alcohol use (Kranzler et al. 2012). The most widely studied medications which purport to show greater efficacy with Type 2 (early-onset) 'alcoholics' are serotonergic agents. Ondansetron (primarily used for nausea in chemotherapy), a selective 5-HT receptor antagonist, has been reported to reduce alcohol craving and consumption more in Type 2 than Type 1 'alcoholics', while persons with either subtype received concurrent cognitive behavioural therapy (CBT). This potentially genetically mediated mechanism (via the SLC6A4 5-HTTLPR polymorphism), however, increased craving in Type 1 (late-onset) 'alcoholics' (see Enoch 2003 for a review). In a study of the selective serotonin reuptake inhibitor (SSRI) antidepressant sertraline, Kranzler et al. (2012) found superior outcomes in the later-onset group given placebo and inferior outcomes in the early-onset group treated with sertraline. These interesting findings require replication.

Early-onset dependent drinkers are less likely to seek alcohol treatment than those with later-onset disorders (Hingson et al. 2006b). Fortunately, approximately 40% of those with adolescent-onset disorders remit by their late 20s and achieve approximately normative social and vocational functioning (Hicks et al. 2010). However, remission studies have largely been limited to males. It is less clear whether cognitive functioning improves with abstinence from alcohol in adolescent-onset cases. Brown et al.'s studies (summarized in Brown and Tapert 2004) have identified modest (~10%) improvements in memory after 3 weeks' abstinence and neurocognitive functioning approximating baseline assessment after a sustained period of abstinence (~4 years). They acknowledge that doing this type of research is challenging in adolescents because their brains are more plastic and additional imaging work is required to inform treatment.

The most common substance use factors associated with risk of alcohol dependence in large cross-sectional and prospective studies are regular drinking, drinking to intoxication and having a family history of substance use disorders. Individual genes predict age of onset of alcohol dependence weakly. Even the most recent age of onset GWAS does not allow us to predict risk with greater accuracy than we can by using a comprehensive family and personal history. Consequently, for an adolescent with a strong family history of substance dependence who has initiated drinking early, the optimal clinical advice is to recommend sustained abstinence. Any comorbid mental health and behavioural problems should also be formally treated to reduce risk of early-onset alcohol use disorders.

9.6 Possible Applications in Prevention

There is an intuitive appeal to stratifying young people by risk markers associated with early alcohol initiation and delivering interventions that target these specific risk factors. Novel prevention approaches that have targeted high-risk groups have been effective (Dietrich et al. 2016), with benefits in some studies extending 3 years post intervention (Newton et al. 2016). Central to these interventions are the assumptions that these risk factors have a causal role in alcohol use disorders and that they can be modified.

Too few studies are available yet that compare the effectiveness of targeted vs universal (generic) prevention approaches to alcohol use disorders. When these studies have been compared, few prospective differences in harmful drinking patterns have been found (e.g. Teesson et al. 2017). Current data do not provide clear guidance on what risk factors are most effective in targeting which prevention approaches to delay alcohol use, or indeed, on whether delaying onset of alcohol use will reduce rates of adult alcohol problems (Maimaris and McCambridge 2014). This is an ongoing area of research and one that will see much more sophisticated research design attempts to disentangle causal factors and risk profiles that inform treatment and prevention approaches.

9.7 Policy Levers

Based on available research, there is modest evidence to support international drinking guidelines that recommend delaying alcohol initiation as a stand-alone policy to reduce subsequent problem drinking. This policy can be justified regardless of whether early initiation is a cause of later alcohol dependence or simply an early marker of increased genetic and other risks of developing alcohol dependence. If the relationship is causal, then delaying initiation may reduce the prevalence of alcohol dependence in adulthood. If it is not causal, delaying initiation of use may still reduce the duration of heavy drinking and perhaps the severity of alcohol dependence that does develop later in adulthood. It may also have the public health benefits of reducing alcohol-related harms, such as accidents, injuries, assaults and suicides during adolescence and young adulthood.

Much more effective public policies with stronger evidence are available that not only may delay the age of onset of alcohol use and reduce alcohol problems, but also have a substantial impact on the overall alcohol-attributable disease burden. These policies make alcohol more expensive by using taxation to increase its price and make alcohol less accessible to adolescents (and adults) by imposing restrictions on the sale and promotion of alcohol. These policies are more effective (Babor et al. 2010; Connor and Hall 2015) and cost-effective but politically unpopular and strenuously opposed by the alcohol industry which prefers ineffective policies such as industry self-regulation and public education about 'responsible drinking'.

Conclusions

Early age of onset of drinking and of alcohol-related problems is associated with developing adult alcohol use disorders. Measurement challenges and methodological limitations weaken the case for earlier use playing a causal role in the onset of future alcohol-related problems. Individuals who initiate drinking earlier than their peers are at elevated risk of developing future alcohol and behavioural disorders for other reasons. Early onset of more regular drinking or drinking to intoxication may be more strongly associated with future alcohol problems than early first use of any alcohol. It remains unclear what the relative contributions are of genetic and concurrent behavioural and psychiatric factors to age on onset of drinking and alcohol use disorders. This uncertainty has, in part, limited the use of age of onset in treatment and prevention. For individuals with early-onset alcohol use or dependence and a strong family history of substance use disorders, abstinence-orientated interventions are a conservative but prudent approach. It is unlikely that the policy to delay age of drinking onset will be effective as a stand-alone intervention, but it may be effective when combined with taxing alcohol more heavily and restricting the sale and promotion of alcohol to young people.

Acknowledgements We would like to thank Sarah Yeates for her editorial assistance in preparing this chapter for publication.

References

Alati R. Should we revisit the 'age at first drink' concept in alcohol research? Addiction. 2016;111:970–1.

Babor T, Caetano R, Casswell S, Edwards G, Giesbrecht N, Graham K, et al. Alcohol: no ordinary commodity: research and public policy. 2nd ed. Oxford: Oxford University Press; 2010.

Babor TF, Hofmann M, DelBoca FK, Hesselbrock V, Meyer RE, Dolinsky ZS, et al. Types of alcoholics, I. Evidence for an empirically derived typology based on indicators of vulnerability and severity. Arch Gen Psychiatry. 1992;49:599–608.

Birrell L, Newton NC, Teesson M, Slade T. Early onset mood disorders and first alcohol use in the general population. J Affect Disord. 2016;200:243–9.
Brown SA, Tapert SF. Adolescence and the trajectory of alcohol use: basic to clinical studies. Ann N Y Acad Sci. 2004;1021:234–44.
Charach A, Yeung E, Climans T, Lillie E. Childhood attention-deficit/hyperactivity disorder and future substance use disorders: comparative meta-analyses. J Am Acad Child Adolesc Psychiatry. 2011;50:9–21.
Chen YC, Prescott CA, Walsh D, Patterson DG, Riley BP, Kendler KS, et al. Different phenotypic and genotypic presentations in alcohol dependence: age at onset matters. J Stud Alcohol Drugs. 2011;72:752–62.
Chorlian DB, Rangaswamy M, Manz N, Wang JC, Dick D, Almasy L, et al. Genetic and neurophysiological correlates of the age of onset of alcohol use disorders in adolescents and young adults. Behav Genet. 2013;43:386–401.
Cloninger CR. Neurogenetic adaptive mechanisms in alcoholism. Science. 1987;236:410–6.
Compton MT, Chien VH, Bollini AM. Associations between past alcohol, cannabis, and cocaine use and current schizotypy among first-degree relatives of patients with schizophrenia and non-psychiatric controls. Psychiatry Q. 2009;80:143–54.
Connor JP, Young RM, Lawford BR, Ritchie TL, Noble EP. D(2) dopamine receptor (DRD2) polymorphism is associated with severity of alcohol dependence. Eur Psychiatry. 2002;17:17–23.
Connor JP, Young RM, Saunders JB, Lawford BR, Ho R, Ritchie TL, et al. The A1 allele of the D2 dopamine receptor gene region, alcohol expectancies and drinking refusal self-efficacy are associated with alcohol dependence severity. Psychiatry Res. 2008;160:94–105.
Connor JP, Hall WD. Alcohol burden in low-income and middle-income countries. Lancet. 2015;386:1922–4.
Connor JP, Haber PS, Hall WD. Seminar: alcohol use disorders. Lancet. 2016;387:988–98.
Crews FT, Vetreno RP, Broadwater MA, Robinson DL. Adolescent alcohol exposure persistently impacts adult neurobiology and behavior. Pharmacol Rev. 2016;68:1074–109.
Crum RM, Storr CL, Ialongo N, Anthony JC. Is depressed mood in childhood associated with an increased risk for initiation of alcohol use during early adolescence? Addict Behav. 2008;33:24–40.
Dawson DA, Goldstein RB, Chou SP, Ruan WJ, Grant BF. Age at first drink and the first incidence of adult-onset DSM-IV alcohol use disorders. Alcohol Clin Exp Res. 2008;32:2149–60.
De Bellis MD, Narasimhan A, Thatcher DL, Keshavan MS, Soloff P, Clark DB. Prefrontal cortex, thalamus, and cerebellar volumes in adolescents and young adults with adolescent-onset alcohol use disorders and comorbid mental disorders. Alcohol Clin Exp Res. 2005;29:1590–600.
Dietrich T, Rundle-Thiele S, Schuster L, Connor JP. A systematic literature review of alcohol education programmes in middle and high school settings (2000-2014). Health Educ. 2016;116:50–68.
Donovan JE. Adolescent alcohol initiation: a review of psychosocial risk factors. J Adolesc Health. 2004;35:529.e7–18.
Enoch MA. Pharmacogenomics of alcohol response and addiction. Am J Pharmacogenomics. 2003;3:217–32.
Ewing JA. Detecting alcoholism. The CAGE questionnaire. JAMA. 1984;252:1905–7.
Gorka SM, Shankman SA, Olino TM, Seeley JR, Kosty DB, Lewinsohn PM. Anxiety disorders and risk for alcohol use disorders: the moderating effect of parental support. Drug Alcohol Depend. 2014;140:191–7.
Grant BF, Dawson DA. Age at onset of alcohol use and its association with DSM-IV alcohol abuse and dependence: results from the National Longitudinal Alcohol Epidemiologic Survey. J Subst Abus. 1997;9:103–10.
Grant BF, Goldstein RB, Saha TD, Chou SP, Jung J, Zhang H, et al. Epidemiology of DSM-5 alcohol use disorder: results from the National Epidemiologic Survey on Alcohol and Related Conditions III. JAMA Psychiat. 2015;72:757–66.
Gruber E, DiClemente RJ, Anderson MM, Lodico M. Early drinking onset and its association with alcohol use and problem behavior in late adolescence. Prev Med. 1996;25:293–300.

Guttmannova K, Bailey JA, Hill KG, Lee JO, Hawkins JD, Woods ML, et al. Sensitive periods for adolescent alcohol use initiation: predicting the lifetime occurrence and chronicity of alcohol problems in adulthood. J Stud Alcohol Drugs. 2011;72:221–31.

Guttmannova K, Hill KG, Bailey JA, Lee JO, Hartigan LA, Hawkins JD, et al. Examining explanatory mechanisms of the effects of early alcohol use on young adult alcohol dependence. J Stud Alcohol Drugs. 2012;73:379–90.

Hasin DS, O'Brien CP, Auriacombe M, Borges G, Bucholz K, Budney A, et al. DSM-5 criteria for substance use disorders: recommendations and rationale. Am J Psychiatry. 2013;170:834–51.

Hawkins JD, Graham JW, Maguin E, Abbott R, Hill KG, Catalano RF. Exploring the effects of age of alcohol use initiation and psychosocial risk factors on subsequent alcohol misuse. J Stud Alcohol. 1997;58:280–90.

Heath AC, Whitfield JB, Martin NG, Pergadia ML, Goate AM, Lind PA, et al. A quantitative-trait genome-wide association study of alcoholism risk in the community: findings and implications. Biol Psychiatry. 2011;70:513–8.

Hicks BM, Iacono WG, McGue M. Consequences of an adolescent onset and persistent course of alcohol dependence in men: adolescent risk factors and adult outcomes. Alcohol Clin Exp Res. 2010;34:819–33.

Hingson RW, Heeren T, Winter MR. Age at drinking onset and alcohol dependence: age at onset, duration, and severity. Arch Pediatr Adolesc Med. 2006a;160:739–46.

Hingson RW, Heeren T, Winter MR. Age of alcohol-dependence onset: associations with severity of dependence and seeking treatment. Pediatrics. 2006b;118:e755–63.

Hu H, Eaton WW, Anthony JC, Wu LT, Cottler LB. Age of first drunkenness and risks for all-cause mortality: a 27-year follow-up from the epidemiologic catchment area study. Drug Alcohol Depend. 2017;176:148–53.

Joos L, Schmaal L, Goudriaan AE, Fransen E, Van den Brink W, Sabbe BG, et al. Age of onset and neuropsychological functioning in alcohol dependent inpatients. Alcohol Clin Exp Res. 2013;37:407–16.

Kapoor M, Wang JC, Wetherill L, Le N, Bertelsen S, Hinrichs AL, et al. Genome-wide survival analysis of age at onset of alcohol dependence in extended high-risk COGA families. Drug Alcohol Depend. 2014;142:56–62.

Kapoor M, Chou YL, Edenberg HJ, Foroud T, Martin NG, Madden PA, et al. Genome-wide polygenic scores for age at onset of alcohol dependence and association with alcohol-related measures. Transl Psychiatry. 2016;6:e761.

King KM, Chassin L. A prospective study of the effects of age of initiation of alcohol and drug use on young adult substance dependence. J Stud Alcohol Drugs. 2007;68:256–65.

Kranzler HR, Feinn R, Armeli S, Tennen H. Comparison of alcoholism subtypes as moderators of the response to sertraline treatment. Alcohol Clin Exp Res. 2012;36:509–16.

Kuntsche E, Rossow I, Simons-Morton B, Bogt TT, Kokkevi A, Godeau E. Not early drinking but early drunkenness is a risk factor for problem behaviors among adolescents from 38 European and North American countries. Alcohol Clin Exp Res. 2013;37:308–14.

Kuntsche E, Rossow I, Engels R, Kuntsche S. Is 'age at first drink' a useful concept in alcohol research and prevention? We doubt that. Addiction. 2016;111:957–65.

Le Strat Y, Grant BF, Ramoz N, Gorwood P. A new definition of early age at onset in alcohol dependence. Drug Alcohol Depend. 2010;108:43–8.

Maimaris W, McCambridge J. Age of first drinking and adult alcohol problems: systematic review of prospective cohort studies. J Epidemiol Community Health. 2014;68:268–74.

Mason WA, Spoth RL. Sequence of alcohol involvement from early onset to young adult alcohol abuse: differential predictors and moderation by family-focused preventive intervention. Addiction. 2012;107:2137–48.

Meier MH, Caspi A, Houts R, Slutske WS, Harrington H, Jackson KM, et al. Prospective developmental subtypes of alcohol dependence from age 18 to 32 years: implications for nosology, etiology, and intervention. Dev Psychopathol. 2013;25:785–800.

Menary KR, Corbin WR, Chassin L. Associations between early internalizing symptoms and speed of transition through stages of alcohol involvement. Dev Psychopathol. 2017;29(4):1455–67.

Morean ME, Kong G, Camenga DR, Cavallo DA, Connell C, Krishnan-Sarin S. First drink to first drunk: age of onset and delay to intoxication are associated with adolescent alcohol use and binge drinking. Alcohol Clin Exp Res. 2014;38:2615–21.

National Health and Medical Research Council. Australian guidelines to reduce health risks from drinking alcohol. Canberra: Commonwealth of Australia; 2009.

Newton NC, Conrod PJ, Slade T, Carragher N, Champion KE, Barrett EL, et al. The long-term effectiveness of a selective, personality-targeted prevention program in reducing alcohol use and related harms: a cluster randomized controlled trial. J Child Psychol Psychiatry. 2016;57:1056–65.

Noble EP. The D2 dopamine receptor gene: a review of association studies in alcoholism and phenotypes. Alcohol. 1998;16:33–45.

Noble EP. Addiction and its reward process through polymorphisms of the D2 dopamine receptor gene: a review. Eur Psychiatry. 2000;15:79–89.

Ohannessian CM, Finan LJ, Schulz J, Hesselbrock V. A long-term longitudinal examination of the effect of early onset of alcohol and drug use on later alcohol abuse. Subst Abus. 2015;36: 440–4.

Palmer RH, McGeary JE, Francazio S, Raphael BJ, Lander AD, Heath AC, et al. The genetics of alcohol dependence: advancing towards systems-based approaches. Drug Alcohol Depend. 2012;125:179–91.

Pilatti A, Godoy JC, Brussino SA, Pautassi RM. Patterns of substance use among Argentinean adolescents and analysis of the effect of age at first alcohol use on substance use behaviors. Addict Behav. 2013;38:2847–50.

Pinto E, Reggers J, Gorwood P, Boni C, Scantamburlo G, Pitchot W, et al. The TaqI A DRD2 polymorphism in type II alcohol dependence: a marker of age at onset or of a familial disease? Alcohol. 2009;43:271–5.

Pitkanen T, Lyyra AL, Pulkkinen L. Age of onset of drinking and the use of alcohol in adulthood: a follow-up study from age 8-42 for females and males. Addiction. 2005;100:652–61.

Prescott CA, Kendler KS. Age at first drink and risk for alcoholism: a noncausal association. Alcohol Clin Exp Res. 1999;23:101–7.

Rehm J, Mathers C, Popova S, Thavorncharoensap M, Teerawattananon Y, Patra J. Global burden of disease and injury and economic cost attributable to alcohol use and alcohol-use disorders. Lancet. 2009;373:2223–33.

Rehm J, Room R. Cultural specificity in alcohol use disorders. Lancet. 2015. https://doi.org/10.1016/S0140-6736(15)00123-3.

Rossow I, Kuntsche E. Early onset of drinking and risk of heavy drinking in young adulthood—a 13-year prospective study. Alcohol Clin Exp Res. 2013;37(Suppl 1):E297–304.

Rothman EF, Edwards EM, Heeren T, Hingson RW. Adverse childhood experiences predict earlier age of drinking onset: results from a representative US sample of current or former drinkers. Pediatrics. 2008;122:e298–304.

Sanchez ZM, Santos MG, Pereira AP, Nappo SA, Carlini EA, Carlini CM, et al. Childhood alcohol use may predict adolescent binge drinking: a multivariate analysis among adolescents in Brazil. J Pediatr. 2013;163:363–8.

Sartor CE, Lynskey MT, Bucholz KK, Madden PA, Martin NG, Heath AC. Timing of first alcohol use and alcohol dependence: evidence of common genetic influences. Addiction. 2009;104:1512–8.

Sartor CE, Bucholz KK, Nelson EC, Madden PA, Lynskey MT, Heath AC. Reporting bias in the association between age at first alcohol use and heavy episodic drinking. Alcohol Clin Exp Res. 2011;35:1418–25.

Sartor CE, Jackson KM, McCutcheon VV, Duncan AE, Grant JD, Werner KB, et al. Progression from first drink, first intoxication, and regular drinking to alcohol use disorder: a comparison of African American and European American youth. Alcohol Clin Exp Res. 2016;40:1515–23.

Schmid B, Blomeyer D, Treutlein J, Zimmermann US, Buchmann AF, Schmidt MH, et al. Interacting effects of CRHR1 gene and stressful life events on drinking initiation and progression among 19-year-olds. Int J Neuropsychopharmacol. 2010;13:703–14.

Seppa K, Sillanaukee P, Koivula T. The efficiency of a questionnaire in detecting heavy drinkers. Br J Addict. 1990;85:1639–45.

Teesson M, Newton NC, Slade T, Carragher N, Barrett EL, Champion KE, et al. Combined universal and selective prevention for adolescent alcohol use: a cluster randomized controlled trial. Psychol Med. 2017;47(10):1761–70.

Vega WA, Aguilar-Gaxiola S, Andrade L, Bijl R, Borges G, Caraveo-Anduaga JJ, et al. Prevalence and age of onset for drug use in seven international sites: results from the international consortium of psychiatric epidemiology. Drug Alcohol Depend. 2002;68:285–97.

Wadolowski M, Hutchinson D, Bruno R, Aiken A, Clare P, Slade T, et al. Early adolescent alcohol use: are sipping and drinking distinct? Alcohol Clin Exp Res. 2015;39:1805–13.

Warner LA, White HR. Longitudinal effects of age at onset and first drinking situations on problem drinking. Subst Use Misuse. 2003;38:1983–2016.

Warner LA, White HR, Johnson V. Alcohol initiation experiences and family history of alcoholism as predictors of problem-drinking trajectories. J Stud Alcohol Drugs. 2007;68:56–65.

Ystrom E, Kendler KS, Reichborn-Kjennerud T. Early age of alcohol initiation is not the cause of alcohol use disorders in adulthood, but is a major indicator of genetic risk. A population-based twin study. Addiction. 2014;109:1824–32.

The Age of Onset of Personality Disorders

10

Andrew M. Chanen and Katherine N. Thompson

10.1 Personality and Personality Disorder

Personality can be broadly defined as an individual's unique variation on the general evolutionary design for human nature (McAdams and Pals 2006) and takes the form of multiple dispositional styles and traits across the entire structure of the person (Millon 2016). Personality disorder (or personality pathology) occurs when this personality structure prevents the individual from achieving adaptive solutions to universal life tasks (Livesley 2011). Such tasks include achieving stable and integrated representations of oneself and others; developing the capacity for intimacy, attachment, and affiliation; and developing the capacity to function adaptively in the social group through prosocial behaviour and/or cooperative relationships. Importantly, these characteristics are relatively pervasive (displayed across a range of situations and contexts) and relatively stable across time and situations. This notion of relative pervasiveness and stability recognises the considerable body of research that demonstrates the changing nature of normal and abnormal personality across the life course (Newton-Howes et al. 2015). Consequently, personality

A. M. Chanen (✉)
Orygen, The National Centre of Excellence in Youth Mental Health,
Melbourne, VIC, Australia

Centre for Youth Mental Health, The University of Melbourne, Melbourne, VIC, Australia

Orygen Youth Health, Melbourne, VIC, Australia
e-mail: andrew.chanen@orygen.org.au

K. N. Thompson
Orygen, The National Centre of Excellence in Youth Mental Health,
Melbourne, VIC, Australia

Centre for Youth Mental Health, The University of Melbourne, Melbourne, VIC, Australia
e-mail: katherine.thompson@unimelb.edu.au

G. de Girolamo et al. (eds.), *Age of Onset of Mental Disorders*,
https://doi.org/10.1007/978-3-319-72619-9_10

disorder can be conceptualised from a life-course developmental perspective, arising from the interaction of biological and environmental factors that work to contribute to the risk, or protect against the onset, of these disorders.

10.2 Personality Disorders

Personality disorders were only operationally defined with the publication of the DSM-III (APA 1980), which listed ten personality disorder categories, divided into three clusters, based upon clinical description. Cluster A comprised paranoid, schizoid, and schizotypal personality disorders. Cluster B comprised antisocial, borderline, histrionic, and narcissistic. Cluster C comprised avoidant, dependent, and obsessive-compulsive personality disorders. This development led to an exponential rise in research and publications in this area (Blashfield and McElroy 1987), principally relating to borderline and antisocial personality disorders. This basic structure has persisted, largely unchanged, into the DSM-5, which defines personality disorder as an enduring, pervasive, and inflexible pattern of thoughts, emotions, and behaviour that markedly differ from societal expectations (APA 2013).

Although the DSM-5 (APA 2013) has continued the tradition of categorical personality disorder diagnosis, using polythetic criteria, there is general agreement among the field that the DSM categorical approach to classification of personality disorder is conceptually and psychometrically flawed (Bernstein et al. 2007). It is widely acknowledged (including in the alternative model in DSM-5 Section III) that the threshold for distinguishing patients with and without personality disorder is arbitrary and that there is no strict demarcation between 'cases' and 'non-cases' (Clark 2007; Herpertz et al. 2017). This issue is especially salient for the notion of onset of personality disorder because the absence of a distinct threshold for 'caseness' also implies that there is no distinct point of 'onset' (Thompson et al. 2017). Moreover, although the DSM-5 states that personality disorder begins in adolescence or early adulthood, it provides no background, discussion, or guidance regarding diagnosis in this age group.

The issue of caseness and onset has been highlighted by research evidence suggesting that the presence of subthreshold features of personality disorder has clinically significant harmful consequences, such as substantially more mental health service use, poorer education and employment, lower income and more reliance on welfare, and a greater number of co-occurring mental disorders (Ellison et al. 2016; Thompson et al. 2017; Zimmerman et al. 2012, 2013). While a person can achieve 'remission' of personality disorder (i.e. have fewer than the required number of criteria for a categorical diagnosis), poor social and occupational functioning continues with little improvement, and in some cases, relapse occurs (Gunderson et al. 2011; Zanarini et al. 2012).

An awareness of the complexities of diagnosis is fundamental to defining onset of illness and gives support for the argument that early intervention for personality disorder requires inclusion of 'subthreshold' forms of the disorder (Chanen and McCutcheon 2013).

The International Classification of Diseases (ICD) has tended to follow the DSM in the classification of mental disorders. The ICD-10 (WHO 1992) attempted to coordinate with the DSM-IV (APA 1994) personality disorder categories but without operationally defined polythetic criteria. This is likely to change with the ICD-11, which is expected to introduce a trait-based, dimensional model of personality disorder (Herpertz et al. 2017; Tyrer et al. 2015).

10.3 Prevalence Among Adults and Young People

A number of studies have reported population prevalence rates of personality disorder in adults, but comparatively fewer have been reported in children and youth. Epidemiological studies in adults report a mean population prevalence of 10.6% for personality disorder, ranging across countries from 4.4% of people in the UK (Coid et al. 2006) to 13.4% in Norway (Torgersen et al. 2001). Between 9.0 and 15.7% of people in the USA have a personality disorder (Lenzenweger 2008; Quirk et al. 2015b; Zanarini et al. 2011), and a WHO Mental Health Survey covering Western Europe reported a rate of 6.1% (Quirk et al. 2015b). A review of adult epidemiological studies reported that Cluster A personality disorders have a prevalence rate of 1.6–6.8% (paranoid, schizoid, schizotypal), Cluster B a rate of 1.2–6.1% (antisocial, borderline, histrionic, narcissistic), and Cluster C a rate of 1.6–10.6% (avoidant, dependent, obsessive-compulsive, passive-aggressive) (Lenzenweger 2008).

The Children in the Community Study remains the most comprehensive prospective study of personality disorder beginning in childhood through to adulthood (Bernstein et al. 1993; Cohen et al. 2005). The estimated prevalence of DSM-III-R personality disorder (excluding antisocial personality disorder) in this sample was 17.2%, with the most prevalent disorder being narcissistic and the least prevalent being schizotypal. This study found the prevalence of personality disorder peaked at age 12 for boys and age 13 for girls. When additional prospective follow-up waves through to age 33 years were taken into account, these researchers estimated the point prevalence of any current DSM-IV (APA 1994) personality disorder (including depressive and passive-aggressive personality disorders) to be between 12.7 and 14.6% through adolescence and young adulthood. The estimated lifetime prevalence of personality disorder at mean age 33 years was 28.2%.

Other large community studies have reported varying rates of personality disorder in children and young adults. In a study of 11-year-old children, 3.2% meet criteria for borderline personality disorder (Zanarini et al. 2011). Research in young adults aged 20–29 years found 9.4% had narcissistic personality disorder (Stinson et al. 2008), and 5.7% had schizotypal personality disorder (Pulay et al. 2009), and these rates reduced with age.

Clinical studies among adolescents have found prevalence rates of between 6 and 17% in community and primary care settings (Lewinsohn et al. 1997), between 41 and 64% in psychiatric outpatients (Feenstra et al. 2011; Grilo et al. 1998), and between 36 and 88% in youth justice samples (Gosden et al. 2003; Kongerslev et al.

2012, 2015). These prevalence estimates are similar to those reported for adults (Zimmerman et al. 2008), making personality disorders among the most common disorders in child and youth mental health.

10.4 Temperament, Personality, and Personality Disorder

Traditionally, each of the research domains of childhood temperament, childhood personality, normal personality, and personality disorder has been separate. However, increasing dialogue among these areas has challenged some long-held assumptions about normal and abnormal personality. For example, it has been well established that there is substantial overlap across childhood temperament, personality and personality disorder traits (De Clercq et al. 2006; Shiner 2009; Tackett et al. 2013) and that personality and personality disorder traits in childhood have some continuity with those in adulthood (O'Connor 2002; Shiner 2009). Also, normal and abnormal personality are now known to change trajectory across the lifespan (Cohen et al. 2008; Hallquist and Lenzenweger 2013; Morey et al. 2007), rather than being highly stable. Personality pathology can also change with treatment, particularly during acute episodes (Stoffers-Winterling et al. 2012). Even characteristic traits can change over time when facilitated by effective treatments, which might take effect by hastening delayed maturational processes (Newton-Howes et al. 2015).

10.5 Normal Versus Maladaptive Personality Traits over the Life Course

The study of normal-range personality has converged on the five-factor model (Markon et al. 2005). These traits account for a significant amount of the variance in both normal-range personality and personality pathology (Kushner et al. 2011; Samuel and Widiger 2008) and demonstrate a similar higher-order structure for these personality dimensions in children, adolescents, and adults (Mervielde et al. 2005; Tackett et al. 2012).

Until recently, most pathological personality trait measures were developed for adult populations and adapted for use in younger age groups (De Fruyt and De Clercq 2014; Kushner et al. 2013). These measures have demonstrated similar associations between normal and pathological personality traits from adolescence through to adulthood (and old age), supporting an overarching structural framework across the lifespan (De Fruyt and De Clercq 2014). This suggests many layers of continuity by demonstrating connections between adult and child trait covariance (Markon et al. 2005; Tackett et al. 2012), connections between normal and pathological personality trait covariance (Markon et al. 2005; Samuel and Widiger 2008), and overlap between different personality pathology trait measures (Kushner et al. 2013). This demonstrates the unifying potential for dimensional approaches to personality pathology across age and development.

The five-factor model traits are observable in early childhood (Tackett et al. 2012) and provide a coherent framework for comprehending the relationships among personality pathology and other forms of mental disorder across the lifespan (De Clercq and De Fruyt 2012; Tackett et al. 2012). The most obvious of these is the link between childhood or adolescent conduct disorder and antisocial personality. Another is the link between childhood neuroticism and social phobia, generalised anxiety disorder, and avoidant personality disorder (De Clercq and De Fruyt 2012). Paranoid, borderline, and antisocial personality disorders are also linked with earlier low conscientiousness and low agreeableness, along with high neuroticism and attention deficit and hyperactivity disorder (De Clercq and De Fruyt 2012). When De Fruyt, De Clercq, and colleagues operationalised this system, it became evident that the distinction between temperament and personality becomes blurred and less meaningful (De Clercq and De Fruyt 2012; De Fruyt and De Clercq 2014). This has given rise to the suggestion of using trait description within childhood mental health assessment (De Clercq and De Fruyt 2012).

The Dimensional Personality Symptom Item Pool (DIPSI) has been used to investigate personality traits in children (De Clercq et al. 2006; Decuyper et al. 2015). These traits have been found to be grouped into externalising and internalising behaviours, with four lower-order factors of disagreeableness, compulsivity, emotional instability, and introversion (De Clercq et al. 2006; Tackett et al. 2013). When the factor structure of personality disorder was investigated among adolescents with borderline personality disorder, two main factors were found, one internally oriented (emptiness, affective instability, paranoid ideation, avoidance of abandonment) and the other externally oriented (impulsivity, inappropriate anger, unstable relationships, suicidal or self-mutilating behaviour) (Speranza et al. 2012). These findings are comparable with studies of adults that have used Livesley's (1998) Dimensional Assessment of Personality Pathology-Basic Questionnaire (DAPP-BQ), which yielded a four-factor structure comprising emotional dysregulation, inhibitedness, dissocial behaviour, and compulsivity. Livesley suggested that this phenotypic approach to personality disorder is advantageous because it results in a large number of building blocks that have specific effects together, with a few factors with widespread effects, thereby explaining the complex variation in the structure of personality and personality disorder (Livesley 1998).

10.6 Temporal Stability of Personality Disorder

Longitudinal studies support the continuity of individual personality differences from early childhood to young adulthood in the general population (Caspi and Silva 1995), although the strength of associations between individual differences in early childhood and adulthood is only weak to moderate. Traits tend to stabilise from childhood into later adulthood (De Fruyt et al. 2006; Roberts and DelVecchio 2000). For example, there is an increase in conscientiousness, emotional stability, and agreeableness and a decrease in openness with age (Roberts et al. 2006). The exception to this is the brief shift to less maturity in the transition between childhood and adolescence and the subsequent upswing in regulation in later adolescence (Soto et al. 2011). Successful navigation through this stage to maturity into young adulthood is necessary to maintain a trajectory that is consistent with normal-range personality development.

Recent meta-analytic data show that personality is moderately stable during childhood. Over time it becomes more 'viscous' (Ferguson 2010; Srivastava et al. 2003) but never ceases to change, with personality stability increasing from adolescence through to emerging adulthood and slowing in its rate of change after age 30 years. The five-factor model dimensions of personality already show substantial stability across community (De Fruyt et al. 2006) and clinical (De Bolle et al. 2009) samples of children and adolescents. Importantly for the assessment of personality pathology in adolescence, there is no sudden increase in the stability of traits across the normal-abnormal range during the transition from the teenage years to young adulthood (Roberts and DelVecchio 2000). Rank-order stability of pathological personality traits is largely identical in adolescence and adulthood (de Clercq et al. 2009; Johnson et al. 2000), dispelling earlier notions that personality disorder was too inconsistent during adolescence to diagnose, research, and/or treat.

Much of the evidence regarding stability and change of personality pathology from childhood to adulthood is based upon the work of the Children in Community (CIC) study (Cohen et al. 2005). The CIC study identified that personality disorder features peak in the early teens and declines linearly from the mid-teens to late 20s (Johnson et al. 2000). This decline partly reflects a normative decrease in dependency, impulsivity, and attention seeking and a normative increase in self-control and social competence. In the CIC study, personality disorder features were moderately stable, which corresponds with comparable studies among adults, conducted over similar time intervals. CIC adolescents with diagnosed personality disorder tended to have elevated personality disorder features during early adulthood, suggesting continuity of personality disorder from adolescence to adulthood. Furthermore, among the CIC sample, 21% of participants experienced *increases* in personality pathology during this maturational period. Overall, the CIC's findings indicate that child and adolescent personality pathology is the strongest predictor of young adult personality disorder, over and above other common mental state disorders. Decreases in personality disorder features were more rapid among individuals who initially had lower levels of personality disorder symptoms (Crawford et al. 2005; de Clercq et al. 2009), giving rise to a broadening gap between individuals with high and those with low personality disorder features in the transition from adolescence to emerging adulthood.

Likewise, the prospective Pittsburgh ['high-risk'] Girls Study found that the mean level of borderline personality disorder features was stable across the period from ages 14 to 17 years (Stepp et al. 2014). Additionally, the authors found that an increase in borderline personality disorder symptoms in 1 year predicted an increase in these symptoms in the next year (Stepp et al. 2014).

These CIC and Pittsburgh Girls Study findings are supported by clinical research, such as that conducted among 15–18-year-old treatment-seeking outpatients, who were assessed against personality disorder criteria using the DSM-IV SCID II interview (Chanen et al. 2004). This study found that 74% of adolescents who met criteria for a personality disorder at baseline still met criteria after 2 years. Rank order and mean level stability were high for antisocial and schizoid personality disorder; moderate for borderline, schizotypal and histrionic personality disorder; and low for the other remaining personality disorders (Chanen et al. 2004).

Although traits are largely consistent across the normal-abnormal range, they also remain dynamic throughout life, with the greatest magnitude of change in mean trait levels occurring during young adulthood (age 20–40 years), not childhood or adolescence (Roberts et al. 2006). Individuals with personality pathology tend to show greater change, which is usually, but not always, in the direction of improvement over time, which can be interspersed by periods of 'relapse' and 'remission' (Gunderson et al. 2011). Intervention and treatment can hasten time to remission of symptoms (Gunderson et al. 2011).

10.7 Functional Impairment

Despite the waxing and waning course of personality disorder that generally leads to attenuation of pathological traits over time, social and occupational functioning tends to remain poor and relatively stable (Skodol 2008; Skodol et al. 2005). Among young people in particular, this can have a catastrophic effect on their ability to successfully transition into adult role functioning (Chanen 2015), with diminished capacity to form intimate relationships, achieve independence, learn life skills, and form a clear identity.

Although poor social and occupational functioning (adaptive functioning) is a requirement for the general diagnosis of personality disorder in the DSM-5 (APA 2013), it is neither included in the specific operational diagnostic criteria nor has it been routinely or consistently studied in personality disorder. Furthermore, common measures of functioning that are used in personality disorder research do not specifically or comprehensively assess maladaptive social and occupational functioning. In fact, frequently used measures, such as the Social and Occupational Assessment Scale (Goldman et al. 1992) and the Global Assessment of Functioning Scale (APA 2000), only provide a single global impression score.

Among 15–18-year-old outpatients, those with personality disorder have been found to have significantly poorer adaptive functioning, compared with outpatients with no personality disorder (Chanen et al. 2007). Among those with personality disorder, those with borderline personality disorder are the worst functioning, in terms of more school truancy, poorer relationships with family and peers, and poor self-care. When these findings are situated in the context of normal development, they suggest that young people with personality disorders are at high risk of unsuccessfully transitioning to adult role functioning (Chanen 2015). These findings are further supported by a systematic review (Winsper et al. 2015) of clinical and psychosocial outcomes for borderline personality disorder in childhood and adolescence, which found that borderline personality disorder in people less than 19 years of age predicted long-term problems in interpersonal functioning and educational, occupational, and financial impairment.

It is therefore not surprising that adults with features of personality disorder have persistently poor adaptive functioning, which continues long after they no longer meet the DSM-5 diagnostic criteria for any particular personality disorder. This is reflected in the 10-year follow-along findings from the Collaborative Longitudinal Personality Disorders Study, which compared patients with borderline, avoidant, obsessive-compulsive, and schizotypal personality disorders and patients with major depression (Gunderson et al. 2011). Of these groups, the patients with borderline personality disorder were the least likely to be employed at the 10-year mark. These results concur with the McLean Study of Adult Development, which found that patients with borderline personality disorder had poorer functioning than patients with other personality disorders, as indicated by lower school or work performance and attendance, and greater reliance on disability benefits (Zanarini et al. 2005a, b).

Poor functioning spans not only social and occupational functioning but also poor physical health and functioning. For example, the National Epidemiologic Survey on Alcohol and Related Conditions in the USA reported borderline, narcissistic, schizoid, schizotypal, and obsessive-compulsive personality disorders were all associated with cardiovascular disease among young adults (Quirk et al. 2015a). Borderline, paranoid, antisocial, and avoidant personality disorders were associated with arthritis. Schizotypal, schizoid, and paranoid personality disorders were associated with diabetes, and borderline, narcissistic, antisocial, and schizotypal personality disorders were associated with gastrointestinal disease.

Therefore, while it is clear that although poor functioning is an important component of personality disorder, it is inadequately understood. There is some evidence to suggest that poor functioning might be comprised of three components: wellbeing, social and interpersonal functioning, and basic functioning (Ro and Clark 2013). It seems clear that an additional component of personality functioning should also be incorporated into general functioning (Clark and Ro 2014), but this requires further research for clarification.

10.8 Risk Factors, Precursor Signs and Symptoms

Heritability estimates for DSM-IV personality disorders are relatively high and comparable to those of other forms of mental disorder, such as bipolar disorder and schizophrenia (Kendler et al. 2007; Torgersen et al. 2012). Estimates range from 0.55 for schizoid, 0.63 for histrionic, 0.66 for paranoid, 0.67 for borderline, 0.69 for antisocial, 0.71 for narcissistic, to 0.72 for schizotypal (Kendler et al. 2007; Torgersen et al. 2012). Although high, these rates still suggest a prominent role for family and other environmental factors.

Historically, developmental studies of personality disorder tended to focus upon early childhood experiences and their influence upon adult psychopathology, without reference to the potential developmental processes that might mediate or even reverse such pathways (Chanen and Kaess 2012; Newton-Howes et al. 2015). It has become clear that a range of signs and symptoms precede the clinical onset of personality disorder. These include childhood temperament and early-onset mental state and behavioural problems (Chanen and Thompson 2014). A lifespan perspective recognises the non-specific and complex relationship between genes and environment taking into account their reciprocal effects and other mediating factors, such as environmental influences, coping mechanisms, protective factors, and cognitive processing of experiences (Newton-Howes et al. 2015; Rutter et al. 2006). In so doing, genes and environment interact to perpetuate continuity and discontinuity of precursor signs and symptoms from childhood to adult life (Schulenberg et al. 2004).

Distal precursors to schizoid and schizotypal personality disorder include perinatal exposure to influenza and prenatal exposure to malnutrition and stress (Raine 2006). Other precursors that have been prospectively associated with personality disorders include low socioeconomic status, parental conflict and illness or death, and welfare support (Cohen et al. 2005). Aspects of parenting that have been found to be important include the presence of parental mental illness (i.e. features of personality disorder or other disorders), low emotional closeness between parent and child, the use of harsh punishment, and maladaptive parenting and family functioning (Cohen 2008; Cohen et al. 2005, 2008; Johnson et al. 2006). Adverse events that have been associated with the development of personality disorder include childhood abuse and neglect (Cohen et al. 2008; Johnson et al. 2001), school expulsion, poor educational achievement, a lack of life goals, and low IQ (Cohen et al. 2005).

Temperamental characteristics, mental health, and behavioural problems have been observed in children and reported by mothers, which prospectively predict the development of personality disorder (Chanen and McCutcheon 2013). These include symptoms of depression and anxiety, attention deficit and hyperactivity disorder, behaviour problems (oppositional defiant disorder and conduct disorder), and substance use disorders (Bernstein et al. 1996; Cohen 2008; Cohen et al. 2005; Kasen et al. 1999, 2001; Lewinsohn et al. 1997; Stepp et al. 2012; Thatcher et al. 2005; Zoccolillo et al. 1992).

When personality disorders and other forms of mental illness co-occur during adolescence, the combination of these disorders increases the chance of personality disorder being present in young adulthood (Kasen et al. 1999). For example, when a disruptive behaviour disorder co-occurs together with a personality disorder in adolescence, individuals were 24.6 times more likely to continue to have a Cluster A personality disorder in adulthood, 12.5 times more likely to have a Cluster B disorder, and 16.3 times more likely to have a Cluster C disorder. Similarly, the odds ratios for persistence of Cluster A with co-occurring anxiety disorder were 16.9. When major depression co-occurred with a personality disorder, the chance of continuity into adult personality disorder was 20.5 for Cluster A, 19.1 for Cluster B, and 16.0 for Cluster C.

Prospective follow-up studies have reported risk factors and precursor signs and symptoms for specific personality disorders (Cohen et al. 2008). Schizotypal personality disorder was associated with cumulative trauma, stressful life events, low socioeconomic status, low intelligence, parenting problems, and male gender (Cohen et al. 2008). In comparison, borderline personality disorder was also associated with these factors but was not specific to gender but was specific to maternal parenting issues (Cohen et al. 2008). Antisocial personality disorder was associated with low closeness to one or both parents, the tendency for mothers to control through guilt, parental antisocial behaviour, and exposure to punishment that was coercive and controlling (Cohen et al. 2005).

It is important to note that these observed childhood antecedents of personality disorder are non-specific, as children with these early behavioural problems, adverse life experiences, and mental state pathology can subsequently develop other personality or mental state disorders (Burke et al. 2010; Chanen and Thompson 2014; Frick and Viding 2009; Helgeland et al. 2005; Rutter 2012). It is therefore incorrect to assume that childhood symptoms of mental illness and behavioural problems are directly related to the later development of a specific personality disorder. Notwithstanding the above, the strongest predictor of adult personality disorder remains the presence of personality disorder features during childhood and adolescence (Chanen and Kaess 2012; Cohen et al. 2005; Crawford et al. 2005).

Importantly, some mediating factors for personality disorder have been found to be protective and to ameliorate other contributing factors. Such 'discontinuity factors' include positive parenting by mothers in response to verbal and physical aggression or dysphoric mood, which has been associated with a decrease in borderline personality disorder pathology during adolescence (Whalen et al. 2014). Similarly, prevention and early intervention that reduces the symptoms of personality disorder during adolescence and youth have been demonstrated to be effective (Chanen and McCutcheon 2013). Little else is known about prospective factors that build resilience and contribute to the discontinuity of personality disorders (Paris et al. 2014; Skodol et al. 2007), which would assist in the development and application of clinical interventions (Newton-Howes et al. 2015).

10.9 Personality Disorder Begins in Childhood and Adolescence

Researchers and especially clinicians have tended to adopt an ambivalent stance towards the notion of 'onset' of personality disorder. On the one hand, since the publication of the DSM-III in 1980 (APA 1980), there has been general acknowledgement that personality disorder 'begins' in childhood and adolescence. On the other hand, the DSM-5 and ICD-10 sections on disorders of childhood and adolescence still do not mention personality disorder.

The evidence summarised above suggests that there is substantial overlap across childhood temperament, personality and personality disorder traits, along with both continuity and change in the trajectory of such traits across the lifespan. If personality disorder is defined to occur when an individual's personality structure prevents them from achieving adaptive solutions to universal life tasks, then clearly such maladaptation can occur in regard to developmental tasks across the lifespan. This might be related to early tasks, such as developing the capacity for attachment, or prosocial and cooperative functioning in groups. However, it might also occur in relation to more complex tasks of later life such as identity formation, developing a capacity for intimate relationships, or caring for others.

A key problem hindering diagnosis is the lack of developmentally congruent personality disorder criteria, or developmentally appropriate illustrations of the current DSM-5 personality disorder criteria (Chanen et al. 2008b). Although the DSM-5 and ICD-10 use scientifically unjustified wording (Chanen and McCutcheon 2008; De Clercq and De Fruyt 2012) that dissuades from the use of personality disorder diagnoses in individuals under the age of 18 years (except for antisocial personality disorder), it is clinical mythology that diagnosis is prohibited. Actually, DSM-5 only requires that features of personality disorder be present for 1 year in adolescents. This period is likely to be too short to accurately distinguish a mental state from a trait disorder (Newton-Howes et al. 2015).

While maladaptive personality traits are observable during childhood, it is arguable that the more severe forms of personality disorder become clinically apparent during the transition between childhood and adulthood, when children are emotionally, cognitively, and socially ready to integrate knowledge and experience about themselves and others into a cohesive self and when 'adaptive failure' has greater personal and social consequences. While personality disorder represents a failure of adaptation in the transition from childhood to adulthood, it also has the potential to foster vicious cycles that will further disrupt the complex developmental tasks associated with this phase of life and the achievement of adult role functioning. Advances in understanding the neural substrates underpinning cognitive, emotional, and social development (Casey et al. 2008) suggested that this period of development that extends from puberty to the middle 20s lays the foundations for adult role functioning. The later phase of this transition is largely a period of exploration of and change in roles, with the goal of self-sufficiency, rather than merely accomplishing demographic transitions (Arnett 2000). The identification of this distinct, coherent, and extended developmental phase (usually termed 'youth') suggests that the term 'adolescent personality disorder' is an inadequate concept (Chanen 2015). Rather, a more rational and developmental approach to defining, studying, and treating personality disorder would distinguish personality disorder in childhood, youth (combining adolescence and emerging adulthood), adulthood, and old age (Chanen 2015; Newton-Howes et al. 2015; Tackett et al. 2009).

Despite the scientific evidence for the validity of personality disorder in childhood and youth, the diagnosis remains prohibited in this age group among many clinicians and clinical service cultures (Chanen and McCutcheon 2008). The above evidence suggests that such views are unwarranted, but many clinicians avoid the diagnosis in order to 'protect' their patients from the adversities associated with the label, especially stigma and discrimination among health professionals (Chanen and McCutcheon 2013). Although this stigma is undeniable, delaying appropriate diagnosis for this reason risks colluding with this stigma and introducing diagnostic delay (Chanen 2015), which carries clinical risks. There is burgeoning evidence to suggest that many of the harms associated with personality disorder emerge early in the course of the disorder and failure to diagnose and treat at the earliest opportunity is likely to restrict appropriate intervention, increase the chances of inappropriate and/or harmful intervention, and worsen outcomes (Chanen 2015; Chanen et al. 2017).

10.10 Implications for Prevention and Early Intervention

The ‘onset’ or clinical manifestation of personality disorder from childhood to emerging adulthood is earlier than previously acknowledged in the literature, and this has important implications for prevention and early intervention.

First, personality disorder is a legitimate differential diagnosis of common mental disorders in young people, especially when there are multiple “comorbidities” (Chanen 2015). It has been suggested that many precursor signs and symptoms that are prospectively associated with personality disorder in young people (e.g. disruptive behaviour disorders, substance use disorder, non-suicidal self-injury, anxiety, and depression) are spuriously defined as mental state pathology in children and later relabelled as personality pathology in adult life (Chanen and Kaess 2012). This is likely due to lack of recognition that many aspects of these disorders are underpinned by traits such as impulsivity, affective instability, or hyper-aggression (Chanen 2015).

Second, similar to other mental disorders, early clinical phenotypes for personality disorder are overlapping and non-specific (Chanen et al. 2016; Hartmann et al. 2017). This means that prevention and early intervention for personality disorder cannot be conducted separately from other disorders and needs to be integrated with preventive strategies for the full range of mental disorders (Chanen et al. 2016). ‘Clinical staging’ (McGorry 2013; McGorry and van Os 2013) offers an integrative framework to guide the assessment of individual patients and the choice of an intervention that is proportionate to the phase and stage of illness for that individual (Chanen et al. 2016). This approach differs markedly from conventional diagnostic practice in personality disorder, which usually ensures ‘late intervention’, when functional impairments and iatrogenic harm are well established (Chanen 2015).

Exemplar preventive programmes for personality disorder already exist, although they are not always recognised as such because of ambivalence about personality disorder diagnosis in children and young people. For example, the Communities That Care System is a universal prevention programme (directed towards the whole population) that targets antisocial behaviour and delinquency (Hawkins and David Hawkins 2012). Intervention was provided to fifth grade students and resulted in a decrease in violent and delinquent behaviour that was sustained until grade 10 (Hawkins and David Hawkins 2012) but waned by grade 12, 3 years post intervention (Hawkins et al. 2014). The Nurse Family Partnership programme is an exemplar selective intervention programme (directed towards individuals with risk factors for personality disorder), which targets low-income mothers and their newborn to 2-year-old children. This programme has showed lasting benefits for both mothers and their children in regard to crime and employment (Olds 2008). Indicated prevention (directed towards those with subthreshold features of personality disorder) and early intervention (for first-presentation disorder) are well established. The Helping Young People Early (HYPE) programme is a manualised programme that specifically targets borderline/severe personality disorder (Chanen et al. 2009b) and which improves borderline personality pathology, general psychopathology, and social functioning (Chanen et al. 2008a, 2009a).

Conclusion

Personality disorder (or personality pathology) occurs when an individual's personality structure prevents them from achieving adaptive solutions to universal life tasks appropriate to their developmental age and stage. There is substantial overlap among childhood temperament, personality and personality disorder traits. These childhood traits show continuity with those in adulthood, but they remain dynamic across the lifespan. Although maladaptive personality traits are observable during childhood, the more severe forms of personality disorder usually become clinically apparent during the transition between childhood and adulthood. The dimensional nature of personality pathology means that there is neither a strict boundary between 'cases' and 'non-cases' nor a distinct point of 'onset'. Specific confusion arises with regard to children and adolescents because of the spurious distinction between personality and mental state pathology when describing many common mental disorders in these age groups.

Despite the waxing and waning course of personality disorder that generally leads to attenuation of pathological traits over time, social and occupational functioning tends to remain poor and relatively stable. One possible mechanism for this is that personality disorder has the potential to foster vicious circles that will further disrupt the complex developmental tasks associated with this phase of life and the achievement of adult role functioning.

Despite strong scientific evidence supporting the validity of personality disorder in childhood and adolescence, the diagnosis remains taboo in this age group among many clinicians and clinical service cultures. Such views are unfounded, and personality disorder is a legitimate differential diagnosis of common mental disorders in young people. However, in common with other mental disorders, early clinical phenotypes for personality disorder are overlapping and non-specific, meaning that prevention and early intervention for personality disorder cannot be conducted separately from other disorders. Exemplar preventive programmes for personality disorder already exist, but, in order to make significant progress, it is essential that prevention for personality disorder is integrated with prevention efforts for the full range of mental disorders.

References

APA. Diagnostic and statistical manual of mental disorders. 3rd ed. Washington, DC: American Psychiatric Association; 1980.

APA. Diagnostic and statistical manual of mental disorders. 4th ed. Washington, DC: American Psychiatric Association; 1994.

APA. Diagnostic and statistical manual of mental disorders. 4th ed., Text Revision. Washington, DC: American Psychiatric Association; 2000.

APA. Diagnostic and statistical manual of mental disorders. 5th ed. Washington, DC: American Psychiatric Association; 2013.

Arnett JJ. Emerging adulthood. A theory of development from the late teens through the twenties. Am Psychol. 2000;55(5):469–80.

Bernstein DP, Cohen P, Skodol A, Bezirganian S, Brook JS. Childhood antecedents of adolescent personality disorders. Am J Psychiatry. 1996;153(7):907–13.

Bernstein DP, Cohen P, Velez CN, Schwab-Stone M, Siever LJ, Shinsato L. Prevalence and stability of the DSM-III-R personality disorders in a community-based survey of adolescents. Am J Psychiatry. 1993;150(8):1237–43.

Bernstein DP, Iscan C, Maser J, Boards of Directors of the Association for Research in Personality Disorders, & International Society for the Study of Personality Disorders. Opinions of personality disorder experts regarding the DSM-IV personality disorders classification system. J Personal Disord. 2007;21(5):536–51.

Blashfield RK, McElroy RA. The 1985 journal literature on the personality disorders. Compr Psychiatry. 1987;28(6):536–46.

Burke JD, Waldman I, Lahey BB. Predictive validity of childhood oppositional defiant disorder and conduct disorder: implications for the DSM-V. J Abnorm Psychol. 2010;119(4):739–51.

Casey BJ, Jones RM, Hare TA. The adolescent brain. Ann N Y Acad Sci. 2008;1124:111–26.

Caspi A, Silva PA. Temperamental qualities at age three predict personality traits in young adulthood: longitudinal evidence from a birth cohort. Child Dev. 1995;66(2):486–98.

Chanen AM. Borderline personality disorder in young people: are we there yet? J Clin Psychol. 2015;71(8):778–91.

Chanen AM, Berk M, Thompson KN. Integrating early intervention for borderline personality disorder and mood disorders. Harv Rev Psychiatry. 2016;24(5):330–41.

Chanen AM, Jackson HJ, McCutcheon LK, Jovev M, Dudgeon P, Yuen HP, et al. Early intervention for adolescents with borderline personality disorder using cognitive analytic therapy: randomised controlled trial. Br J Psychiatry. 2008a;193(6):477–84.

Chanen AM, Jackson HJ, McCutcheon LK, Jovev M, Dudgeon P, Yuen HP, et al. Early intervention for adolescents with borderline personality disorder: quasi-experimental comparison with treatment as usual. Aust N Z J Psychiatry. 2009a;43(5):397–408.

Chanen AM, Jackson HJ, McGorry PD, Allot KA, Clarkson V, Yuen HP. Two-year stability of personality disorder in older adolescent outpatients. J Personal Disord. 2004;18(6):526–41.

Chanen AM, Jovev M, Jackson HJ. Adaptive functioning and psychiatric symptoms in adolescents with borderline personality disorder. J Clin Psychiatry. 2007;68(2):297–306.

Chanen AM, Jovev M, McCutcheon L, Jackson H, McGorry P. Borderline personality disorder in young people and the prospects for prevention and early intervention. Curr Psychiatr Rev. 2008b;4(1):48–57.

Chanen AM, Kaess M. Developmental pathways to borderline personality disorder. Curr Psychiatry Rep. 2012;14(1):45–53.

Chanen AM, McCutcheon L. Prevention and early intervention for borderline personality disorder: current status and recent evidence. Br J Psychiatry Suppl. 2013;54:s24–9.

Chanen AM, McCutcheon LK. Personality disorder in adolescence: the diagnosis that dare not speak its name. Personal Ment Health. 2008;2(1):35–41.

Chanen AM, McCutcheon LK, Germano D, Nistico H, Jackson HJ, McGorry PD. The HYPE clinic: an early intervention service for borderline personality disorder. J Psychiatr Pract. 2009b;15(3):163–72.

Chanen AM, Sharp C, Hoffman P, Global Alliance for Prevention and Early Intervention for Borderline Personality Disorder. Prevention and early intervention for borderline personality disorder: a novel public health priority. World Psychiatr. 2017;16(2):215–6.

Chanen AM, Thompson KN. Borderline personality and mood disorders: risk factors, precursors, and early signs in childhood and youth. In: Choi-Kain L, Gunderson J, editors. Borderline personality and mood disorders. New York: Springer; 2014. p. 155–74.

Clark LA. Assessment and diagnosis of personality disorder: perennial issues and an emerging reconceptualization. Annu Rev Psychol. 2007;58:227–57.

Clark LA, Ro E. Three-pronged assessment and diagnosis of personality disorder and its consequences: personality functioning, pathological traits, and psychosocial disability. Personal Disord. 2014;5(1):55–69.

Cohen P. Child development and personality disorder. Psychiatr Clin North Am. 2008;31(3):477–93.

Cohen P, Chen H, Gordon K, Johnson J, Brook J, Kasen S. Socioeconomic background and the developmental course of schizotypal and borderline personality disorder symptoms. Dev Psychopathol. 2008;20(2):633–50.

Cohen P, Crawford TN, Johnson JG, Kasen S. The children in the community study of developmental course of personality disorder. J Personal Disord. 2005;19(5):466–86.

Coid J, Yang M, Tyrer P, Roberts A, Ullrich S. Prevalence and correlates of personality disorder in Great Britain. Br J Psychiatry. 2006;188:423–31.

Crawford TN, Cohen P, Johnson JG, Kasen S, First MB, Gordon K, Brook JS. Self-reported personality disorder in the children in the community sample: convergent and prospective validity in late adolescence and adulthood. J Personal Disord. 2005;19(1):30–52.

De Bolle M, De Clercq B, Van Leeuwen K, Decuyper M, Rosseel Y, De Fruyt F. Personality and psychopathology in Flemish referred children: five perspectives of continuity. Child Psychiatry Hum Dev. 2009;40(2):269–85.

De Clercq B, De Fruyt F. A Five-Factor Model framework for understanding childhood personality disorder antecedents. J Pers. 2012;80(6):1533–63.

De Clercq B, De Fruyt F, Van Leeuwen K, Mervielde I. The structure of maladaptive personality traits in childhood: a step toward an integrative developmental perspective for DSM-V. J Abnorm Psychol. 2006;115(4):639–57.

de Clercq B, van Leeuwen K, van den Noortgate W, de Bolle M, de Fruyt F. Childhood personality pathology: dimensional stability and change. Dev Psychopathol. 2009;21(3):853–69.

Decuyper M, De Clercq B, Tackett JL. Assessing maladaptive traits in youth: an English-language version of the Dimensional Personality Symptom Itempool. Personal Disord. 2015;6(3):239–50.

De Fruyt F, Bartels M, Van Leeuwen KG, De Clercq B, Decuyper M, Mervielde I. Five types of personality continuity in childhood and adolescence. J Pers Soc Psychol. 2006;91(3):538–52.

De Fruyt F, De Clercq B. Antecedents of personality disorder in childhood and adolescence: toward an integrative developmental model. Annu Rev Clin Psychol. 2014;10:449–76.

Ellison WD, Rosenstein L, Chelminski I, Dalrymple K, Zimmerman M. The clinical significance of single features of borderline personality disorder: anger, affective instability, impulsivity, and chronic emptiness in psychiatric outpatients. J Personal Disord. 2016;30(2):261–70.

Feenstra DJ, Busschbach JJV, Verheul R, Hutsebaut J. Prevalence and comorbidity of axis I and axis II disorders among treatment refractory adolescents admitted for specialized psychotherapy. J Personal Disord. 2011;25(6):842–50.

Ferguson CJ. A meta-analysis of normal and disordered personality across the life span. J Pers Soc Psychol. 2010;98(4):659–67.

Frick PJ, Viding E. Antisocial behavior from a developmental psychopathology perspective. Dev Psychopathol. 2009;21(4):1111–31.

Goldman HH, Skodol AE, Lave TR. Revising axis V for DSM-IV: a review of measures of social functioning. Am J Psychiatry. 1992;149(9):1148–56.

Gosden NP, Kramp P, Gabrielsen G, Sestoft D. Prevalence of mental disorders among 15-17-year-old male adolescent remand prisoners in Denmark. Acta Psychiatr Scand. 2003;107(2):102–10.

Grilo CM, McGlashan TH, Quinlan DM, Walker ML, Greenfeld D, Edell WS. Frequency of personality disorders in two age cohorts of psychiatric inpatients. Am J Psychiatry. 1998;155(1):140–2.

Gunderson JG, Stout RL, McGlashan TH, Shea MT, Morey LC, Grilo CM, et al. Ten-year course of borderline personality disorder: psychopathology and function from the Collaborative Longitudinal Personality Disorders study. Arch Gen Psychiatry. 2011;68(8):827–37.

Hallquist MN, Lenzenweger MF. Identifying latent trajectories of personality disorder symptom change: growth mixture modeling in the longitudinal study of personality disorders. J Abnorm Psychol. 2013;122(1):138–55.

Hartmann JA, Nelson B, Spooner R, Paul Amminger G, Chanen AM, Davey CG, et al. Broad clinical high-risk mental state (CHARMS): methodology of a cohort study validating criteria for pluripotent risk. Early Interv Psychiatry. 2017. https://doi.org/10.1111/eip.12483.

Hawkins JD, David Hawkins J. Sustained decreases in risk exposure and youth problem behaviors after installation of the communities that care prevention system in a randomized trial. Arch Pediatr Adolesc Med. 2012;166(2):141.

Hawkins JD, Oesterle S, Brown EC, Abbott RD, Catalano RF. Youth problem behaviors 8 years after implementing the communities that care prevention system: a community-randomized trial. JAMA Pediatr. 2014;168(2):122–9.

Helgeland MI, Kjelsberg E, Torgersen S. Continuities between emotional and disruptive behavior disorders in adolescence and personality disorders in adulthood. Am J Psychiatry. 2005;162(10):1941–7.

Herpertz SC, Huprich SK, Bohus M, Chanen AM, Goodman M, Mehlum L, et al. The challenge of transforming the diagnostic system of personality disorders. J Personal Disord. 2017;31(5):577–89.

Johnson JG, Cohen P, Chen H, Kasen S, Brook JS. Parenting behaviors associated with risk for offspring personality disorder during adulthood. Arch Gen Psychiatry. 2006;63(5):579–87.

Johnson JG, Cohen P, Kasen S, Skodol AE, Hamagami F, Brook JS. Age-related change in personality disorder trait levels between early adolescence and adulthood: a community-based longitudinal investigation. Acta Psychiatr Scand. 2000;102(4):265–75.

Johnson JG, Cohen P, Kasen S, Smailes E, Brook JS. Association of maladaptive parental behavior with psychiatric disorder among parents and their offspring. Arch Gen Psychiatry. 2001;58(5):453–60.

Kasen S, Cohen P, Skodol AE, Johnson JG, Brook JS. Influence of child and adolescent psychiatric disorders on young adult personality disorder. Am J Psychiatry. 1999;156(10):1529–35.

Kasen S, Cohen P, Skodol AE, Johnson JG, Smailes E, Brook JS. Childhood depression and adult personality disorder: alternative pathways of continuity. Arch Gen Psychiatry. 2001;58(3):231–6.

Kendler KS, Myers J, Torgersen S, Neale MC, Reichborn-Kjennerud T. The heritability of cluster A personality disorders assessed by both personal interview and questionnaire. Psychol Med. 2007;37(05):655.

Kongerslev MT, Chanen AM, Simonsen E. Personality disorder in childhood and adolescence comes of age: a review of the current evidence and prospects for future research. Scand J Child Adolesc Psychiatr Psychol. 2015;3(1):31–48.

Kongerslev MT, Moran P, Bo S, Simonsen E. Screening for personality disorder in incarcerated adolescent boys: preliminary validation of an adolescent version of the standardised assessment of personality—abbreviated scale (SAPAS-AV). BMC Psychiatry. 2012;12:94.

Kushner SC, Quilty LC, Tackett JL, Bagby RM. The hierarchical structure of the Dimensional Assessment of Personality Pathology (DAPP-BQ). J Personal Disord. 2011;25(4):504–16.

Kushner SC, Tackett JL, De Clercq B. The joint hierarchical structure of adolescent personality pathology: converging evidence from two approaches to measurement. J Can Acad Child Adolesc Psychiatry. 2013;22(3):199–205.

Lenzenweger MF. Epidemiology of personality disorders. Psychiatr Clin North Am. 2008;31(3):395–403, vi.

Lewinsohn PM, Rohde P, Seeley JR, Klein DN. Axis II psychopathology as a function of Axis I disorders in childhood and adolescence. J Am Acad Child Adolesc Psychiatry. 1997;36(12):1752–9.

Livesley WJ. Suggestions for a framework for an empirically based classification of personality disorder. Can J Psychiatry. 1998;43(2):137–47.

Livesley WJ. An empirically-based classification of personality disorder. J Personal Disord. 2011;25(3):397–420.

Markon KE, Krueger RF, Watson D. Delineating the structure of normal and abnormal personality: an integrative hierarchical approach. J Pers Soc Psychol. 2005;88(1):139–57.

McAdams DP, Pals JL. A new Big Five: fundamental principles for an integrative science of personality. Am Psychol. 2006;61(3):204–17.

McGorry P. Early clinical phenotypes and risk for serious mental disorders in young people: need for care precedes traditional diagnoses in mood and psychotic disorders. Can J Psychiatr. 2013;58(1):19–21.

McGorry P, van Os J. Redeeming diagnosis in psychiatry: timing versus specificity. Lancet. 2013;381(9863):343–5.

Mervielde I, De Clercq B, De Fruyt F, Van Leeuwen K. Temperament, personality, and developmental psychopathology as childhood antecedents of personality disorders. J Personal Disord. 2005;19(2):171–201.

Millon T. What is a personality disorder? J Personal Disord. 2016;30(3):289–306.

Morey LC, Hopwood CJ, Gunderson JG, Skodol AE, Shea MT, Yen S, et al. Comparison of alternative models for personality disorders. Psychol Med. 2007;37(7):983–94.

Newton-Howes G, Clark LA, Chanen AM. Personality disorder across the life course. Lancet. 2015;385(9969):727–34.

O'Connor BP. The search for dimensional structure differences between normality and abnormality: a statistical review of published data on personality and psychopathology. J Pers Soc Psychol. 2002;83(4):962–82.

Olds DL. Preventing child maltreatment and crime with prenatal and infancy support of parents: the nurse-family partnership. J Scand Stud Criminol Crime Prev. 2008;9(S1):2–24.

Paris J, Perlin J, Laporte L, Fitzpatrick M, DeStefano J. Exploring resilience and borderline personality disorder: a qualitative study of pairs of sisters. Personal Ment Health. 2014;8(3):199–208.

Pulay AJ, Stinson FS, Dawson DA, Goldstein RB, Chou SP, Huang B, et al. Prevalence, correlates, disability, and comorbidity of DSM-IV schizotypal personality disorder: results from the wave 2 national epidemiologic survey on alcohol and related conditions. Prim Care Companion J Clin Psychiatry. 2009;11(2):53–67.

Quirk SE, El-Gabalawy R, Brennan SL, Bolton JM, Sareen J, Berk M, et al. Personality disorders and physical comorbidities in adults from the United States: data from the National Epidemiologic Survey on Alcohol and Related Conditions. Soc Psychiatry Psychiatr Epidemiol. 2015a;50(5):807–20.

Quirk SE, Williams LJ, Chanen AM, Berk M. Personality disorder and population mental health. Lancet Psychiatry. 2015b;2(3):201–2.

Raine A. Schizotypal personality: neurodevelopmental and psychosocial trajectories. Annu Rev Clin Psychol. 2006;2:291–326.

Roberts BW, DelVecchio WF. The rank-order consistency of personality traits from childhood to old age: a quantitative review of longitudinal studies. Psychol Bull. 2000;126(1):3–25.

Roberts BW, Walton KE, Viechtbauer W. Patterns of mean-level change in personality traits across the life course: a meta-analysis of longitudinal studies. Psychol Bull. 2006;132(1):1–25.

Ro E, Clark LA. Interrelations between psychosocial functioning and adaptive- and maladaptive-range personality traits. J Abnorm Psychol. 2013;122(3):822–35.

Rutter M. Psychopathy in childhood: is it a meaningful diagnosis? Br J Psychiatry. 2012;200(3):175–6.

Rutter M, Moffitt TE, Caspi A. Gene-environment interplay and psychopathology: multiple varieties but real effects. J Child Psychol Psychiatry. 2006;47(3–4):226–61.

Samuel DB, Widiger TA. A meta-analytic review of the relationships between the five-factor model and DSM-IV-TR personality disorders: a facet level analysis. Clin Psychol Rev. 2008;28(8):1326–42.

Schulenberg JE, Sameroff AJ, Cicchetti D. The transition to adulthood as a critical juncture in the course of psychopathology and mental health. Dev Psychopathol. 2004;16(4):799–806.

Shiner RL. The development of personality disorders: perspectives from normal personality development in childhood and adolescence. Dev Psychopathol. 2009;21(3):715–34.

Skodol AE. Longitudinal course and outcome of personality disorders. Psychiatr Clin North Am. 2008;31(3):495–503, viii.

Skodol AE, Johnson JG, Cohen P, Sneed JR, Crawford TN. Personality disorder and impaired functioning from adolescence to adulthood. Br J Psychiatry. 2007;190:415–20.

Skodol AE, Pagano ME, Bender DS, Shea MT, Gunderson JG, Yen S, et al. Stability of functional impairment in patients with schizotypal, borderline, avoidant, or obsessive-compulsive personality disorder over two years. Psychol Med. 2005;35(3):443–51.

Soto CJ, John OP, Gosling SD, Potter J. Age differences in personality traits from 10 to 65: big five domains and facets in a large cross-sectional sample. J Pers Soc Psychol. 2011;100(2):330–48.

Speranza M, Pham-Scottez A, Revah-Levy A, Barbe RP, Perez-Diaz F, Birmaher B, Corcos M. Factor structure of borderline personality disorder symptomatology in adolescents. Can J Psychiatr. 2012;57(4):230–7.

Srivastava S, John OP, Gosling SD, Potter J. Development of personality in early and middle adulthood: set like plaster or persistent change? J Pers Soc Psychol. 2003;84(5):1041–53.

Stepp SD, Whalen DJ, Pilkonis PA, Hipwell AE, Levine MD. Children of mothers with borderline personality disorder: identifying parenting behaviors as potential targets for intervention. Personal Disord. 2012;3(1):76–91.

Stepp SD, Whalen DJ, Scott LN, Zalewski M, Loeber R, Hipwell AE. Reciprocal effects of parenting and borderline personality disorder symptoms in adolescent girls. Dev Psychopathol. 2014;26(2):361–78.

Stinson FS, Dawson DA, Goldstein RB, Chou SP, Huang B, Smith SM, et al. Prevalence, correlates, disability, and comorbidity of DSM-IV narcissistic personality disorder: results from the wave 2 national epidemiologic survey on alcohol and related conditions. J Clin Psychiatry. 2008;69(7):1033–45.

Stoffers-Winterling JM, Völlm BA, Rücker G, Timmer A, Huband N, Lieb K. Psychological therapies for people with borderline personality disorder. Cochrane Database Syst Rev. 2012;(8):CD005652.

Tackett JL, Balsis S, Oltmanns TF, Krueger RF. A unifying perspective on personality pathology across the life span: developmental considerations for the fifth edition of the Diagnostic and Statistical Manual of Mental Disorders. Dev Psychopathol. 2009;21(03):687.

Tackett JL, Kushner SC, De Fruyt F, Mervielde I. Delineating personality traits in childhood and adolescence: associations across measures, temperament, and behavioral problems. Assessment. 2013;20(6):738–51.

Tackett JL, Slobodskaya HR, Mar RA, Deal J, Halverson CF Jr, Baker SR, et al. The hierarchical structure of childhood personality in five countries: continuity from early childhood to early adolescence. J Pers. 2012;80(4):847–79.

Thatcher DL, Cornelius JR, Clark DB. Adolescent alcohol use disorders predict adult borderline personality. Addict Behav. 2005;30(9):1709–24.

Thompson KN, Jackson HJ, Cavelti M, Betts J, McCutcheon L, Jovev M, Chanen AM. The clinical significance of subthreshold borderline personality disorder features in outpatient youth. J Personal Disord. 2017.

Torgersen S, Kringlen E, Cramer V. The prevalence of personality disorders in a community sample. Arch Gen Psychiatry. 2001;58(6):590–6.

Torgersen S, Myers J, Reichborn-Kjennerud T, Røysamb E, Kubarych TS, Kendler KS. The heritability of Cluster B personality disorders assessed both by personal interview and questionnaire. J Personal Disord. 2012;26(6):848–66.

Tyrer P, Reed GM, Crawford MJ. Classification, assessment, prevalence, and effect of personality disorder. Lancet. 2015;385(9969):717–26.

Whalen DJ, Scott LN, Jakubowski KP, McMakin DL, Hipwell AE, Silk JS, Stepp SD. Affective behavior during mother-daughter conflict and borderline personality disorder severity across adolescence. Personal Disord. 2014;5(1):88–96.

WHO. International classification of diseases, version 10. 10th ed. Geneva: World Health Organisation; 1992.

Winsper C, Marwaha S, Lereya ST, Thompson A, Eyden J, Singh SP. Clinical and psychosocial outcomes of borderline personality disorder in childhood and adolescence: a systematic review. Psychol Med. 2015;45(11):2237–51.

Zanarini MC, Frankenburg FR, Hennen J, Reich DB, Silk KR. Psychosocial functioning of borderline patients and axis II comparison subjects followed prospectively for six years. J Personal Disord. 2005a;19(1):19–29.

Zanarini MC, Frankenburg FR, Hennen J, Reich DB, Silk KR. The McLean Study of Adult Development (MSAD): overview and implications of the first six years of prospective follow-up. J Personal Disord. 2005b;19(5):505–23.

Zanarini MC, Frankenburg FR, Reich DB, Fitzmaurice G. Attainment and stability of sustained symptomatic remission and recovery among patients with borderline personality disorder and axis II comparison subjects: a 16-year prospective follow-up study. Am J Psychiatry. 2012;169(5):476–83.

Zanarini MC, Horwood J, Wolke D, Waylen A, Fitzmaurice G, Grant BF. Prevalence of DSM-IV borderline personality disorder in two community samples: 6,330 English 11-year-olds and 34,653 American adults. J Personal Disord. 2011;25(5):607–19.

Zimmerman M, Chelminski I, Young D. The frequency of personality disorders in psychiatric patients. Psychiatr Clin North Am. 2008;31(3):405–20, vi.

Zimmerman M, Chelminski I, Young D, Dalrymple K, Martinez J. Does the presence of one feature of borderline personality disorder have clinical significance? Implications for dimensional ratings of personality disorders. J Clin Psychiatry. 2012;73(1):8–12.

Zimmerman M, Chelminski I, Young D, Dalrymple K, Martinez J. Is dimensional scoring of borderline personality disorder important only for subthreshold levels of severity? J Personal Disord. 2013;27(2):244–51.

Zoccolillo M, Pickles A, Quinton D, Rutter M. The outcome of childhood conduct disorder: implications for defining adult personality disorder and conduct disorder. Psychol Med. 1992;22(4):971–86.

11 The Age of Onset of Eating Disorders

Angela Favaro, Paolo Busetto, Enrico Collantoni, and Paolo Santonastaso

11.1 Introduction

Eating disorders (EDs) are complex mental disorders characterised by a disturbance of eating-related behaviours and concerns about body weight and shape. They cause significant physical and psychosocial impairment, and are burdened with many psychiatric and medical co-morbidities and high mortality rates. EDs show higher prevalence in industrialised countries and female individuals, with a typical age of onset (AOO) ranging from adolescence to young adulthood.

In the fifth edition of the *Diagnostic and Statistical Manual of Mental Disorders* (DSM) (DSM-5; 2013) the "Feeding and Eating Disorders" section includes three ED diagnoses: anorexia nervosa (AN), bulimia nervosa (BN) and binge eating disorder (BED). Key features of AN are persistent energy intake restriction, body image disturbance, intense fear of gaining weight or becoming fat, or persistent behaviour that interferes with weight gain.

BN features are the presence of recurrent episodes of binge eating, which means excessive food consumption accompanied by a sense of lack of control, recurrent inappropriate compensatory behaviours to prevent weight gain, and undue influence of body shape and weight on self-evaluation.

A. Favaro (✉) · P. Busetto · E. Collantoni · P. Santonastaso
Department of Neuroscience, Psychiatric Clinic, University of Padova, Padova, Italy
e-mail: angela.favaro@unipd.it; paolo.santonastaso@unipd.it

G. de Girolamo et al. (eds.), *Age of Onset of Mental Disorders*,
https://doi.org/10.1007/978-3-319-72619-9_11

BED diagnosis is defined by recurrent episodes of binge eating that must occur, on average, at least once per week for 3 months, in the absence of compensatory behaviours.

Compared to DSM-IV, many significant changes were introduced in DSM-5 diagnostic criteria for ED. Firstly, criteria to make a diagnosis of AN or BN have been broadened. With regard to AN, the weight loss criterion (Criterion A) was modified, excluding specific body mass index (BMI) cut-off values and only requiring a "significantly low" weight; fear of gaining weight or becoming fat (Criterion B) does not necessarily need to be verbalised or acknowledged by the patient but can be inferred from the patient's history, clinical data and observation of persistent behaviours that prevent weight gain; and amenorrhoea is no longer a diagnostic criterion, but is considered among the "signs" of clinically significant malnutrition. With regard to BN, the frequency requirements for binge eating and compensatory behaviours have been reduced from twice to once weekly.

Secondly, BED, previously listed in Appendix B of DSM-IV among the "Eating Disorders Not Otherwise Specified" (EDNOS), has been included as a proper ED diagnosis, with reduced frequency requirements for binge eating, from twice to once weekly, and reduced duration of symptoms requirement from 6 to 3 months.

Besides BED, three new diagnoses, namely avoidant/restrictive food intake disorder (ARFID), pica and rumination disorder, have been added to the "Feeding Disorders" subgroup in order to facilitate symptom detection in early infancy and childhood. ARFID is, together with AN, the most common restrictive disorder in prepubertal patients: it is characterised by food restriction and weight loss due to a lack of interest in eating without body image concerns or fear of gaining weight (Ornstein et al. 2013; Fisher et al. 2014, 2015; Nicely et al. 2014; Norris et al. 2014).

Thirdly, the "Other Specified Feeding and Eating Disorders" (OSFED) category has been added, including sub-threshold diagnoses such as atypical AN, BN (of low frequency and/or limited duration), BED (of low frequency and/or limited duration), purging disorder and night eating syndrome.

11.2 Prevalence and Incidence of Eating Disorders (EDs)

The DSM-5 revision of diagnostic criteria, based on extensive evidence from the literature, aimed to reduce the number of individuals who received an EDNOS diagnosis, which was up to 60% of patients referred to specialised ED units, while increasing the validity of diagnostic groups (Flament et al. 2015; Stice et al. 2013).

Following the introduction of DSM-5, several studies suggest a noteworthy increase in the lifetime prevalence rates of EDs due to the change in diagnostic criteria. For example, in a sample of 3043 children and adolescents aged 11–20 years, the overall prevalence of full-threshold ED was twice as high with DSM-5 (3.8%) than with DSM-IV (1.8%) criteria (Flament et al. 2015). In another study, a 60% increase of AN lifetime prevalence, from 2.2% (DSM-IV) to 3.6% (DSM-5) has been found in a 16- to 20-year-old female population (Mustelin et al. 2016). DSM-5 lifetime prevalence in women was found to be up to 2% for BN (Stice et al. 2013; Flament et al. 2015) and 2% for BED, with a conspicuous reduction of sub-threshold diagnoses (Smink et al. 2013). The incidence rates, up to 490 per 100,000 person-years for AN and 300 per 100,000 person-years for BN, have also been affected by the updated diagnostic criteria (Smink et al. 2013).

In studies adopting DSM-5 criteria, the highest incidence rates are among females aged 14–19 years for AN, with a peak in the 14–15 years old category (Javaras et al. 2015), and among females aged 16–20 years for BN (Stice et al. 2013). In the literature preceding the publication of DSM-5, although an early study (Halmi et al. 1979) described two peaks of incidence in AN—one around 14.5 years and the other around 18 years of age—a study with a very large sample size (1666 patients) found a unique peak at 16 years (Favaro et al. 2009). In BN, although early incidence studies reported that the highest incidence rate was among females aged 20–24 years (Hoek and Van Hoeken 2003), the study by Favaro et al. (2009) found that, once cases with a previous episode of AN were excluded, the peak of AOO was 17 years. Using an admixture analysis, Volpe et al. (2016) found, in both AN and BN, the existence of two groups of patients based on their AOO: a larger group (about 75% of patients) with a mean AOO of 16 years and a smaller group with an AOO of 23–25 years.

While the time trend of ED incidence seems to have reached a plateau in the past three decades, the AOO has been decreasing (Favaro et al. 2009). Studies in paediatric samples reported incidence rates of ED ranging from 1.4 to 3.01 per 100,000 (Madden et al. 2009; Nicholls et al. 2011; Pinhas et al. 2011), promoting a growing awareness of very-early-onset EDs as a clinical reality.

Conversely, data regarding late-onset ED are scarce. In AN, an onset after the age of 25 years is usually considered atypical (Halmi et al. 1979; Fairburn and Harrison 2003; Smink et al. 2013; Stice et al. 2013). The prevalence of ED in late life ranges from 1.8% to 3.6%, including both new-onset and chronic disorders, and BED is the most common full-threshold diagnosis in patients older than 40 years (Luca et al. 2015; Micali et al. 2017).

11.2.1 Transdiagnostic "Migration" Due to DSM-5

A high rate of trans-diagnostic migration among different types of EDs has been described, reinforcing the hypothesis of common pathogenetic mechanisms for AN, BN and other EDs (Fairburn and Harrison 2003). Although the DSM-5 criteria seem to have reduced the crossover percentage compared with DSM-IV, diagnostic instability in ED remains significant. Follow-up studies that adopted DSM-5 criteria reported the following crossover rates: 9–23.4% from AN to BN, 0.5–8.4% from BN to AN, 1–23% from BN to BED, 7.1–20% from BED to BN, and nearly no shifting (< 1%) from AN to BED and vice versa (Castellini et al. 2011; Ekeroth et al. 2013; Fichter et al. 2017; Stice et al. 2013). Roughly one-third of the individuals presenting a full-threshold ED diagnosis at baseline shift to a sub-threshold or EDNOS diagnosis (Ekeroth et al. 2013; Stice et al. 2013).

Considering the high rate of trans-diagnostic migration, it is important to emphasise that diagnostic assessment of a patient with an ED should always include the assessment of the "current" episode and a retrospective evaluation of previous episodes, similar to what is recommended for bipolar disorders. Patients with previous episodes of EDs and those with higher weight suppression are more prone to gaining weight more rapidly and this point has considerable clinical importance, since patients who gain weight rapidly are more at risk of worsening their body dissatisfaction and being less compliant, with a higher risk of relapse or dropping out of treatment.

11.2.2 Aetiopathogenetic Pathways and Age of Onset (AOO) Definitions in EDs

There are few descriptions of and no systematic studies regarding the phenomenology and possible pathways that lead to the onset of EDs. Usually, patients describe body uneasiness as the first symptom, followed by behaviours aimed at decreasing caloric intake. In most cases, dieting or avoidance of certain types of food (carbohydrates, fats, etc.) are used, although in a minority of patients more pathological compensatory behaviours, such as self-induced vomiting or purging, are employed as a first attempt to control energy intake. According to cognitive–behavioural theories, which have proven to be the most influential for their therapeutic implications, two psychological mechanisms underlie restriction: a need to feel in control, pursued through eating, and over-evaluation of body shape and weight (Fairburn and Harrison 2003). The consequent restriction is highly reinforcing, resulting in a perpetuation of the vicious cycle and facilitating the onset of other maintenance factors such as social withdrawal, higher binge eating frequency (promoted by restraint) and negative effects of the loss of control (i.e. secondary negative self-evaluation and need for an even stricter self-control). Finally, in BN and BED, the onset of binge eating is usually preceded by weight loss or reduced caloric intake; however, sometimes, especially in BED, binge eating is the first symptom.

Knowledge of pathogenetic pathways and the course of disease are essential to provide a correct definition of AOO. Most clinical and epidemiological studies did not provide a clear statement regarding the AOO definition employed. There are alternative possible definitions of AOO, the most common being: (1) age of the first symptom; (2) age of first ascertainment (when receiving a medical diagnosis); or (3) age of first fulfilment of all diagnostic criteria (usually retrospectively). All these definitions have intrinsic advantages and limitations.

The age of the first symptom is usually easier to recollect and characterises the beginning of the pathological process; however, very often the first symptom is a very common (not necessarily pathological) behaviour, such as caloric restraint or avoidance of some foods, which is not distinguishable from dieting in a "non-pathological" way. The second definition, age of first ascertainment, has the advantage of representing the result of a medical/psychological assessment, but very often ascertainment is late, since many patients are referred months or even years after the beginning of the ED. Longitudinal studies performed in large cohorts of community samples are usually in the condition to use this definition, and probably provide the most reliable evaluation of age at onset. The third definition is probably the most widely used (Favaro et al. 2009; Volpe et al. 2016) in clinical studies and represents an attempt to reliably recollect the beginning of the disordered, defined as the co-existence of all the diagnostic criteria. This process is usually (but not always) easy when dealing with pathological behaviour (first episode of binge eating or vomiting or purging) or history of weight, but not at all easy when dealing with cognitive processes, especially in patients with high levels of denial or in very young patients. In some patients, frequency of binge eating/purging behaviour can be sub-threshold for a period of time before fulfilling the diagnostic criteria and, in these cases, the exact AOO is not easily defined. Similarly, in patients who did not check their body weight, history of weight is also very unreliable.

In clinical samples, it should be recommended that "AOO" is used to describe the onset of the first episode of an ED and not simply the onset of the current episode. For example, in a patient with a current episode of BN and a previous episode of AN, the AOO should be the age at which the patient fulfilled all the criteria for AN for the first time and not the AOO of binge eating.

In many mental disorders, the time elapsed between onset and ascertainment of the diagnosis is considered to have a prognostic value. In the field of EDs, no study to date has explored the impact of the time from onset to ascertainment as a prognostic factor. In addition, ascertainment is not always followed by the beginning of effective treatment, due to the high levels of denial and refusal of treatment that characterise EDs, and particularly AN.

11.3 AOO of EDs in a Large Italian Sample

In a previous study (Favaro et al. 2009) conducted in a large cohort of 2459 patients with DSM-IV-based full diagnosis of an ED (1666 patients with lifetime AN and 793 with lifetime BN without previous episodes of AN), we found that the distribution of AOO in the two groups was very similar, with a normal distribution of AOO and a unique peak in both cases (16 years in AN and 17 years in BN). Both disorders exhibited their typical onset during adolescence, since 71% of AN and 65% of BN subjects were already affected before the age of 20 years. This previous study was the first to explore the possibility of a change in the AOO of EDs, analysing data according to year of birth: a trend towards a progressively decreasing AOO in both AN and BN cases emerged, even after restricting our analyses to subjects born between 1970 and 1981 and to those with an onset before 25 years, to obtain more reliable data and avoid cohort effects due to time of collection of data (Favaro et al. 2009). An analysis of correlates of AOO found significant effects of age at menarche, socioeconomic status and parity (having siblings was shown to have a protective effect).

Here, we analyse for the first time a larger sample of the same cohort of patients (those referred to the ED Unit of Padova Hospital, Padova, Italy). However, we also include patients who completed the baseline diagnostic assessment (present and lifetime diagnosis) between 1993 and 2016 ($n = 3164$). Diagnostic assessment was performed by means of the Structured Clinical Interview from DSM-IV ("Eating Disorders" section); in addition, all patients were assessed by means of a semi-structured clinical interview that included information about history of weight, body attitudes and lifetime eating psychopathology. All these data allowed lifetime diagnoses to be reformulated according to DSM-5.

Using DSM-IV criteria, the sample was composed of 1154 patients with lifetime AN, 866 with lifetime BN without previous episodes of AN, 304 with BED and 840 with EDNOS. In contrast, using DSM-5, the sample included 1827 patients with lifetime AN, 823 with lifetime BN without previous AN, 315 with BED and 199 with EDs otherwise specified (atypical AN, sub-threshold BN, sub-threshold BED and purging disorder).

The age range at presentation was 13–59 years for AN cases, 14–66 years for BN, 15–60 years for BED and 12–59 years for EDNOS. AOO of EDs is described in Table 11.1.

Table 11.1 Age of onset of eating disorders according to DSM-IV and DSM-5 diagnostic criteria

Lifetime diagnosis	*n*	Mean [years (SD)]	Range (years)	Onset before 16 years [*n* (%)]	Onset after 20 years [*n* (%)]	Onset after 25 years [*n* (%)]
DSM-IV criteria						
DSM-IV anorexia nervosa	1154	18.2 (5.1)	10–53	344 (30)	227 (20)	76 (7)
DSM-IV bulimia nervosa	866	19.1 (5.7)	9–57	210 (24)	245 (28)	97 (11)
DSM-IV binge eating disorder	304	25.4 (11.5)	6–60	59 (19)	169 (56)	121 (40)
DSM-IV ED OS	840	19.5 (6.8)	8–56	223 (26)	233 (28)	112 (13)
DSM-5 criteria						
DSM-5 anorexia nervosa	1827	18.3 (5.2)	10–56	534 (29)	375 (20)	127 (7)
DSM-5 bulimia nervosa	823	19.6 (6.5)	9–57	196 (24)	255 (31)	116 (14)
DSM-5 binge eating disorder	315	25.7 (11.5)	6–60	61 (19)	178 (56)	129 (41)
DSM-5 ED OS	199	20.0 (6.9)	8–56	45 (23)	66 (33)	34 (17)

DSM-IV Diagnostic and Statistical Manual of Mental Disorders, Fourth Edition, *DSM-5* Diagnostic and Statistical Manual of Mental Disorders, Fifth Edition, *ED OS* eating disorder otherwise specified, *SD* standard deviation

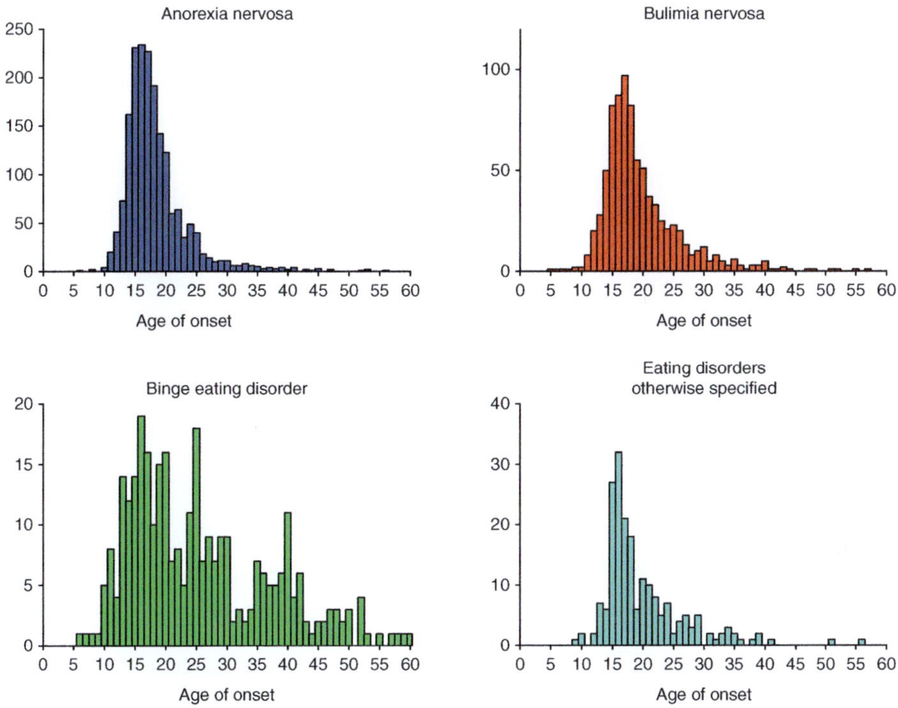

Fig. 11.1 Distribution of age of onset in *Diagnostic and Statistical Manual of Mental Disorders, Fifth Edition* (DSM-5) anorexia nervosa, bulimia nervosa, binge eating disorders and eating disorders otherwise specified

In the cohort analysed here, we found that the distribution of AOO in AN and BN groups were very similar, with a normal distribution of AOO and a unique peak in both cases (16 years in AN and 17 years in BN). A normal distribution (peak at 16 years) was also present in the EDs otherwise specified group, but not in the BED group (mode is 16 years, but other peaks seem to be present). Distribution of AOO is shown in Fig. 11.1.

All EDs (except for BED) exhibited their typical onset during adolescence, since 80% of AN, 69% of BN and 67% of subjects with EDs otherwise specified were already affected before the age of 20 years. For BED, in contrast, an AOO after 20 years is quite common (56% of cases).

Analysing the trends of AOO according to year of birth (Fig. 11.2), a progressive decrease in AOO is evident, as was shown in our previous study. In Table 11.2, we reported the estimated risk of having an onset before the age of 16 years in subjects with AN and BN according to DSM-5 diagnosis in those subjects born between 1970 and 1990. No significant cohort effect (increase of risk with more recent generations) has been observed in BED and EDs otherwise specified (not shown). In this subsample, the year of birth showed a significant negative correlation with AOO in all four groups (using DSM-5 diagnoses): AN (n = 1827;

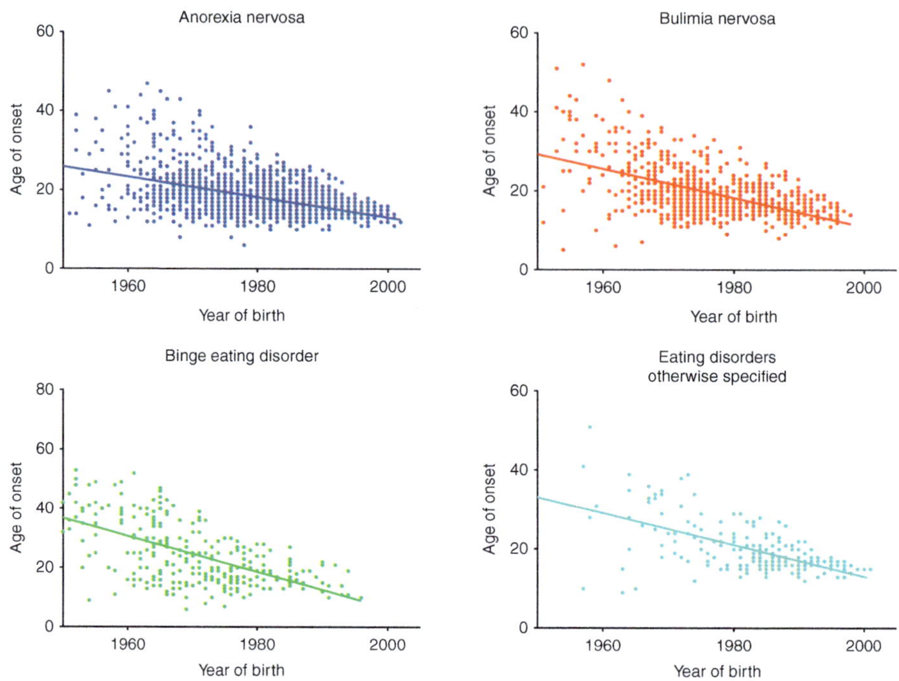

Fig. 11.2 Relationship between age of onset and year of birth in *Diagnostic and Statistical Manual of Mental Disorders, Fifth Edition* (DSM-5) anorexia nervosa, bulimia nervosa, binge eating disorders and eating disorders otherwise specified

rho = −0.43; $p < 0.001$), BN ($n = 823$; rho = −0.47; $p < 0.001$), BED ($n = 315$; rho = −0.58; $p < 0.001$) and EDs otherwise specified ($n = 199$; rho = −0.52; $p < 0.001$).

11.3.1 DSM-5 Diagnostic Criteria and Their Implications for the AOO in the Italian Sample

Our data show that the introduction of DSM-5 causes a significantly different distribution of ED diagnoses, with a substantial increase of AN cases and a decrease of EDs otherwise specified. However, the "migration" of patients from one diagnosis to another does not imply a modification in patterns of AOO. The average AOO in patients grouped according to DSM-IV diagnoses is very similar to that in patients grouped according to DSM-5 (Table 11.1). The only relevant difference is a somewhat greater variability (i.e. standard deviations in Table 11.1) in AOO of DSM-5 than in DSM-IV BN patients. It is noteworthy that AOO in BED substantially differs from AOO of all the other groups: it is significantly higher and has a different distribution, characterised by more than one peak.

Although the DSM-5 modifications in diagnostic criteria leads to substantial changes in the number of patients with a full ED diagnosis, we confirm a trend towards a decreasing AOO in new generations in both AN and BN, but not in BED. The decrease of AOO was linear in AN cases born from 1970 to 1987 and seems to be stabilising in those born after 1988. In BN, a more irregular trend is observable (Table 11.2). Further studies analysing large cohorts from different treatment centres and different geographical areas are needed to fully understand this phenomenon. The implications of our findings in terms of long-term outcome and risk of altering developmental trajectories of bone mass, height (Favaro et al. 2007) and the central nervous system remain to be explored and understood, although we know that an earlier AOO has a more deleterious impact on these specific aspects of general health (Favaro et al. 2007; Hall et al. 2008). Our previous study found that AOO was significantly predicted by an earlier age at menarche, absence of siblings and a high socioeconomic status. However, the socio-cultural and biological factors

Table 11.2 Pattern of presentation in *Diagnostic and Statistical Manual of Mental Disorders, Fifth Edition* (DSM-5) anorexia nervosa and bulimia nervosa cases according to year of birth

		Age at presentation (years)	AOO (years)	AOO < 16 years		
Years	*n*	Mean (SD)	Mean (SD)	*n* (%)	OR (95% CI)	*p*-Value
Anorexia nervosa						
1970–1972	166	27.6 (5.9)	20.1 (5.0)	23 (14)	1.0	
1973–1975	212	24.4 (4.9)	18.8 (4.0)	33 (16)	1.1 (0.6–2.0)	0.642
1976–1978	239	22.5 (4.6)	17.8 (3.8)	62 (26)	2.2 (1.3–3.7)	0.004
1979–1981	220	22.0 (4.5)	17.4 (3.5)	66 (30)	2.7 (1.6–4.5)	<0.001
1982–1984	176	21.3 (4.3)	17.4 (3.4)	59 (34)	3.1 (1.8–5.4)	<0.001
1985–1987	148	20.8 (3.7)	16.7 (3.2)	56 (38)	3.8 (2.2–6.6)	<0.001
1988–1990	141	19.8 (2.8)	17.0 (2.9)	42 (30)	2.6 (1.5–4.7)	0.001
All[a]	1302	22.7 (5.1)	17.9 (3.9)	341 (26)		
Bulimia nervosa**						
1970–1972	104	28.2 (6.1)	19.9 (4.8)	15 (14)	1.0	=
1973–1975	121	25.9 (5.3)	19.2 (4.4)	24 (20)	1.5 (0.7–3.0)	0.287
1976–1978	115	23.8 (4.6)	18.0 (4.1)	27 (24)	1.8 (0.9–3.6)	0.092
1979–1981	73	22.8 (4.7)	17.6 (3.7)	24 (33)	2.9 (1.4–6.1)	0.004
1982–1984	65	21.9 (3.6)	17.8 (3.1)	14 (22)	1.6 (0.7–3.6)	0.235
1985–1987	53	21.5 (3.7)	17.5 (3.9)	14 (26)	2.1 (0.9–4.8)	0.071
1988–1990	64	20.4 (3.0)	16.2 (3.1)	27 (42)	4.3 (2.1–9.1)	<0.001
All[a]	595	24.1 (5.4)	18.3 (4.2)	145 (24)		

AOO age of onset, *CI* confidence interval, *OR* odds ratio, *SD* standard deviation
[a]Subjects born before 1970 and after 1990 were excluded

that are causing these changes, as well as their scientific and clinical implications, remain to be adequately explored by future studies.

11.4 AOO in Other Large Samples of EDs

The literature regarding AOO in EDs is difficult to review and interpret due to the paucity of studies specifically designed to explore this issue. In addition, available literature that describes large samples of patients with EDs addressing other characteristics or different aims (epidemiology, risk factors, genetic associations, etc.) are also difficult to interpret for a series of reasons, such as: (1) the lack of a precise definition of AOO (see Sect. 11.2.2) in large multicentre studies; and (2) in most countries, the organisation of ED units is based on age at referral, with separate units for adolescents and adults and, therefore, data collected in these units are biased (in adolescent units, late-onset patients are lacking; in adult units, early-onset patients who recover before the age of 18 years are lacking). More reliable information can be achieved via large-scale epidemiological studies when (a) a large age range is considered; (b) lifetime (and not only present) diagnoses are assessed; and (c) AOO is reported.

For example, the National Comorbidity Survey Replication (Hudson et al. 2007), which assessed 9282 adults, defined AOO using the CIDI (Composite International Diagnostic Interview) criteria and considered lifetime diagnoses. The mean AOO was 18.9 (standard error [SE] = 0.8) for BN, 19.7 (SE = 1.3) and 25.4 (SE = 1.2) years for BED, whereas the medians were 18.0 (25–75% quartiles, 16–22), 18.0 (25–75% quartiles, 14–22) and 21.0 (25–75% quartiles, 17–32) years, respectively. A similar large-scale epidemiological study conducted in Europe, the ESEMeD-WMH (European Study of the Epidemiology of Mental Disorders–World Mental Health) project (Preti et al. 2009) unfortunately did not report AOO. However, another study performed in Switzerland (Mohler-Kuo et al. 2016), which adopted the same instruments on a representative sample of 10,038 residents aged 15–60 years, reported the following: mean AOO was 18.0 (SE = 0.5) for AN, 17.8 (SE = 0.4) for AN according to DSM-5 criteria, and 21.2 (SE = 0.8) years for BN, whereas the medians were 18 (25–75% quartiles, 15–20), 17 (25–75% quartiles, 16–19.5) and 18 (25–75% quartiles, 15–25) years, respectively. These figures are in line with the AOO reported by Hudson et al. (2007) and in our Italian cohort (Favaro et al. 2009).

It is of note that the only large-scale epidemiological study, performed in a cohort of 10,123 adolescents aged 13–18 years (Swanson et al. 2011), found a median (25–75% quartiles) AOO of 12.3 (11.2–13) for AN, 12.4 (11.1–13.5) for BN and 12.6 (10–14.3) years for BED. The low AOO observed in this study, considering that the prevalence rates of EDs in adolescents were only slightly lower than those reported for adult cohorts, suggests that, without a clear definition of AOO, retrospective assessments in adults could possibly overestimate the AOO of these conditions (Swanson et al. 2011).

11.5 Prognostic Implications of the AOO in EDs

Few data are available on the prognostic role of AOO in EDs. According to the literature (Steinhausen 2002), early AOO is a favourable prognostic factor in AN, although some observations suggest that a prepubertal onset may confer a worse course of disorder (Zipfel et al. 2015). It would probably be more appropriate to consider "typical" AOO—instead of "early" AOO—as a positive prognostic factor, since both extremes of AOO seem to be associated with negative outcomes in AN. The onset of AN before puberty is reported to be a very poor outcome condition and associated with more severe medical complications and often requires medical admission. In addition, the consequences of severe malnutrition on neurodevelopmental trajectories are not known.

Globally, prospective studies that evaluate the outcome of adolescent patients with AN seem to indicate that approximately 70% achieve remission (Jagielska and Kacperska 2017). This observation has important therapeutic implications, since it confirms the importance of early recognition of symptoms of EDs and early treatment. In a recent review, Treasure et al. (2015) support the importance of a staging model to map the course of EDs to design treatment programmes tailored to the phase of the disorder. The opportunity to consider the clinical and neurobiological characteristics of EDs from a longitudinal perspective seems to be important in order to design more specific and effective therapeutic interventions.

The presence of stronger evidence that supports the effectiveness of specific psychotherapeutic programmes in adolescent patients with AN compared with adult patients, together with the observation of a worse prognosis in patients with a later onset of the disorder, suggest the opportunity to provide early treatment in adolescent patients, but also to design new therapeutic programmes to improve the outcome of adult patients. Fewer data are available regarding the role of age as a predictive factor in BN and in BED.

Conclusions

A review of the available literature shows that few studies to date have addressed in a specific way the topic of AOO in EDs. Studies performed on a large Italian cohort show a trend towards a decreasing AOO in new generations, particularly in AN, that seems to be reaching a stabilisation in patients born after 1988. However, these findings need to be confirmed in other cohorts and their prognostic implications need to be explored. Although in other psychiatric disorders, such as schizophrenia and mood disorders, timing and rapidity of symptom onset have been examined as potential prognostic factors, no studies to date have fully explored these issues in EDs (Solmi et al. 2018).

While large-scale epidemiological studies show a concordance in average and median AOO of lifetime EDs in adult and late-adolescent populations, a study in an adolescent cohort (Swanson et al. 2011) underscored the possibility of a recall bias in adult patients, which would lead to an overestimation of AOO. This is a further confirmation of the need for a shared definition of AOO in the field of EDs. In addition, the study of Swanson et al. (2011) showed that adolescents with EDs had higher than expected prevalence rates and high levels of psychiatric co-morbidity, role impairment and suicidality, all of which represent major public health concerns. Further studies analysing large cohorts from different geographical areas are needed to fully understand the phenomenology of AOO in EDs.

Acknowledgments The authors declare that they have no conflict of interest. The study was performed without any external financial help.

References

American Psychiatric Association. Task Force on DSM 5. Diagnostic and statistical manual of mental disorders DSM-5. Washington, DC: American Psychiatric Association; 2013.

Castellini G, Lo Sauro C, Mannucci E, Ravaldi C, Rotella CM, Faravelli C, et al. Diagnostic crossover and outcome predictors in eating disorders according to DSM-IV and DSM-V proposed criteria: a 6-year follow-up study. Psychosom Med. 2011;73:270–9. https://doi.org/10.1097/PSY.0b013e31820a1838.

Ekeroth K, Clinton D, Norring C, Birgegård A. Clinical characteristics and distinctiveness of DSM-5 eating disorder diagnoses: findings from a large naturalistic clinical database. J Eat Disord. 2013;1:31. https://doi.org/10.1186/2050-2974-1-31.

Fairburn CG, Harrison PJ. Eating disorders. Lancet. 2003;361:407–16. https://doi.org/10.1016/S0140-6736(03)12378-1.

Favaro A, Tenconi E, Degortes D, Soave M, Zanetti T, Nardi MT, et al. Association between low height and eating disorders: cause or effect? Int J Eat Disord. 2007;40:549–53. https://doi.org/10.1002/eat.20409.

Favaro A, Caregaro L, Tenconi E, Bosello R, Santonastaso P. Time trends in age at onset of anorexia nervosa and bulimia nervosa. J Clin Psychiatry. 2009;70:1715–21. https://doi.org/10.4088/JCP.09m05176blu.

Fichter MM, Quadflieg N, Crosby RD, Koch S. Long-term outcome of anorexia nervosa: results from a large clinical longitudinal study. Int J Eat Disord. 2017:1–13. https://doi.org/10.1002/eat.22736.

Fisher MM, Rosen DS, Ornstein RM, Mammel KA, Katzman DK, Rome ES, et al. Characteristics of avoidant/restrictive food intake disorder in children and adolescents: a "new disorder" in DSM-5. J Adolesc Health. 2014;55:49–52. https://doi.org/10.1016/j.jadohealth.2013.11.013.

Fisher M, Gonzalez M, Malizio J. Eating disorders in adolescents: how does the DSM-5 change the diagnosis? Int J Adolesc Med Health. 2015;27:437–41. https://doi.org/10.1515/ijamh-2014-0059.

Flament MF, Buchholz A, Henderson K, Obeid N, Maras D, Schubert N, et al. Comparative distribution and validity of DSM-IV and DSM-5 diagnoses of eating disorders in adolescents from the community. Eur Eat Disord Rev. 2015;23:100–10. https://doi.org/10.1002/erv.2339.

Hall CH, Hewitt G, Stevens SL. Assessment and management of bone health in adolescents with anorexia nervosa. Part two: bone health in adolescents with anorexia nervosa. J Pediatr Adolesc Gynecol. 2008;21:221–4.

Halmi KA, Casper RC, Eckert ED, Goldberg SC, Davis JM. Unique features associated with age of onset of anorexia nervosa. Psychiatry Res. 1979;1:209–15. https://doi.org/10.1016/0165-1781(79)90063-5.

Hoek HW, Van Hoeken D. Review of the prevalence and incidence of eating disorders. Int J Eat Disord. 2003;34:383–96. https://doi.org/10.1002/eat.10222.

Hudson JI, Hiripi E, Pope HG Jr, Kessler RC. The prevalence and correlates of eating disorders in the National Comorbidity Survey Replication. Biol Psychiatry. 2007;61:348–58.

Jagielska G, Kacperska I. Outcome, comorbidity and prognosis in anorexia nervosa. Psychiatr Pol. 2017;51:205–18. https://doi.org/10.12740/PP/64580.

Javaras KN, Runfola CD, Thornton LM, Agerbo E, Birgegård A, Norring C, et al. Sex- and age-specific incidence of healthcare-register-recorded eating disorders in the complete Swedish 1979-2001 birth cohort. Int J Eat Disord. 2015;48:1070–81. https://doi.org/10.1002/eat.22467.

Luca A, Luca M, Calandra C. Eating disorders in late-life. Aging Dis. 2015;6:48–55. https://doi.org/10.14336/AD.2014.0124.

Madden S, Morris A, Zurynski YA, Kohn M, Elliot EJ. Burden of eating disorders in 5-13-year-old children in Australia. Med J Aust. 2009;190:410–4.

Micali N, Martini MG, Thomas JJ, Eddy KT, Kothari R, Russell E, et al. Lifetime and 12-month prevalence of eating disorders amongst women in mid-life: a population-based study of diagnoses and risk factors. BMC Med. 2017;15:12. https://doi.org/10.1186/s12916-016-0766-4.

Mohler-Kuo M, Schnyder U, Dermota P, Wei W, Milos G. The prevalence, correlates, and help-seeking of eating disorders in Switzerland. Psychol Med. 2016;46:2749–58.

Mustelin L, Silén Y, Raevuori A, Hoek HW, Kaprio J, Keski-Rahkonen A. The DSM-5 diagnostic criteria for anorexia nervosa may change its population prevalence and prognostic value. J Psychiatr Res. 2016;77:85–91. https://doi.org/10.1016/j.jpsychires.2016.03.003.

Nicely TA, Lane-Loney S, Masciulli E, Hollenbeak CS, Ornstein RM. Prevalence and characteristics of avoidant/restrictive food intake disorder in a cohort of young patients in day treatment for eating disorders. J Eat Disord. 2014;2:21. https://doi.org/10.1186/s40337-014-0021-3.

Nicholls DE, Lynn R, Viner RM. Childhood eating disorders: British National Surveillance Study. Br J Psychiatry. 2011;198:295–301. https://doi.org/10.1192/bjp.bp.110.081356.

Norris ML, Robinson A, Obeid N, Harrison M, Spettigue W, Henderson K. Exploring avoidant/restrictive food intake disorder in eating disordered patients: A descriptive study. Int J Eat Disord. 2014;47:495–9. https://doi.org/10.1002/eat.22217.

Ornstein RM, Rosen DS, Mammel KA, Callahan ST, Forman S, Jay MS, et al. Distribution of eating disorders in children and adolescents using the proposed DSM-5 criteria for feeding and eating disorders. J Adolesc Health. 2013;53:303–5. https://doi.org/10.1016/j.jadohealth.2013.03.025.

Pinhas L, Morris A, Crosby RD, Katzman DK. Incidence and age-specific presentation of restrictive eating disorders in children. Arch Pediatr Adolesc Med. 2011;165:895. https://doi.org/10.1001/archpediatrics.2011.145.

Preti A, de Girolamo G, Vilagut G, Alonso J, de Graaf R, Bruffaerts R, et al. The epidemiology of eating disorders in six European countries: results of the EDEMeD-WMH project. J Psychiatr Res. 2009;43:1125–32. https://doi.org/10.1016/j.jpsychires.2009.04.003.

Smink FRE, van Hoeken D, Hoek HW. Epidemiology, course, and outcome of eating disorders. Curr Opin Psychiatry. 2013;26:543–8. https://doi.org/10.1097/YCO.0b013e328365a24f.

Solmi M, Gallicchio D, Collantoni E, Meneguzzo P, Zanetti T, Degortes D, et al. The impact of weight suppression and weight loss speed on baseline clinical characteristics and response to treatment. Int J Eat Disord. 2018;51(6):542–8.

Steinhausen H-C. The outcome of anorexia nervosa in the 20th century. Am J Psychiatry. 2002;159:1284–93. https://doi.org/10.1176/appi.ajp.159.8.1284.

Stice E, Marti CN, Rohde P. Prevalence, incidence, impairment, and course of the proposed DSM-5 eating disorder diagnoses in an 8-year prospective community study of young women. J Abnorm Psychol. 2013;122:445–57. https://doi.org/10.1037/a0030679.

Swanson SA, Crow SJ, Le Grange D, Swendsen J, Merikangas KR. Prevalence and correlates of eating disorders in adolescents. Results from the National Comorbidity Survey Replication Adolescent Supplement. Arch Gen Psychiatry. 2011;68:714–23. https://doi.org/10.1001/archgenpsychiatry.2011.22.

Treasure J, Stein D, Maguire S. Has the time come for a staging model to map the course of eating disorders from high risk to severe enduring illness? An examination of the evidence. Early Interv Psychiatry. 2015;9:173–84. https://doi.org/10.1111/eip.12170.

Volpe U, Tortorella A, Manchia M, Monteleone AM, Albert U, Monteleone P. Eating disorders: what age at onset? Psychiatry Res. 2016;238:225–7. https://doi.org/10.1016/j.psychres.2016.02.048.

Zipfel S, Giel KE, Bulik CM, Hay P, Schmidt U. Anorexia nervosa: aetiology, assessment, and treatment. Lancet Psychiatry. 2015;2:1099–111. https://doi.org/10.1016/S2215-0366(15)00356-9.

The Age of Onset of Attention-Deficit Hyperactivity Disorder

12

David Coghill, Phillip Asherson, Stephen V. Faraone, and Luis A. Rohde

12.1 The Age of Onset of Attention Deficit Hyperactivity Disorder

What is the age of onset (AOO) of attention deficit/hyperactivity disorder (ADHD)? Until recently this would have been seen by most as a relatively simple question and with a typical response going something like "ADHD is a neurodevelopmental disorder that starts early in life and certainly before the age of 7 years". However several recent lines of research have led us to question this received wisdom and indeed opened up the possibility that ADHD can also onset much later in life and, perhaps, even arise de novo in adulthood. This chapter reviews the literature, highlighting the early history, the changes over time in the formal diagnostic criteria for AOO, issues

D. Coghill (✉)
Departments of Paediatrics and Psychiatry, University of Melbourne, Parkville, VIC, Australia

Murdoch Children's Research Institute, Melbourne, VIC, Australia

Royal Children's Hospital, Melbourne, VIC, Australia
e-mail: david.coghill@unimelb.edu.au

P. Asherson
MRC Social Genetic and Developmental Psychiatry (SGDP), Institute of Psychiatry, London, UK
e-mail: philip.asherson@kcl.ac.uk

S. V. Faraone
Departments of Psychiatry and of Neuroscience and Physiology, SUNY Upstate Medical University, Syracuse, NY, USA
e-mail: sfaraone@childpsychresearch.org

L. A. Rohde
Department of Psychiatry, Federal University of Rio Grande do Sul, Porto Alegre, Brazil

Hospital de Clínicas de Porto Alegre, Porto Alegre, Brazil

G. de Girolamo et al. (eds.), *Age of Onset of Mental Disorders*,
https://doi.org/10.1007/978-3-319-72619-9_12

relating to the stability of ADHD symptoms across development and the recent evidence for a possible adult-onset ADHD.

12.1.1 A Historical Perspective

Whilst the contemporary concept of ADHD, as appears in the *Diagnostic and Statistical Manual of Mental Disorders* (DSM) and hyperkinetic disorder as described in the *International Classification of Diseases* (ICD), is relatively recent, most authors agree that the notion of a disorder characterised by excessive, impairing and pervasive inattention, impulsivity and overactivity has been described in the literature since at least the nineteenth century (Lange et al. 2010). In these early descriptions, there was general agreement that these problems typically start early in a person's life. Sir Alexander Crichton, a Scottish physician, is credited as the first author to describe a disorder very similar to ADHD. In the second of his three book series entitled *An Inquiry Into the Nature and Origin of Mental Derangement: Comprehending a Concise System of the Physiology and Pathology of the Human Mind and a History of the Passions and Their Effects* (Crichton 2008), Crichton included a chapter entitled "On Attention and its Diseases". In this chapter he describes a disorder of attention with several symptoms of inattention and distractibility that resonate strongly with the current descriptions of ADHD. Crichton's description does not fully match our current concept of ADHD. He does not, for instance, explicitly mention hyperactivity although he does allude to a condition he describes as "the fidgets". He also clearly indicates an early onset and comments on the developmental nature of these problems saying that "When born with a person it becomes evident at a very early period of life, and has a very bad effect, inasmuch as it renders him incapable of attending with constancy to any one object of education. But it seldom is in so great a degree as totally to impede all instruction; and what is very fortunate, it is generally diminished with age."

Just over a century later in his lectures to the Royal College of Physicians of London entitled "On Some Abnormal Psychical Conditions in Children", Sir George Still described several groups of children with what he termed "abnormal defects of moral control". Within these, there was a group of children who many have considered to represent an early description of ADHD. This group, whose symptoms are very similar to those of ADHD and whose problems were noted not to be associated with either intellectual impairment or physical disease, was described by Still as having a "history of severe cerebral disturbance in early infancy" (Still 2006). Seven of the nine cases where AOO was commented on were said to have demonstrated symptoms before the age of 7 years.

Some 30 years later, the German physicians Franz Kramer and Hans Pollnow also stressed the early onset of symptoms in their report "On a hyperkinetic disease of infancy" (Kramer and Pollnow 1932); the main symptoms in their cases were again very similar to our current concept of ADHD. These cases described by Kramer and Pollnow had a peak AOO at 6 years of age with some cases starting as early as 3 or 4 years.

Around the same time, several groups of researchers started to focus on the idea that hyperactivity was a consequence of brain damage, particularly to the frontal lobes, and the concept of "minimal brain damage" became increasingly popular (Kessler 1980). Much of the focus within this concept was on various forms of brain damage that were assumed to have occurred prenatally or very early in life and that were evidenced by behavioural rather than neurological evidence. By the 1960s, however, this concept of brain damage started to be criticised by a number of researchers and clinicians (Birch 1964; Rapin 1964). These authors were unhappy with the suggestion that every child presenting with abnormal behaviour was assumed to have some form of brain damage, particularly where there was no neurological evidence to support this. As a consequence there was a shift from the concept of "minimal brain damage" to one of "minimal brain dysfunction" (Conners 2000). However the notion of early onset was still very much enshrined within this concept, whereby the brain dysfunction was still seen as a response to neurological factors such are pre- and perinatal "cerebral hypoxic lesions" rather than environmental or social factors (Towbin 1978). This concept of minimal brain dysfunction, whilst including many of those who would now be deemed to have ADHD, was however much more general, and it too was soon criticised on the grounds that it was too broad and heterogeneous. It was therefore relatively quickly abandoned and replaced by multiple more specific descriptive labels such as "hyperactivity", "learning disability", "dyslexia" and "language disorders" (Lange et al. 2010). In 1968, a definition of a disorder characterised by hyperactivity was incorporated into DSM-II (Association 1968). This disorder, named "hyperkinetic reaction of childhood", was described very briefly as a disorder "characterized by overactivity, restlessness, distractibility, and short attention span", and whilst there was not yet any specific guidance about AOO, it was noted that this disorder was found "especially in young children" and that "the behaviour usually diminishes by adolescence".

Interestingly, several of these early descriptions also highlighted the presence of emotional instability alongside the hyperactivity, impulsivity and inattention. Whilst this was also included in the early DSM descriptions, it was dropped in DSM-IV due to a lack of specificity. It is however still recognised that many individuals with ADHD also have problems with emotional instability and that this is a prominent feature of ADHD in adults.

Notwithstanding the changes in the conceptualisation noted above, there was always a general agreement that symptoms of the disorder, we now recognise as ADHD, tend to start early in life. More recently there has also been a focus on the concept of neurodevelopmental disorders. Whilst some disorders such as schizophrenia that are known to have a neurodevelopmental trajectory do not necessarily manifest symptoms during childhood, there is a clear expectation within DSM-5/ICD-10 that a neurodevelopmental disorder should have an onset during infancy or childhood. It was therefore not surprising that those seeking to define ADHD within the diagnostic manuals started to focus more on trying to define AOO more explicitly. Unfortunately this took place without the generation of any clear empirical evidence to guide those making decisions. As a consequence, when specific AOO criteria were introduced into the definition of attention deficit disorder in DSM-III (American

Psychiatric 1980), these were based solely on clinical experience. The DSM-III committee introduced an AOO criterion, Criterion B, into the diagnostic criteria. Criterion B required symptoms to be present before the age of 7 years. A significant factor in prompting this decision was to avoid the potential misdiagnosis of those children who presented with hyperactivity, impulsivity and inattention arising as a reaction to the stresses associated with starting school (Barkley and Biederman 1997; Applegate et al. 1997). With the publication of DSM-IV, Criterion B was modified to require the presence of impairment as well as symptoms before age 7 years. Again no empirical evidence was put forward to support this amendment, and the consequences of these decisions will be addressed later in the chapter.

12.1.2 How Early in Life Can We Diagnose ADHD?

Whilst much of the discussion and debate about AOO in ADHD has focussed on whether ADHD can present beyond early childhood, it is important to acknowledge that most individuals who will meet criteria for ADHD at some point in their life have had at least some symptoms from early on in life. The diagnostic process during the school years, whilst not always straightforward, is relatively well described and is a part of core business for many child psychiatrists, child psychologists and paediatricians. During the assessment process, it often becomes clear that symptoms were apparent during the preschool period and, not uncommonly, during infancy. Whilst these differences may be easy to identify with hindsight, it is actually much more difficult to define the boundaries of normal levels of activity, impulsivity and attention during the preschool years due to there being far greater variability in these characteristics during this period of development. Defining clinical levels of hyperactivity and impulsivity is challenging during the preschool period, and population-based studies show that this group of symptoms are in fact very common among typically developing preschoolers (Smidts and Oosterlaan 2007). Because hyperactive-impulsive symptoms are so common in the preschool years, it is challenging to define extreme levels. This problem has been solved by several rating scales (Smith and Corkum 2007), but clinicians lacking such tools may not be able to make such norm-based evaluations. It is, however, generally agreed that it is, in some cases at least, possible to make a diagnosis of ADHD during the preschool period, at least for those aged 4 years and older. Evidence for the validity of diagnosing ADHD in preschoolers comes from studies of clinically referred preschoolers who go on to be formally diagnosed as having ADHD. For example, such cases have rates of ADHD symptom levels four to eight times higher during the preschool period than age matched, non-ADHD peers (Kadesjo et al. 2001). In addition the levels of impairment reported in preschoolers with a diagnosis of ADHD has been shown to be similar to that reported for school age children with ADHD (Wilens et al. 2002). Preschoolers with ADHD are also reported to be less academically ready for school entry, to have poorer fine motor skills and to be less socially skilled relative to healthy controls (DuPaul et al. 2001). Preschool ADHD also has a significant impact on family functioning with increased levels of expulsion from preschool, greater difficulty maintaining babysitters and childcare with higher levels of parents missing work and less personal time (Barkley 2006).

Several studies of the stability and predictive validity of preschool diagnoses of ADHD (e.g. Lahey et al. 2004, 2005; Posner et al. 2007; Tandon et al. 2011) support a relatively strong continuity of ADHD from preschool into school age. For example, Lahey et al. (2004) followed up, annually for 3 years, two cohorts of children from two sites who were aged between 4 and 6 years of age when first seen. Almost all of those children who met full diagnostic criteria for ADHD at the first visit continued to meet full criteria over the next 3 years. They also continued to show marked functional impairments relative to healthy controls. These findings all held true after differences in intelligence, other mental health symptoms and demographic characteristics were controlled for. Whilst there was a clear continuity of overall ADHD status, this was not true for ADHD subtypes.

Neuropsychological studies have also provided some support for the validity and continuity of preschool ADHD, although the precise nature of the deficits remains uncertain. Some studies have shown that executive functioning deficits are associated with ADHD symptoms in children as young as 3–5 years of age (Sonuga-Barke et al. 2003) and that preschoolers with ADHD show poorer inhibitory control than healthy controls (Dalen et al. 2004). Other groups have found that preschoolers with high levels of inattention and hyperactivity/impulsivity perform more poorly than healthy controls not only on these tasks with high executive demand but also on more basic tasks with a much lower executive load (Berwid et al. 2005; Marks et al. 2005), suggesting a more global cognitive impairment associated with ADHD rather than specific deficits in executive functioning.

Evidence-based clinical guidelines have started to include guidance on the assessment and management of ADHD in preschoolers, and there are specialist sections in the most recent versions of both the UK NICE (NICE 2008) and American Academy of Pediatrics (Subcommittee on Attention-Deficit/Hyperactivity et al. 2011) guidelines. Both highlight the validity of diagnosing preschool ADHD but also note the particular challenges associated with determining the presence of key symptoms during this period of rapid development and the need to try and access good-quality and reliable collateral information when there is no teacher to provide a report.

Validity for the concept of ADHD as an early-onset condition, with continuity of aetiological influences across the lifespan, is supported by population twin studies that have investigated heritability and continuity of genetic influences on ADHD at different ages. Investigating maternal reports of child ADHD symptoms in 2-, 3- and 4-year-olds, estimated heritability at each age lies in the range of 0.78–0.81 (Price et al. 2005). Furthermore, genetic influences were found to underlie 91% of the stable variance of ADHD symptoms during this developmental stage. These findings demonstrated that even in children as young as 2 years of age ADHD can be measured in a reliable way, since heritability estimates cannot be greater than reliability of test-retest reliability of the phenotype. Further, a continuity of genetic influences explained stability of ADHD from ages 2 to 4. Other studies, which investigated older children and adolescents in the age ranges of 8–13 years (Larsson et al. 2004) and 13–20 years (Chang et al. 2013), drew similar conclusions. Heritability for ADHD was similar for infants, adolescents and adults, with continuity of genetic influences explaining the stability of ADHD across development. In addition, these studies all showed evidence for new genetic effects at the different ages, consistent with the effects of maturational processes on ADHD, potentially leading to individual differences for AOO, and different levels of compensatory mechanisms (Faraone et al. 2015). In the adult years, studies using self-ratings of ADHD symptoms showed much lower heritability estimates in the region of 30–40%. However both parent ratings of young adult ADHD and heritability for the clinical diagnosis of ADHD in adults showed similar high heritability to that seen in younger children (Brikell et al. 2015). These findings indicate marked rater effects, with self-ratings not showing the same strong relationship to genetic influences as either parent ratings or full diagnostic assessments. These rater effects were further validated in follow-up studies of children with ADHD into young adulthood that showed greater concordance between parent ratings of ADHD and cognitive performance deficits than self-ratings (Du Rietz et al. 2016). Overall these studies indicate that a continuity of genetic influences into young adulthood accounts for the developmental stability of ADHD, with new genetic effects at different ages potentially leading to individual differences in developmental trajectories.

12.2 Defining and Refining the AOO Criteria for ADHD

Joseph Biederman was the first to publically question the validity of the DSM-IV AOO criterion which required both symptoms and impairment to be present before the age of 7 years. He along with Russel Barkley (Barkley and Biederman 1997) reviewed the evidence available to support this position. Whilst they acknowledged that the empirical and conceptual evidence did support the notion of ADHD as a disorder that typically onsets early in life, there was no support for the selection of age 7 years as the AOO for either symptoms or impairment as the basis for valid diagnoses. Kieling et al. (2010) systematically reviewed the literature on studies that investigated the age at onset criterion for ADHD. They identified 31 studies reporting original data meeting their inclusion criteria. They highlighted the DSM-IV field trials (Applegate et al. 1997) which found differences in AOO depending on subtype, with the inattentive group exhibiting a later onset. There were also differences with respect to impairment. Whilst almost all of those with the predominantly hyperactive-impulsive subtype met both the AOO symptom and impairment criterion, 18% of those with combined type ADHD and 43% with the predominantly inattentive type did not show signs of impairment before the age of 7 years. This same study also demonstrated that, for the combined and inattentive subtypes, the requirement for impairment before age 7 years reduced the accuracy of identification of currently impaired cases of ADHD and reduced the levels of agreement between the research diagnosis and clinicians' judgments, with an increase in the rate of false negative diagnoses. Clinicians validated 75% of cases meeting symptom criteria but lacking the onset criterion. The authors also pointed out that concerns about the validity of the age of onset are likely to increase with age and as the period of time that must be recalled increases. The review also highlights a series of studies from a group in

Boston that examined later-onset (defined as symptoms and impairment after 7 years of age) ADHD. All of these studies highlighted the similarities between those who did not meet the AOO criterion and those who did. These similarities were seen across a broad range of factors including neuropsychological profile, comorbidity, personality traits, substance use and current levels of impairment (Faraone et al. 2006a, c, 2007, 2009). Similarly two independent studies reported that response to treatment with stimulant medication was similar between cases that did and did not meet the Criterion B AOO criterion (Biederman et al. 2006; Reinhardt et al. 2007).

Several prospective cohort studies, which are by their nature unbiased by memory recall, also confirmed the similarities between early- and late-onset ADHD groups in terms of both psychopathology and impairment (Barkley et al. 1990, 2008; Todd et al. 2008). Also a large cross-sectional population survey of adults found that whilst only 50% of individuals with current clinical features of ADHD recalled an onset before age 7 years, 95% recalled an onset before age 12 and 99% before age 16 (Kessler et al. 2005). Prospective data have also highlighted poor recall of AOO, with nearly one-half of a group of children who were assessed and diagnosed with ADHD and as meeting AOO criteria as children were not reported as meeting the onset criterion in later life when this was reassessed retrospectively (Barkley et al. 2008). In contrast to these findings, Kieling et al. did not identify any studies that reported significant findings which differentiated children with onset of ADHD before and after 7 years of age (Kieling et al. 2010).

Summing up their systematic review, Kieling et al. suggest that a review of the AOO criterion as defined in DSM-IV was both prudent and necessary (Kieling et al. 2010). Their preliminary recommendation was to raise the age of onset criterion from 7 to 12 years which they felt would minimise the number of false negative diagnoses, which are particularly likely to occur for those cases where assessment is conducted later in life whilst at the same time reaffirming ADHD as a disorder of childhood onset. Barkley and Biederman went further suggesting that we should dispense with a precise AOO criterion completely until such time as an empirical justification can be detailed for a precise and valid cut-off, generously broadening the criterion to include onset of symptoms during the entire childhood and adolescent years (Barkley and Biederman 1997). Other authors voiced concerns that extending the upper limit would increase the prevalence of the disorder and result in children whose problems are a reaction to the increased demands and stresses associated with school entry, rather than as a consequence of a neurodevelopmental disorder per se, receiving a diagnosis of ADHD (Polanczyk et al. 2010).

Polanczyk et al. (2010) set out to test the potential impact of raising the AOO criterion to 12 on the prevalence of ADHD at age 12 and to assess whether the change would result in changes to the clinical and cognitive features, impairment profile and risk factors associated with the disorder. They focused on symptoms rather than impairment arguing that there is no empirical evidence to support that using impairment actually improves predictive validity compared to using symptom data alone and in fact highlight data that suggests it may actually be a less reliable approach (Barkley and Biederman 1997; Applegate et al. 1997; Barkley et al. 2008). They used data from the Environmental Risk (E-Risk) Longitudinal Twin Study, which tracked a nationally representative sample of 2232 British twins drawn from a larger birth register of twins born in England and Wales in 1994 to 1995. The results were fascinating. Data were available on 1979 children. Of these, only 547 (27.6%) never had ADHD symptoms, 68 (3.4%) met the full ADHD criteria for ADHD with onset before 7 years, whilst 1183 (59.8%) had ADHD symptoms that started before age 7 years but did not meet diagnostic criteria for ADHD and 181 (9.1%) had ADHD symptoms that started between 7 and 12 years but did not meet diagnostic criteria for ADHD. Only 2 of the 181 children with symptoms starting between 7 and 12 years of age met full diagnostic criteria for ADHD as defined by DSM-IV (excepting the AOO criterion). From this they estimated that extending the AOO criterion up to before age 12 would only increase the prevalence estimate by 0.1%. Similar to previous studies, the children who first manifested ADHD symptoms between ages 7 and 12 were not significantly different with respect to their clinical correlates or risk factors from those who manifested symptoms before age 7.

On first reading these results one might ask: if raising the AOO criterion only yields a very small number of additional cases, then what is the benefit of the change? However as described previously, a significant proportion of adolescents and adults who otherwise appear to meet full ADHD criteria do not remember suffering from their first ADHD symptoms until after age 7 even if they in fact did. The Polanczyk data suggest that this may be more a problem of remembering than of later symptom onset. However, by insisting that the earlier AOO criterion is met many of these individuals would be denied a diagnosis and probably also treatment.

12.2.1 Into the Present: Changes to the AOO Criterion in DSM-5

Although the changes to the ADHD diagnostic criteria made by the DSM-5 committee were generally quite conservative, they did agree that the AOO criterion needed to change. The requirement for impairment was dropped, and it is now only required that "several symptoms" (with or without impairment) are present before the age of 12 years (Association 2013). It is essential to note here that the requirement is for several symptoms, not the full syndrome which has never been the case. It is, as has always been the case, possible for the full syndrome to emerge later in life. It will of course be important to monitor the impact of these changes on both epidemiological and administrative prevalence rates. Whilst the study of Polanczyk et al. (2010) suggested that the increase from 7 to 12 years was unlikely to result in significant changes for childhood ADHD, a subsequent study which assessed the impact of these changes in a US sample reported a 47% increase in prevalence from 7.38% up to 10.84% (Vande Voort et al. 2014). In this study the youth with later AOO did not differ from those with an earlier onset in terms of severity and patterns of comorbidity; they were however more likely to come from lower income and ethnic minority families. A caveat of this study is that AOO was assessed retrospectively and is therefore likely to be subject to recall bias. In another multisite clinical study of adult patients with substance use disorders, the rise in rates of diagnosis ranged from 0 to

1.9% across seven sites (van de Glind et al. 2014). Whilst there are no data to suggest temporal trends in AOO in recent decades, the changes from DSM-IV to DSM-5 will artificially modify the AOO upwards. It is also the case that over the years as clinicians have become more confident in diagnosing first adolescents and then adults the age of diagnosis in clinical datasets has risen. This increase in age at recognition and diagnosis should not be confused with an increase in the AOO. Overall it does however seem likely that, as a result of the changes to the AOO criterion, both the epidemiological prevalence and the rates of diagnosis in adolescents and adults will rise. By how much remains unclear, and whether this is really an issue when one considers that whilst the impairment requirement has been dropped from the AOO criterion, the presence of impairment remains integral to making a diagnosis.

The dropping of the impairment requirement from the AOO criterion does seem sensible. Clinicians working in the ADHD field will be very familiar with the adolescent or adult who had at least some very clear ADHD symptoms from an early age (often with more emerging over time) but for whom these were not impairing until later in life when as the demands of life increase, for example, with a change from primary to high school or from high school to college, university or work. In such cases, the usual clinical formulation is to recognise that, until the change in situation, there was adequate scaffolding to prevent the ADHD symptoms from causing significant impairment. Such scaffolding could be a result of a strong family, a supportive school environment, high intelligence or a combination of these or other positive factors in the person's life. Under the DSM-IV criteria, such a person would not have been eligible for a diagnosis of ADHD even though the available data suggests that they would be indistinguishable from those with similar current symptoms and impairments but who had a diagnosis by virtue of their impairment starting earlier in life.

Dropping the impairment requirement from the AOO criterion in no way diminishes the importance of impairment to the diagnostic process. Indeed, in view of the many studies that support a dimensional perspective of ADHD (Coghill and Sonuga-Barke 2012) and the continuous nature of ADHD symptoms across the population (Kuntsi et al. 2014; Levy et al. 1997), it is clear that the key determinant of caseness is the presence of clinically significant impairment. Whilst the presence of impairment is a defining characteristic of many mental disorders, it is particularly important for trait-like disorders such as ADHD where the symptoms are not necessarily a reflection of a change from a premorbid state (Asherson et al. 2016).

We are unaware of any studies that have specifically looked for differences in AOO of ADHD in different parts of the world. Epidemiological studies suggest that observed differences in overall prevalence are likely to be due to methodological differences between studies rather than actual differences in prevalence (Polanczyk et al. 2007). This is also likely to be the case for AOO. Those countries where ICD-10, which retains an earlier cut-off for the AOO criterion, is the predominant classification system will have datasets with earlier onset than those using DSM-5. We are also unaware of any specific data regarding differences in AOO between the sexes. ADHD is two to three times more common in boys than in girls and much more likely to present with inattentive rather than hyperactive-impulsive symptoms

(Hinshaw 2002; Polanczyk et al. 2007). As inattention is more difficult to accurately identify early in life, it is possible that the AOO in girls will be somewhat later than for boys, but without data this remains speculative.

12.3 Can ADHD Onset in Adulthood?

For many years, ADHD was thought of as a childhood disorder that in most, if not all cases, is remitted by adulthood. This notion has been strongly challenged in recent years, and it is now generally accepted that a significant proportion of those with ADHD continue to have symptoms and impairment into adulthood. A meta-analysis of studies that followed up children with ADHD into adulthood estimated the persistence of ADHD to be 65%: 15% of children continued to meet full diagnostic criteria by the age of 25 years, with a further 50% having some residual ADHD symptoms that were causing continuing impairments (Faraone et al. 2006b). Long-term follow-up of children from the MTA study using a norm-based threshold of four symptoms rather than DSM criteria reported that 60% of this group demonstrated symptom persistence with 41% meeting both symptom and impairment criteria as adults (mean age 24.7 years). A recent European study found that around 86% of 17-year-olds who had been initially assessed and diagnosed 6 years earlier still met full DSM-5 criteria for an ADHD diagnosis (van Lieshout et al. 2016a). Two other European follow-up studies of children meeting DSM-IV ADHD combined type criteria, from child mental health clinics in Southeast England and the Netherlands, with an average follow-up period of around 6 years, found far higher persistence rates of ADHD in young adulthood, in the region of 80% (Cheung et al. 2015; Van Lieshout et al. 2016b).

Taken together these data provide strong support for the persistence of ADHD into adulthood in a significant proportion of cases. In general the higher persistence rates from more recent studies support the data from cross-sectional epidemiological surveys in adults which suggest rates of ADHD in adults of around 3–4 % (Fayyad et al. 2007). The wording in DSM-5 does however still emphasise that ADHD should be considered as a neurodevelopmental disorder that begins in childhood, with the minimum requirement that several symptoms of ADHD should be present before the age of 12 years. With this comes the expectation that, when ADHD is seen in adults, it represents a continuation of the childhood disorder.

Whilst we have already explained why DSM-5 raised the AOO criterion to 12, four recent epidemiological studies from New Zealand (Dunedin), Brazil (1993 Pelotas) and the UK (2 studies: E-Risk, ALSPAC) have challenged the core notion that ADHD always reflects a childhood-onset neurodevelopmental disorder and introduced the idea that the ADHD syndrome can arise de novo in adulthood (Moffitt et al. 2015; Caye et al. 2016; Agnew-Blais et al. 2016; Riglin et al. 2016). Unlike previous studies that have followed up clinically diagnosed cases into adulthood, these three studies analysed data from population-based prospective cohorts followed up into either late adolescence or adulthood. The findings were unexpected and have prompted intense discussion and debate as to how they should be interpreted. The main findings from the studies are summarised in Table 12.1.

Table 12.1 Persistence, remission and emergence of ADHD across three population cohorts

Study	Sample	Sample size	Age at child assessment	Age at adult assessment	Number (prevalence) with ADHD at child assessment	Number (prevalence) with ADHD at adult assessment	Number (%) with remitted ADHD[a]	Number (%) with persistent ADHD[b]	Number (%) with late-onset ADHD[c]
Moffitt et al. (2015)	Dunedin Birth Cohort (New Zealand)	1037	11, 13, 15 years	38 years	61 (5.9%)	31 (3%)	58 (95%)	3 (5%)	28 (90%)
Caye et al. (2016)	1993 Pelotas Birth Cohort (Brazil)	5249	11 years	18–19 years	393 (8.9%)	492 (12.2%)	288 (73%)	60 (15%)	416 (85%)
Agnew-Blais et al. (2016)	Environmental Risk (E-Risk) Longitudinal Twin Study (United Kingdom)	2232	5, 7, 10, 12 years	18 years	247 (12.1%)	166 (8.1%)	193 (78%)	54 (22%)	112 (67%)
Riglin et al. (2016)	Avon Longitudinal Study of Parents and Children (ALSPAC) Study (United Kingdom)	4824	7 years	17 years	476 (9.9%)	228 (4.8%)	370 (78%)	106 (22%)	122 (53%)

[a]"Remitted ADHD" refers to those with ADHD as a child but not as an adult (% is the percentage of those with ADHD as a child who have remitted)
[b]"Persistent ADHD" refers to those with ADHD as a child and as an adult (% is the percentage of those with ADHD as a child who also have ADHD as an adult)
[c]"Late-onset ADHD" refers to those who did not have ADHD as a child but do as an adult (% is the percentage of those with ADHD as an adult who did not have ADHD as a child)

With respect to persistence rates of full threshold ADHD, it was notable that whilst the observed rates in the Brazilian (15%) and the two UK studies (both 22%) were very similar to those reported in the previous meta-analysis (Faraone et al. 2006b), those for the New Zealand study (5%) were much lower than expected. In part this may reflect the fact that participants in the Brazilian and UK studies were still in their teens at the time of the "adult" assessment, whilst those in the New Zealand study were 38 years old. However, the rates of persistence for the New Zealand study were much lower than the 22% found for the clinical sample followed up in the New York longitudinal study of children diagnosed with ADHD, who were a similar age at follow-up (Mannuzza et al. 1991). It seems likely that this, at least in part, reflects inherent differences between clinical and population-based cohorts; however it will be important to consider other potentially important factors (Castellanos 2015). Also these findings all refer to persistence as defined by meeting all DSM diagnostic criteria, and rates would be higher if those with sub-threshold impairing symptoms were included.

The key finding however from across all four studies, and the one that has sparked the greatest interest and controversy, was that, despite there being some continuity from childhood to adulthood, the majority of those adults who met criteria for ADHD (ignoring the AOO requirement) did not appear to have met full categorical criteria for ADHD as children (New Zealand 90%; Brazil 88%; UK, E-Risk 67%; UK, ALSPAC 53%).

There were several potentially important similarities and differences in all three samples between the childhood- and adult-onset cases. In the New Zealand study, whilst the childhood- and adult-onset groups had similar levels of parent-reported ADHD symptoms as adults and showed similar levels of impairment in adulthood, the adult-onset group had lower levels of self-reported symptoms and did not have neuropsychological deficits in either childhood or adulthood (Moffitt et al. 2015). Whilst it is also reported in the New Zealand study that those in the adult-onset group did not show association with the polygenic risk for childhood ADHD, this was a very low powered analysis, and the findings may be misleading (Moffitt et al. 2015). In the ALSPAC study, the mean polygenic risk scores for ADHD differed between the four identified groups (low ADHD, variance = −0.035 [$p = 0.018$]; childhood-limited ADHD, variance = 0.043 [$p = 0.061$]; persistent ADHD, variance = 0.252 [$p = 0.102$]; and adolescent-onset ADHD, 0.101 [0.104]; $p = 0.03$) with higher polygenic risk for ADHD in the persistent compared with the low ADHD subgroup and intermediate risk scores for the childhood-limited and adolescent-onset ADHD groups. This suggests that, in addition to explaining initial levels of ADHD symptoms in childhood, the common genetic variants associated with ADHD diagnosis also contribute to the persistence of ADHD symptoms in the general population. It does not, however, seem that these gene variants are associated with symptoms that arise later in life. These later-onset symptoms may however be associated with different genetic variants and/or they may be more environmentally determined. In the Brazilian study, both those with childhood- and adult-onset also had similar levels of impairment as adults, irrespective of whether or not they still met diagnostic criteria (Caye et al. 2016).

The Brazilian study was also able to confirm that the adult ADHD impairments were not explained by the presence of comorbid disorders (Caye et al. 2016). In the UK E-Risk study, those with late-onset ADHD showed fewer externalising problems and higher IQ scores in childhood compared to those with persistent ADHD but had comparable levels of ADHD symptoms and impairment and similarly elevated rates of mental health disorders (Agnew-Blais et al. 2016). It was also the case that in at least three of these studies many of the "adult-onset" cases appear to have had neurodevelopmental roots. Compared with controls, the adult-onset ADHD subjects in the New Zealand group had more teacher-rated symptoms of ADHD and more conduct disorder in childhood and were more likely to have had a combined parent-teacher report of ADHD symptom onset prior to age 12 years. In the UK study, those in the adult-onset ADHD group also had elevated rates of childhood ADHD symptoms, which is in line with DSM-5, and higher rates of conduct disorder and oppositional defiant disorder in childhood. Also in line with DSM-5 and the notion of emergent ADHD in children with subthreshold ADHD, the Brazilian study found that only 38% of the participants who went on to have adult-onset ADHD were defined as "neurotypical" with respect to ADHD and conduct disorder symptoms in childhood.

Three of the four studies all propose striking conclusions: perhaps the most moderate is from the UK E-Risk study "that adult ADHD is more complex than a straight forward continuation of the childhood disorder", whilst the Brazilian study proposed that we should consider whether child and adult ADHD are "distinct syndromes"; and the New Zealand study that adult ADHD is "not a neurodevelopmental disorder". Several commentators have suggested that such conclusions are premature (Faraone and Biederman 2016; Asherson et al. 2016). In their editorial, which accompanied the publication of the Brazilian and UK E-Risk studies, Faraone and Biederman highlight several of the methodological issues that need to be considered when interpreting the findings of these three studies (Faraone and Biederman 2016). In three studies the reported prevalence rates for adult-onset ADHD (Brazil, 10.3%; UK E-Risk, 5.5%; and New Zealand, 2.7%) were higher than for childhood-onset adult ADHD (Brazil, 1.5%; UK E-Risk, 2.6%; and New Zealand, 0.3%). For the Brazilian study, the overall prevalence of ADHD in adults (12.2%) was higher than that for children (8.9%). These patterns do not fit with the rest of the ADHD literature. If, as concluded by the New Zealand study, adult ADHD with childhood onset is very rare, then it is difficult to see how is it possible that a meta-analysis of epidemiologic studies of adult ADHD with childhood onset reports a prevalence of 2.5% (Simon et al. 2009). Likewise, there are a great many neuropsychological, neuroimaging, treatment and family studies that would not have been possible if adult ADHD with childhood onset were a rare condition. Faraone and Biederman also point to a study of clinically referred adults who retrospectively reported childhood symptoms (Chandra et al. 2016). Based on clinical features and familial transmission, that study concluded that onsets of ADHD in late adolescence and early adulthood were valid.

Faraone and Biederman propose several potential reasons why the rarity of adult ADHD with childhood onset may have been overestimated by the three studies discussed above (Faraone and Biederman 2016). There is of course the potential for recall bias in the adult studies. Another possibility, highlighted by the authors of the Brazilian study, is the phenomenon known as the "false positive paradox", whereby for low prevalence conditions, even when false positive rates are low, most diagnoses in a population study will be false. For example, given Simon and colleagues' meta-analytic estimate that the prevalence of adult ADHD with childhood onset is 2.5%, if the false positive rate of diagnosis is 5%, then two-thirds of the diagnoses in a population study will be false (Simon et al. 2009). As the false positive paradox is dependent on the sensitivity and specificity of the assessment methods, it can vary considerably when these are varied. This is particularly relevant for the two studies that used a screening questionnaire (the Strengths and Difficulties Questionnaire) rather than a diagnostic interview, as the basis for either the initial (Brazilian study) or all (UK ALSPAC) clinical assessments. It is also a potential factor for the New Zealand, Brazilian and UK E-Risk studies where different approaches to assessment were used at different time points with child diagnoses all based on parent and/or teacher reports, whilst adult diagnoses were based on self-report. Clear differences between these approaches have been identified, and several lines of evidence have suggested that informant reports (e.g. parents) are more accurate than self-report (Sibley et al. 2012; Hoza et al. 2004). Studies have also reported that current symptoms of ADHD were under-reported by adults who had ADHD in childhood and over-reported by adults who did not (Sibley et al. 2012) and that the prevalence of persistent ADHD is higher when the diagnosis is based on parent report than on self-report (Cheung et al. 2016). As such it is likely that the three population-based studies may have underestimated the persistence of ADHD and overestimated the prevalence of adult-onset ADHD. Another important limitation of these studies is that three of the four (Brazilian, UK E-Risk and ALSPAC) were only followed up into the late teens with no or limited data in between the child and "adult" assessments making it difficult to argue these data as evidence for an adult onset of ADHD. It is not yet clear if AOO in general or the proposed *adult onset* more specifically is associated with differences in treatment response. This was not addressed by the four community-based studies described above, and current data has yet to show any difference based on AOO.

Despite these issues, the authors of three of the population studies suggested that there are two separate but phenotypically similar syndromes, one with childhood onset and another with later onset of ADHD symptoms and impairments. Whilst some have argued that these data suggest the presence of distinct developmental trajectories and potentially separable causal pathways and underlying pathophysiologies for the early- and late-onset presentations, these suggestions, based almost entirely on findings from the New Zealand cohort, must be regarded as extremely speculative at this time, and alternative hypotheses have been put forward. Faraone and Biederman propose that these apparent adult-onset cases may be better understood as "subthreshold cases" of childhood ADHD (Faraone and Biederman 2016). This concept has been alluded to earlier in the chapter and refers to those cases whereby the onset of symptoms and impairment are separated in time, sometimes by many years. It is argued that in such cases the impairment is delayed by the presence of either strong intellectual abilities or the presence of effective scaffolding at home and in school. Impairment becomes apparent when this scaffolding is removed.

In this sense, it is important to keep in mind that the current understanding of most chronic conditions in medicine is that the clinical phenotype arises out of intricate and complex interactions between biological and environmental factors (Bousquet et al. 2014). Those factors exert protective or harmful pressures. The clinical syndrome is a result of the interplay of those pressures. For example, type 2 diabetes is clearly affected by environmental pressure, especially obesogenic factors. However, we know that obesity is not necessary nor sufficient to cause type 2 diabetes, because biological pressures, like genetic predisposition, are essential components of the equation (Alonso-Magdalena et al. 2011). Considering the complex phenotype of chronic diseases, type 1 diabetes would arise from a very high biological pressure, depending very little of the environmental pressure to reach a diagnostic threshold on blood glucose levels. Type 2 diabetes, on the other hand, arises much later in life exactly due to the fact that it depends moderately of biological and environmental pressures. An analogous situation might be suggested for ADHD with childhood and late onsets. Other models can be proposed, and clearly much further study is required before the field accepts adult-onset ADHD as a separate entity from childhood-onset ADHD. In the meanwhile, the results from these population studies remind us that a group of individuals may have their phenotypic presentation emerging more strongly and associated with impairment only later after childhood. This group might be smaller than initially suggested by these studies but higher than expected before; however it is our view that it is unlikely to account for a substantial fraction of adult ADHD patients seen in clinical settings.

12.4 Conclusions and Clinical Relevance

ADHD is recognised as a heterogeneous disorder at all levels of analysis and, perhaps unsurprisingly, it would appear that AOO is no different. In most cases seen in clinical settings, onset of symptoms is reported as starting early in life, sometimes very early. In young children it can be difficult to be certain about the diagnosis until around the time of starting formal education, and many clinicians will prefer to give a provisional diagnosis in the preschool period. It has become increasingly clear in recent years that there are individuals who, despite having onset of ADHD symptoms early in life, may not meet diagnostic thresholds for symptom count or impairment until later in life, often adolescence but sometimes adulthood. These shifts into greater levels of symptoms and impairment are often associated with major life transitions such as from primary to secondary school or from high school into higher education, work or when moving from the family home into independent living. In addition, recent epidemiological studies have opened up the possibility that there may be adult-onset forms of ADHD that reflect distinct aetiological conditions from the childhood-onset version and perhaps not even a neurodevelopmental disorder.

Taken together we suggest that it is always the case that recognition of ADHD as early as possible after onset is preferable and that this, if appropriate treatment and support is offered, is likely to result in more positive outcomes and less secondary impairments and disability. For most this will mean recognition during childhood or adolescence, but for some this will be later in life. ADHD appearing early in life that is not recognised or treated is likely to be associated with a wide range of negative outcomes both from the core ADHD symptoms and secondary comorbid disorders. If ADHD genuinely onsets later in life (i.e. symptoms if present have truly not been impairing up until this point in time), then, as long as it is recognised, believed and treated relatively promptly, this may limit other negative outcomes developing. However when adults with later-onset ADHD are not identified correctly (and perhaps disbelieved), then outcomes are unlikely to be good. However, because of the many methodological and interpretive issues with the current studies, the concept of adult-onset ADHD must be considered as preliminary hypotheses that now require further rigorous testing and investigation. In the meanwhile, clinicians faced with apparent cases of adult-onset ADHD should be cautious before making a diagnosis. This includes being strict about the implementation of impairment and chronicity criteria and considering treating comorbid disorders first.

References

Agnew-Blais JC, Polanczyk GV, Danese A, Wertz J, Moffitt TE, Arseneault L. Evaluation of the persistence, remission, and emergence of attention-deficit/hyperactivity disorder in young adulthood. JAMA Psychiat. 2016;73:713–20.

Alonso-Magdalena P, Quesada I, Nadal A. Endocrine disruptors in the etiology of type 2 diabetes mellitus. Nat Rev Endocrinol. 2011;7:346–53.

American Psychiatric Association. Diagnostic and statistical manual of mental disorders. Washington, DC: American Psychiatric Association; 1980.

Applegate B, Lahey BB, Hart EL, Biederman J, Hynd GW, Barkley RA, et al. Validity of the age-of-onset criterion for ADHD: a report from the DSM-IV field trials. J Am Acad Child Adolesc Psychiatry. 1997;36(9):1211–21.

Asherson P, Buitelaar J, Faraone SV, Rohde LA. Adult attention-deficit hyperactivity disorder: key conceptual issues. Lancet Psychiatry. 2016;3:568–78.

American Psychiatric Association. Diagnostic and statistical manual of mental disorders (DSM-II). 2nd ed. Washington, DC: American Psychiatric Association; 1968.

American Psychiatric Association. Diagnostic and statistical manual of mental disorders DSM 5. 5th ed. Washington, DC: American Psychiatric Association; 2013.

Barkley R, Murphy KR, Fischer M. ADHD in adults: what the science says. New York: Guilford; 2008.

Barkley RA. ADHD in adults: developmental course and outcome of children with ADHD, and ADHD in clinic-referred adults. In: Barkley RA, editor. Attention-deficit hyperactivity disorder, a handbook for diagnosis and treatment. 3rd ed. New York: Guilford Press; 2006.

Barkley RA, Biederman J. Toward a broader definition of the age-of-onset criterion for attention-deficit hyperactivity disorder. J Am Acad Child Adolesc Psychiatry. 1997;36:1204–10.

Barkley RA, Fischer M, Edelbrock CS, Smallish L. The adolescent outcome of hyperactive children diagnosed by research criteria: I. An 8-year prospective follow-up study. J Am Acad Child Adolesc Psychiatry. 1990;29:546–57.

Berwid OG, Curko Kera EA, Marks DJ, Santra A, Bender HA, Halperin JM. Sustained attention and response inhibition in young children at risk for Attention Deficit/Hyperactivity Disorder. J Child Psychol Psychiatry. 2005;46:1219–29.

Biederman J, Mick E, Spencer T, Surman C, Hammerness P, Doyle R, et al. An open-label trial of OROS methylphenidate in adults with late-onset ADHD. CNS Spectr. 2006;11:390–6.

Birch HG. Brain damage in children: the biological and social aspects. Baltimore: Williams & Wilkins; 1964.

Bousquet J, Jorgensen C, Dauzat M, Cesario A, Camuzat T, Bourret R, et al. Systems medicine approaches for the definition of complex phenotypes in chronic diseases and ageing. From concept to implementation and policies. Curr Pharm Des. 2014;20:5928–44.

Brikell I, Kuja-Halkola R, Larsson H. Heritability of attention-deficit hyperactivity disorder in adults. Am J Med Genet B Neuropsychiatr Genet. 2015;168:406–13.

Castellanos FX. Is adult-onset ADHD a distinct entity? Am J Psychiatry. 2015;172:929–31.

Caye A, Rocha TB, Anselmi L, Murray J, Menezes AM, Barros FC, et al. Attention-deficit/hyperactivity disorder trajectories from childhood to young adulthood: evidence from a birth cohort supporting a late-onset syndrome. JAMA Psychiat. 2016;73:705–12.

Chandra S, Biederman J, Faraone SV. Assessing the validity of the age at onset criterion for diagnosing ADHD in DSM-5. J Atten Disord. 2016. https://doi.org/10.1177/1087054716629717. http://journals.sagepub.com/doi/abs/10.1177/1087054716629717?url_ver=Z39.88-2003&rfr_id=ori:rid:crossref.org&rfr_dat=cr_pub%3dpubmed. Accessed 30/07/2018.

Chang Z, Lichtenstein P, Asherson PJ, Larsson H. Developmental twin study of attention problems: high heritabilities throughout development. JAMA Psychiat. 2013;70:311–8.

Cheung CH, Rijdijk F, McLoughlin G, Faraone SV, Asherson P, Kuntsi J. Childhood predictors of adolescent and young adult outcome in ADHD. J Psychiatr Res. 2015;62:92–100.

Cheung CH, Rijsdijk F, McLoughlin G, Brandeis D, Banaschewski T, Asherson P, et al. Cognitive and neurophysiological markers of ADHD persistence and remission. Br J Psychiatry. 2016;208:548–55.

Coghill D, Sonuga-Barke EJ. Annual research review: categories versus dimensions in the classification and conceptualisation of child and adolescent mental disorders—implications of recent empirical study. J Child Psychol Psychiatry. 2012;53:469–89.

Conners CK. Attention-deficit/hyperactivity disorder: historical development and overview. J Atten Disord. 2000;3:173–91.

Crichton A. An inquiry into the nature and origin of mental derangement: on attention and its diseases. J Atten Disord. 2008;12:200–4; discussion 205–6.

Dalen L, Sonuga-Barke EJ, Hall M, Remington B. Inhibitory deficits, delay aversion and preschool AD/HD: implications for the dual pathway model. Neural Plast. 2004;11:1–11.

Du Rietz E, Cheung CH, McLoughlin G, Brandeis D, Banaschewski T, Asherson P, et al. Self-report of ADHD shows limited agreement with objective markers of persistence and remittance. J Psychiatr Res. 2016;82:91–9.

Dupaul GJ, McGoey KE, Eckert TL, Vanbrakle J. Preschool children with attention-deficit/hyperactivity disorder: impairments in behavioral, social, and school functioning. J Am Acad Child Adolesc Psychiatry. 2001;40:508–15.

Faraone SV, Asherson P, Banaschewski T, Biederman J, Buitelaar JK, Ramos-Quiroga JA, et al. Attention-deficit/hyperactivity disorder. Nat Rev Dis Primers. 2015;1:15020.

Faraone SV, Biederman J. Can attention-deficit/hyperactivity disorder onset occur in adulthood? JAMA Psychiatry. 2016;73:655–6.

Faraone SV, Biederman J, Doyle A, Murray K, Petty C, Adamson JJ, et al. Neuropsychological studies of late onset and subthreshold diagnoses of adult attention-deficit/hyperactivity disorder. Biol Psychiatry. 2006a;60:1081–7.

Faraone SV, Biederman J, Mick E. The age-dependent decline of attention deficit hyperactivity disorder: a meta-analysis of follow-up studies. Psychol Med. 2006b;36:159–65.

Faraone SV, Biederman J, Spencer T, Mick E, Murray K, Petty C, et al. Diagnosing adult attention deficit hyperactivity disorder: are late onset and subthreshold diagnoses valid? Am J Psychiatry. 2006c;163:1720–9; quiz 1859.

Faraone SV, Kunwar A, Adamson J, Biederman J. Personality traits among ADHD adults: implications of late-onset and subthreshold diagnoses. Psychol Med. 2009;39:685–93.
Faraone SV, Wilens TE, Petty C, Antshel K, Spencer T, Biederman J. Substance use among ADHD adults: implications of late onset and subthreshold diagnoses. Am J Addict. 2007;16(Suppl 1):24–32; quiz 33–4.
Fayyad J, De Graaf R, Kessler R, Alonso J, Angermeyer M, Demyttenaere K, et al. Cross-national prevalence and correlates of adult attention-deficit hyperactivity disorder. Br J Psychiatry. 2007;190:402–9.
Hinshaw SP. Preadolescent girls with attention-deficit/hyperactivity disorder: I. Background characteristics, comorbidity, cognitive and social functioning, and parenting practices. J Consult Clin Psychol. 2002;70:1086–98.
Hoza B, Gerdes AC, Hinshaw SP, Arnold LE, Pelham WE Jr, Molina BS, et al. Self-perceptions of competence in children with ADHD and comparison children. J Consult Clin Psychol. 2004;72:382–91.
Kadesjo C, Kadesjo B, Hagglof B, Gillberg C. ADHD in Swedish 3- to 7-year-old children. J Am Acad Child Adolesc Psychiatry. 2001;40:1021–8.
Kessler JW. History of minimal brain dysfunctions. In: Rie HE, Rie ED, editors. Handbook of minimal brain dysfunctions: a critical view. New York: Wiley; 1980.
Kessler RC, Berglund P, Demler O, Jin R, Merikangas KR, Walters EE. Lifetime prevalence and age-of-onset distributions of DSM-IV disorders in the National Comorbidity Survey Replication. Arch Gen Psychiatry. 2005;62:593–602.
Kieling C, Kieling RR, Rohde LA, Frick PJ, Moffitt T, Nigg JT, et al. The age at onset of attention deficit hyperactivity disorder. Am J Psychiatry. 2010;167:14–6.
Kramer F, Pollnow H. Uber eine hyperkinetische Erkrankung im Kindesalter. Aus der Psychiatrischen und Nerven-Klinik der Charite´ in Berlin (Direktor: Geh. Med.-Rat Prof. Dr. Bonhoeffer). Mschr Psychiat Neurol. 1932;82:21–40.
Kuntsi J, Pinto R, Price TS, Van Der Meere JJ, Frazier-Wood AC, Asherson P. The separation of ADHD inattention and hyperactivity-impulsivity symptoms: pathways from genetic effects to cognitive impairments and symptoms. J Abnorm Child Psychol. 2014;42:127–36.
Lahey BB, Pelham WE, Loney J, Kipp H, Ehrhardt A, Lee SS, et al. Three-year predictive validity of DSM-IV attention deficit hyperactivity disorder in children diagnosed at 4-6 years of age. Am J Psychiatry. 2004;161:2014–20.
Lahey BB, Pelham WE, Loney J, Lee SS, Willcutt E. Instability of the DSM-IV Subtypes of ADHD from preschool through elementary school. Arch Gen Psychiatry. 2005;62:896–902.
Lange KW, Reichl S, Lange KM, Tucha L, Tucha O. The history of attention deficit hyperactivity disorder. Atten Defic Hyperact Disord. 2010;2:241–55.
Larsson JO, Larsson H, Lichtenstein P. Genetic and environmental contributions to stability and change of ADHD symptoms between 8 and 13 years of age: a longitudinal twin study. J Am Acad Child Adolesc Psychiatry. 2004;43:1267–75.
Levy F, Hay DA, McStephen M, Wood C, Waldman I. Attention-deficit hyperactivity disorder: a category or a continuum? Genetic analysis of a large-scale twin study. J Am Acad Child Adolesc Psychiatry. 1997;36:737–44.
Mannuzza S, Klein RG, Bonagura N, Malloy P, Giampino TL, Addalli KA. Hyperactive boys almost grown up. V. Replication of psychiatric status. Arch Gen Psychiatry. 1991;48:77–83.
Marks DJ, Berwid OG, Santra A, Kera EC, Cyrulnik SE, Halperin JM. Neuropsychological correlates of ADHD symptoms in preschoolers. Neuropsychology. 2005;19:446–55.
Moffitt TE, Houts R, Asherson P, Belsky DW, Corcoran DL, Hammerle M, et al. Is adult ADHD a childhood-onset neurodevelopmental disorder? Evidence from a four-decade longitudinal cohort study. Am J Psychiatry. 2015;172:967–77.
NICE. Attention deficit hyperactivity disorder diagnosis and management of ADHD in children, young people and adults. London: National Institute for Health and Clinical Excellence; 2008.

Polanczyk G, Caspi A, Houts R, Kollins SH, Rohde LA, Moffitt TE. Implications of extending the ADHD age-of-onset criterion to age 12: results from a prospectively studied birth cohort. J Am Acad Child Adolesc Psychiatry. 2010;49:210–6.

Polanczyk G, de Lima MS, Horta BL, Biederman J, Rohde LA. The worldwide prevalence of ADHD: a systematic review and metaregression analysis. Am J Psychiatry. 2007;164:942–8.

Posner K, Melvin GA, Murray DW, Gugga SS, Fisher P, Skrobala A, et al. Clinical presentation of attention-deficit/hyperactivity disorder in preschool children: the Preschoolers with Attention-Deficit/Hyperactivity Disorder Treatment Study (PATS). J Child Adolesc Psychopharmacol. 2007;17:547–62.

Price TS, Simonoff E, Asherson P, Curran S, Kuntsi J, Waldman I, et al. Continuity and change in preschool ADHD symptoms: longitudinal genetic analysis with contrast effects. Behav Genet. 2005;35:121–32.

Rapin I. Brain damage in children. In: Brennemann J, editor. Practice of paediatrics. Hagerstown: Prior; 1964.

Reinhardt MC, Benetti L, Victor MM, Grevet EH, Belmonte-de-Abreu P, Faraone SV, et al. Is age-at-onset criterion relevant for the response to methylphenidate in attention-deficit/hyperactivity disorder? J Clin Psychiatry. 2007;68:1109–16.

Riglin L, Collishaw S, Thapar AK, Dalsgaard S, Langley K, Smith GD, et al. Association of genetic risk variants with attention-deficit/hyperactivity disorder trajectories in the general population. JAMA Psychiat. 2016;73:1285–92.

Sibley MH, Pelham WE, Molina BS, Gnagy EM, Waxmonsky JG, Waschbusch DA, et al. When diagnosing ADHD in young adults emphasize informant reports, DSM Items, and impairment. J Consult Clin Psychol. 2012;80(6):1052–61.

Simon V, Czobor P, Balint S, Meszaros A, Bitter I. Prevalence and correlates of adult attention-deficit hyperactivity disorder: meta-analysis. Br J Psychiatry. 2009;194:204–11.

Smidts DP, Oosterlaan J. How common are symptoms of ADHD in typically developing preschoolers? A study on prevalence rates and prenatal/demographic risk factors. Cortex. 2007;43:710–7.

Smith KG, Corkum P. Systematic review of measures used to diagnose attention-deficit/hyperactivity disorder in research on preschool children. Top Early Childhood Spec Educ. 2007;27:164–73.

Sonuga-Barke EJ, Dalen L, Remington B. Do executive deficits and delay aversion make independent contributions to preschool attention-deficit/hyperactivity disorder symptoms? J Am Acad Child Adolesc Psychiatry. 2003;42:1335–42.

Still GF. Some abnormal psychical conditions in children: excerpts from three lectures. J Atten Disord. 2006;10:126–36.

Subcommittee on Attention-Deficit/Hyperactivity Disorder, Steering Committee on Quality Improvement and Management, Wolraich M, Brown L, Brown RT, Dupaul G, et al. ADHD: clinical practice guideline for the diagnosis, evaluation, and treatment of attention-deficit/hyperactivity disorder in children and adolescents. Pediatrics. 2011;128:1007–22.

Tandon M, Si X, Luby J. Preschool onset attention-deficit/hyperactivity disorder: course and predictors of stability over 24 months. J Child Adolesc Psychopharmacol. 2011;21:321–30.

Todd RD, Huang H, Henderson CA. Poor utility of the age of onset criterion for DSM-IV attention deficit/hyperactivity disorder: recommendations for DSM-V and ICD-11. J Child Psychol Psychiatry. 2008;49:942–9.

Towbin A. Cerebral dysfunction related to perinatal organic damage: clinical—neuropathologic correlations. J Abnorm Psychol. 1978;87:617–35.

van de Glind G, Konstenius M, Koeter MW, van Emmerik-van Oortmerssen K, Carpentier PJ, Kaye S, et al. Variability in the prevalence of adult ADHD in treatment seeking substance use disorder patients: results from an international multi-center study exploring DSM-IV and DSM-5 criteria. Drug Alcohol Depend. 2014;134:158–66.

van Lieshout M, Luman M, Twisk JW, van Ewijk H, Groenman AP, Thissen AJ, et al. A 6-year follow-up of a large European cohort of children with attention-deficit/hyperactivity disorder-combined subtype: outcomes in late adolescence and young adulthood. Eur Child Adolesc Psychiatry. 2016a;25:1007–17.

van Lieshout M, Luman M, Twisk JWR, Groenman AP, Thissen AJ, Faraone SV, et al. A six-year follow up study of a large European cohort of children with attention-deficit/hyperactivity disorder combined subtype: outcomes in late adolescence and young adulthood. Eur Child Adolesc Psychiatry. 2016b;25(9):1007–17.

Vande Voort JL, He JP, Jameson ND, Merikangas KR. Impact of the DSM-5 attention-deficit/hyperactivity disorder age-of-onset criterion in the US adolescent population. J Am Acad Child Adolesc Psychiatry. 2014;53:736–44.

Wilens TE, Biederman J, Brown S, Monuteaux M, Prince J, Spencer TJ. Patterns of psychopathology and dysfunction in clinically referred preschoolers. J Dev Behav Pediatr. 2002;23:S31–6.

The Age of Onset of Dementias 13

Sandra Landwehr, Ralph Brinks, and Annika Hoyer

13.1 Introduction

The burden of mental disorders is continuously increasing worldwide. The World Health Organization (WHO) reported that four of the ten most frequent disorders are caused by mental disorders, and it is estimated that nearly 12% of total global medical expenses is caused by mental disorders (WHO 2001). Therefore, mental disorders are the focus of national and international politics, society and medicine. Dementia as one of the most frequent non-communicable mental disorders is currently a major public health problem which will grow in future. A well-known report from the WHO found that 35.6 million people—an enormous number—were affected across the world in 2011 (WHO 2012).

In general, dementia is a disease of the brain that has a chronic or progressive course. It is associated with a disturbance of multiple higher cortical functions, including memory, thinking, orientation, comprehension, calculation, learning capacity, language and judgement as well as worsening social behaviour and emotional control (WHO 2012).

All authors contributed equally to this chapter.

S. Landwehr (✉)
Kassenärztliche Vereinigung Nordrhein, Düsseldorf, Germany
e-mail: sandra.landwehr@kvno.de

R. Brinks
Hiller Research Unit for Rheumatology, Medical Faculty of the University Hospital Düsseldorf, Düsseldorf, Germany

Institute for Biometry and Epidemiology, German Diabetes Center, Düsseldorf, Germany
e-mail: ralph.brinks@ddz.uni-duesseldorf.de

A. Hoyer
Institute for Biometry and Epidemiology, German Diabetes Center, Düsseldorf, Germany
e-mail: annika.hoyer@ddz.uni-duesseldorf.de

G. de Girolamo et al. (eds.), *Age of Onset of Mental Disorders*,
https://doi.org/10.1007/978-3-319-72619-9_13

Higher age is the most important risk factor for developing dementia. For instance, compared to a 70-year-old woman, a 90-year-old woman has a 13-fold risk of having dementia (Ziegler and Doblhammer 2009). Nearly a quarter of the older population (aged above 65 years) suffer from mental disorders (Ziegler and Doblhammer 2009; Hendrie 1998). Ziegler and Doblhammer (2009) additionally pointed out that epidemiological studies showed incidence rates from 1 per 100 person-years in the age range of 60–64 years to nearly 35–55 per 100 person-years in the age class of 95 years and above, an enormous increase. The increasing prevalence and incidence with age and the well-known population ageing [it is estimated that the world population over the age of 60 years will be 2 billion in 2050 (WHO 2012)] are indicators for the enormous burden of dementia now and in the future. Moreover, this burden is reflected in the fact that Alzheimer's disease and other dementias are listed among the leading diseases in people 60 years and older, with an increasing number of disability-adjusted life-years (DALYs) over time (GBD 2015 DALYs and HALE Collaborators 2016).

Dementia is classified into three major types: Alzheimer's disease, vascular dementia and secondary dementia. Secondary dementia includes frontotemporal dementia (Morbus Pick), dementia with Lewy bodies, Morbus Binswanger, dementia with Parkinson's disease and Huntington's chorea (WHO 2012; Ziegler and Doblhammer 2009). Alzheimer's disease is the most common form, accounting for about 60–70% of all cases (WHO 2012). Alzheimer's disease is diagnosed based on *International Classification of Diseases, Tenth Edition* (ICD-10) criteria, including evidence of a decrease in memory and a considerable impact on daily activities. Additionally, the following conditions should be fulfilled: creeping onset of symptoms and slow degeneration, exclusion of other causes for dementia, and absence of a sudden onset or neurological symptoms such as partial paralysis and facial deficiencies (Weyerer 2005). Vascular dementias are caused by circulation disorders, whereas secondary dementias result from other existing diseases as Huntington's chorea (Weyerer 2005).

The impact of dementia on daily life differs from person to person as each individual is affected in a different way. As pointed out by the WHO (2012), there are three stages of dementia:

- Early stage (years 1–2)
- Second stage (years 2–4 or 5)
- Late stage (years 5 and later).

The later the stage, the more affected the patients are, with eventual total dependence and inactivity.

The enormous loss of quality of life is a substantial problem for dementia patients and their families and caregivers (Bruvik et al. 2012). Additionally, the annual costs of dementia are alarming: these costs are estimated at US$604 billion worldwide and, moreover, are expected to increase in the future even more (WHO 2012).

Due to the increasing healthcare costs and the social and individual burden of dementia, it is of great concern to estimate the exact numbers of new (incident)

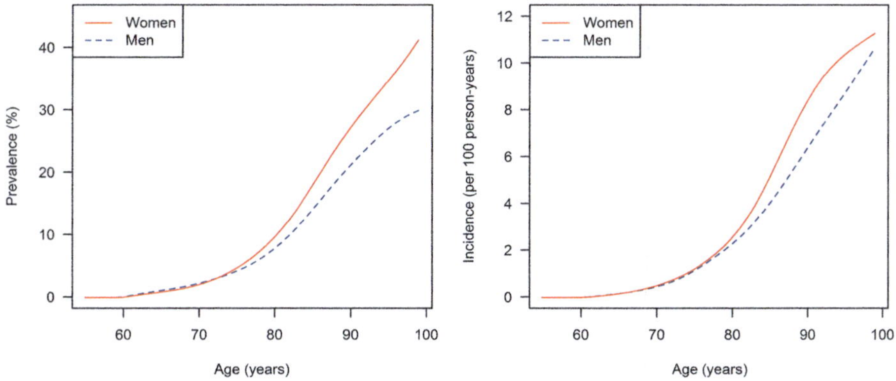

Fig. 13.1 Age-specific prevalence (left) and incidence (right) of dementia for men and women (Ziegler and Doblhammer 2009)

cases and the numbers of all prevalent cases of dementia. As only a small number of epidemiological studies exist on dementia, which is due to methodological problems, high expenses and the huge expenditure of time required, several authors conducted meta-analyses of different studies. Ziegler and Doblhammer (2009) present several meta-analyses that deal with the estimation of incidences and prevalences of dementia. Moreover, the authors present a new study based on data from the German statutory health insurance, which aims to provide new estimates of the incidence and prevalence of dementia in Germany. The estimated age- and sex-specific prevalences from Ziegler and Doblhammer (2009) are shown in the left part of Fig. 13.1. It becomes obvious that the prevalence of dementia increases considerably from under 1% in the age group of 60–64 years for both sexes up to 29.7% and 43.5% in the age groups of around 100 years for men and women, respectively. To compare their findings with other studies, Ziegler and Doblhammer (2009) showed the results of several published studies and meta-analyses: studies from Bickel (2000, 2002), Lopes and Bottino (2002), Fratiglioni and Rocca (2001), Ritchie and Kildea (1995), Ritchie et al. (1992), Hofman et al. (1991) and Jorm et al. (1987) were included. All of these studies report metadata from several time periods, which agree very well with the results of Ziegler and Doblhammer (2009). Only slight differences exist, which are predominantly caused by different definitions of dementia (mild or severe dementia). In general, the findings regarding the age course of prevalence and incidence rate are of the same order of magnitude.

Qiu et al. (2009) published another article on the prevalence of mental disorders, focusing on Alzheimer's disease as the most common type of dementia. Similar to Ziegler and Doblhammer (2009), they found nearly the same prevalence trends of Alzheimer's disease. Moreover, they collected data from studies that were conducted on different countries and continents, including Europe (Lobo et al. 2000), USA (Plassmann et al. 2007), Brazil (Scazufca et al. 2008) and China (Zhang et al. 2005). In summary, there were no large regional differences in the prevalence of dementia or Alzheimer's disease.

The estimated incidence rates mirror the prevalences as women are diagnosed with dementia more often than men. Again, Ziegler and Doblhammer (2009) report on other meta-analyses that estimated incidence rates of dementia: in addition to the studies of Bickel (2000, 2002) that are also used for prevalence comparisons, these are the studies of Fratiglioni et al. (2000), Launer et al. (1999), Jorm and Jolley (1998) and Gao et al. (1998). All of these study findings are in line with the incidence rates reported by Ziegler and Doblhammer (2009), except the study from Jorm and Jolley (1998), which is only due to the case definition that includes a mild form of dementia. Qiu et al. (2009) also provide an overview on incidences of dementia. In addition to Ziegler and Doblhammer (2009), the authors included the study of Kukull et al. (2002), which reports on the incidence of dementia in the USA and results from the Canadian Study of Health and Aging (The Canadian Study of Health and Aging Working Group 2000). All studies come to a similar result, as reported in Ziegler and Doblhammer (2009), that the age-specific incidence rate of dementia is nearly the same in different countries. This holds true within the male and female populations.

As, in general, measuring incidence rates requires long-lasting and expensive studies, age of onset (AOO) has been suggested as an alternative epidemiological measure for disease frequency (Boshuizen and Greenland 1997). In fact, the AOO is a subject of epidemiological research and forms a part of many modelling approaches in the setting of various diseases. It has already played an essential role in building relations between the epidemiological quantities incidence, prevalence and mortality of diseases (Keiding et al. 1990). For example, Keiding et al. (1989) retrospectively estimated diabetes incidence from a cross-sectional population under the assumptions of known mortality rates, a closed population and a known distribution of AOO. The first estimation of the AOO of dementia in the context of an illness–death model was performed by Brinks et al. (2013b).

This chapter is organised as follows: first, statistical methods that allow for an estimation of the AOO at different calendar times are introduced based on the approach of Brinks et al. (2013b). This involves a description of the underlying illness–death model, which can be seen as an easy way to describe analytical relationships between prevalence, incidence and mortality. Based on the illness–death model, mathematical formulas for the calculation of the AOO are then developed, which are used to analyse epidemiological data on dementia from Germany, India and the USA. The chapter concludes with a summary and a discussion of the findings.

13.2 Methods

13.2.1 Illness–Death Model

Based on a state (or, equivalently, compartmental) model, it is possible to derive statistical distributions of AOO from incidence rates. With an approach recently introduced in Brinks et al. (2013a) and Brinks and Landwehr (2014, 2015),

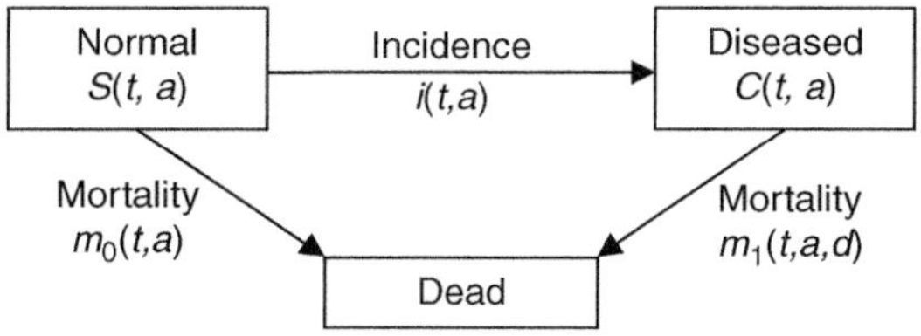

Fig. 13.2 Illness–death model consisting of the three states with the numbers of healthy [$S(t,a)$] and diseased individuals [$C(t,a)$] and incidence, mortality and remission rates, which may depend on up to three timescales

cross-sectional data and information on mortality rates of chronic diseases are sufficient to obtain incidence rates and, hence, their distributions of the AOO.

First, we outline the general form of the model we considered. It consists of the three states *Normal*, *Diseased* and *Dead*, and the numbers of individuals in these states are given as S (susceptibles), C (cases) and D (dead), respectively. We note that the three states should always be understood in terms of a specific disease. This means that, for example, individuals in the *Normal* state are regarded as non-diseased with respect to the disease under consideration and, hence, the compartments are regarded as disjointed in this respect. The model is complemented by the rates that represent the possible transitions between *Normal*, *Diseased* and *Dead*. More precisely, the incidence rate i describes the intensity of the movement of healthy individuals to the *Diseased* state, and the mortality rates m_0 and m_1 the transitions towards the *Dead* state for non-diseased and diseased persons, respectively. In general, all of the rates involved may depend on calendar time t, on the individuals' age a and, for the mortality m_1, also on the disease duration d. This situation is summarised in Fig. 13.2.

In the case of dementia, epidemiological research has empirically shown that the prevalence and the incidence rates do not show calendar time trends. As already mentioned in Sect. 13.1, quite a few references over a large period of time can be found that report age-specific incidence rates of dementia. Empirically, these incidence rates all show similar patterns. This gives us a reason to consider calendar time-independent incidence rates in our model. Even more, observed increasing incidence rates across years are in fact misleading. What we actually see are the effects of an ageing society in many developed countries. Increasing life expectancy and declining (or stable at the most) birth rates lead to declining percentages of the young and middle age groups in many European countries. In this respect, it is not surprising that mortality rates depend on the calendar time, which is the reason we confine ourselves to the time scales age (a) and calendar time (t). Further, in a recent analysis, we have shown that the duration of dementia only plays a minor role [see Example 3.1 in Brinks and Landwehr (2015)].

For a situation in which the rates in the illness–death model do not depend on time t and duration d, Murray and Lopez (1994) developed a two-dimensional system of linear ordinary differential equations (ODEs) of first order that use the rates i, m_0 and m_1 to describe the change in the numbers of S and C in healthy and diseased individuals of age *a*. The ODEs describe the in- and outgoing flows in the states *Normal* and *Diseased*. More specifically, healthy individuals may either contract the disease at rate *i* or die at rate m_0 without ever having contracted the disease. Recently, Brinks et al. (2013a) transformed the ODE system in Murray and Lopez (1994) into a one-dimensional scalar ODE by employing the disease prevalence instead of the total numbers of healthy and diseased individuals. In Brinks and Landwehr (2014, 2015), this approach has been generalised to include all transition rates and all possible time scales, calendar time *t*, age *a* and duration *d*. Besides our approach based on the analytic tool of an ODE, stochastic approaches via Markov models have been introduced in the context of illness–death models applied to dementia (Kapetanakis et al. 2013; Touraine et al. 2016; Rouanet et al. 2016).

As a result of this transformation, we obtain the partial differential equation (Eq. 13.1), which relates the temporal change of the age-specific prevalence $p = C/(S + C)$ to the incidence *i*, mortality (*m*) of the general population—often available from official statistics or lifetables—and the relative mortality $R = m_1/m_0$.

$$\left(\frac{\partial}{\partial t}+\frac{\partial}{\partial a}\right)p=(1-p)\times\left(i-m\frac{p(R-1)}{1+p(R-1)}\right) \tag{13.1}$$

To solve Eq. (13.1), the partial differential equation is transformed into an ODE of Abelian type for which there is only a numerical solution available. The numerical solution can be obtained using the classical Runge-Kutta method, a standard method in numerical analysis. In the special case of non-differential mortality (i.e. $m_1 = m_0$), the partial differential equation has an exact analytical solution (Keiding 1991). Working with the general mortality (*m*) and the relative mortality (*R*) instead of the mortality rates m_1 and m_0 from the illness–death model is advantageous because these numbers are more accessible from epidemiological surveys. Instead of looking for information on age-specific rates of mortality of healthy (m_0) and diseased persons (m_1), it is often easier to obtain age-specific mortality for the entire population—not distinguishing between diseased and non-diseased individuals. Moreover, for many diseases, relative mortality risk *R* is reported in epidemiological studies rather than the two involved rates separately. It turns out that the fraction on the right-hand side of Eq. (13.1) is the population attributable risk (PAR), which in our case indicates the proportion of deaths in a population attributable to dementia. The general definition of the PAR of this well-known epidemiological measure can be found in, for example, Campbell et al. (2007). Equation (13.1) provides an exact and analytical tool to estimate either unknown incidence or prevalence while knowing the other relevant quantities. In particular, using prevalences from cross-sectional data and mortality risks *R* and *m* from epidemiological studies and vital statistics, respectively, Eq. (13.1) provides a way to estimate incidence for which otherwise lengthy and costly follow-up studies would be needed. This is advantageous, especially in low-cost settings (Brinks et al. 2016). The problem of estimating the incidence rates from cross-sectional data has been known since 1934 (Muench 1934). In Landwehr and Brinks (2016), the performance of this prevalence-based incidence estimation technique has been compared with alternative methods that have been known for decades.

13.2.2 Age of Onset (AOO) of a Chronic Disease

Using the definitions of the quantities in the illness–death model (Fig. 13.2), in particular the age-specific incidence i and the prevalence p of the disease, as well as the absolute age-specific numbers of the susceptible and diseased individuals, explicit formulas can be written for the expected age of disease onset. For an arbitrary point in time, t_0, we define a small positive time interval δ from t_0 to $t_0 + \delta$. This leads to an approximation of the number of newly diseased individuals aged a using the following expression:

$$i(t_0,a)S(t_0,a)\delta = i(t_0,a)(1-p(t_0,a))N(t_0,a)\delta \tag{13.2}$$

The quantity $N(t_0,a)$ is the number of people in the general population aged a at time t_0. Since these are either diseased with probability p—which is the prevalence or proportion of diseased persons—or non-diseased with probability $1 - p$, the quantity $(1 - p(t_0,a))N(t_0,a)$ is equal to the number of non-diseased individuals $S(t_0,a)$ aged a at time t_0, which yields Eq. (13.2). The idea behind the replacement of S by N and the prevalence p is the accessibility of data. Prevalence data are often easily available from cross-sectional studies; the number N of people in the general population is accessible from population statistics or census data.

Equation (13.2) is an essential equation, since it allows computation of the number of newly diseased persons across all ages by applying the mathematical tool of integration with respect to age a. From a stochastic viewpoint, we may regard the AOO of a chronic disease at calendar time t_0 as a random variable, the probability density function f_{AOO} of which is constructed with the help of Eq. (13.2). It has the form $f_{\text{AOO}}(t_0,a) = \alpha(t_0)i(t_0,a)(1 - p(t_0,a))N(t_0,a)$, where $\alpha(t_0)$ is a normalising constant given as follows:

$$\alpha(t_0) = \frac{1}{\int_0^\infty i(t_0,a)(1-p(t_0,a))N(t_0,a)\ da}$$

The number $N(t_0,a)$ of people in the general population aged a at time t_0 can be expressed by the (relative) age distribution f_{POP} of the general population, $f_{\text{POP}}(t_0,a) = N(t_0,a)/N_{\text{total}}(t_0)$, where $N_{\text{total}}(t_0)$ is the overall number of people in the general population at time t_0. Combining these quantities yields the following expression for the probability density of the AOO:

$$f_{\text{AOO}}(t_0,a) = \frac{i(t_0,a)\left(1-p(t_0,a)\right) f_{\text{POP}}(t_0,a)}{\int_0^\infty i(t_0,a)\left(1-p(t_0,a)\right) f_{\text{POP}}(t_0,a)\,\mathrm{d}a} \tag{13.3}$$

It is well-known from random variable theory that once the probability density function is known, important statistical quantities such as mean, median, variance, percentiles and so on follow immediately. For example, integrating the density function in Eq. (13.3) across all ages and weighting it with age a gives an explicit expression for the mean AOO at t_0:

$$\overline{\text{AOO}}(t_0) = \frac{\int_0^\infty a\,i(t_0,a)\left(1-p(t_0,a)\right) f_{\text{POP}}(t_0,a)\,\mathrm{d}a}{\int_0^\infty i(t_0,a)\left(1-p(t_0,a)\right) f_{\text{POP}}(t_0,a)\,\mathrm{d}a}$$

Due to the explicit Eq. (13.3) for the density function f_{AOO}, it is possible to obtain percentiles of the distribution of the AOO in a very straightforward way. For instance, the 25th percentile of this distribution, the first quartile, is the age at which the area under the density function in Eq. (13.3) covers 25% of the entire area under a density curve. Here we use Eq. (13.3) to calculate quartiles, mean and median. For more details on the involved equations, the reader is referred to Brinks et al. (2013b).

13.2.3 Age Distributions

For the application of this method to dementia data, we need—besides prevalence and incidence—the age distribution of the considered population. For example, in Germany, the Federal Statistical Office holds information on vital statistics and provides publicly available data on the age distribution. In addition, they (Federal Statistical Office of Germany 2015) provide forecasts of the development of population numbers under various assumptions on birth rates, migration rates and life expectancies.

We aim to compare the AOO of dementia in Germany with India and the USA. These countries were chosen as examples of highly populated countries on three continents. In order to apply Eq. (13.3), the age distributions of these countries are also necessary. It is shown that the selected countries vary in their gender-specific age distributions. For India and the USA, the age distributions

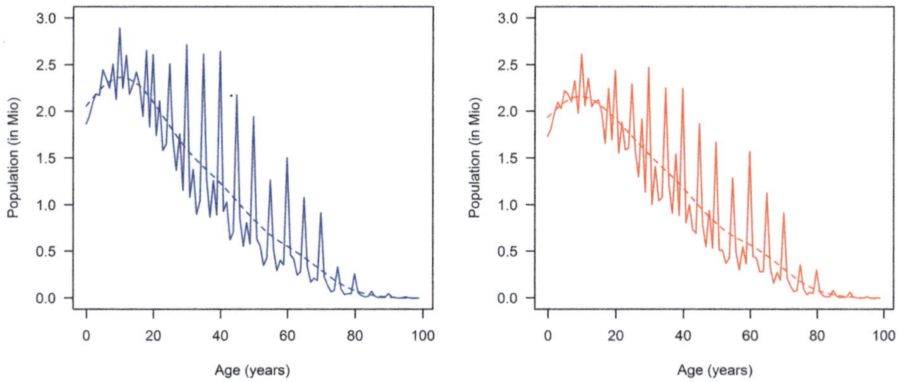

Fig. 13.3 Empirical age distribution of men (left) and women (right) in India according to the 2011 census. The solid lines show the surveyed values from the census. The modelled age distributions are shown as dashed lines

are easily accessible via the internet (U.S. Census Bureau 2014; Office of the Registrar General and Census Commissioner India 2011). However, the Indian data reveal a problem: many people in India give their age rounded up to a number divisible by five or ten, which leads to peaks in the empirically surveyed age distribution (see solid lines in Fig. 13.3). To obtain an age distribution without these possibly artificial effects, we used a spline to smooth out the peaks (Green and Silverman 1994). The results of this smoothing step are shown as dashed lines in Fig. 13.3.

13.2.4 Rates for the Illness–Death Model

Based on the empirical finding that within the group of men and women in virtually all countries the age-specific prevalence (p) and incidence rate (i) are approximately the same (see Sect. 13.1), we use the data from Germany (Ziegler and Doblhammer 2009) to make the cross-country comparisons of AOO via Eq. (13.3). However, it is likely that due to medical progress the future prevalence of dementia will increase for nearly all age groups. For instance, medical progress is likely to reduce the future mortality of diseased persons. This may happen, for example, by improved care and medication for the diseased or by reducing the risk of subsequent complications of dementia. Thus, the prevalence of dementia will probably increase (Brinks and Landwehr 2014). To calculate the increase in the prevalence, we solve the partial differential equation (Eq. 13.1) for the age-specific prevalence p up to the year 2040, as in Brinks and Landwehr (2014). Under the assumption that the age-specific relative mortality (R) in Eq. (13.1) does not change during this period, the expected decrease of the general mortality (m) will lead to an increasing prevalence as described in detail in Brinks and Landwehr (2014).

13.3 Results

13.3.1 Estimated AOO of Dementia in Three Countries

Figure 13.4 shows the relative age distributions (f_{POP}) for men (top row of Fig. 13.4) and women (bottom row) in Germany, India and the USA during the period between 2011 and 2015.

Within each country, the relative distributions of men and women have a similar shape. Compared to the other two countries, Germany has the lowest percentage of people aged below 20 years, and India the highest. While Germany has a maximum in the relative age distribution at the age of about 50 years, India's maximum is at an age of about 10 years. In the age range 10–100 years, the relative age distribution in India is decreasing—roughly speaking—nearly linearly. In the USA, the relative age distribution is relatively flat in the age range 0–60 years and decreases in the age range 60–100 years.

The differences in the relative age distributions shown in Fig. 13.4 lead to different distributions of the AOO of dementia in the three countries according to Eq. (13.3). The results are shown in Fig. 13.5, where the first, second (median) and third quartiles (i.e. the 25th, 50th and 75th percentiles) of the AOO of dementia for men and women in the three countries in the associated years are depicted as horizontal bars. The quartiles of the AOO of dementia for men and women in the three countries are also given in Table 13.1.

In each of the three countries, the median AOO of dementia is higher in women than in men. The same holds true for the other two quartiles. The effects of the higher incidence of dementia in women, when compared with men, seem to outperform the effect of the higher prevalence (p) in women (which leads to a lower factor $1 - p$) in each of the countries [see Eq. (13.3)]. The differences between the countries are more interesting. Within each sex stratum, the differences between the three countries shown in Fig. 13.5 are an effect of the differences of the age distributions shown in Fig. 13.4.

Note that within each sex stratum, we have assumed that the age-specific prevalences (p) and incidence rates (i) are the same in all three countries. Thus, differences between the distributions of AOO in Eq. (13.3) can only be due to differences in the age distribution f_{POP} of the different countries.

13.3.2 Differences in AOO of Dementia Over Time

As the age distributions change over time, the AOO will change according to Eq. (13.3). The effect of the changing age distribution is examined for Germany over the period from year 2000 to 2040. Figure 13.6 shows the age distributions of the male and female population in Germany in the years 2000 (solid line) and 2040 (dashed) according to the official population projection of the Federal Statistical Office of Germany. One can easily see how the maximum age distribution in 2000 at the age of about 40 years in men and women becomes the peak at about 80 years of age in

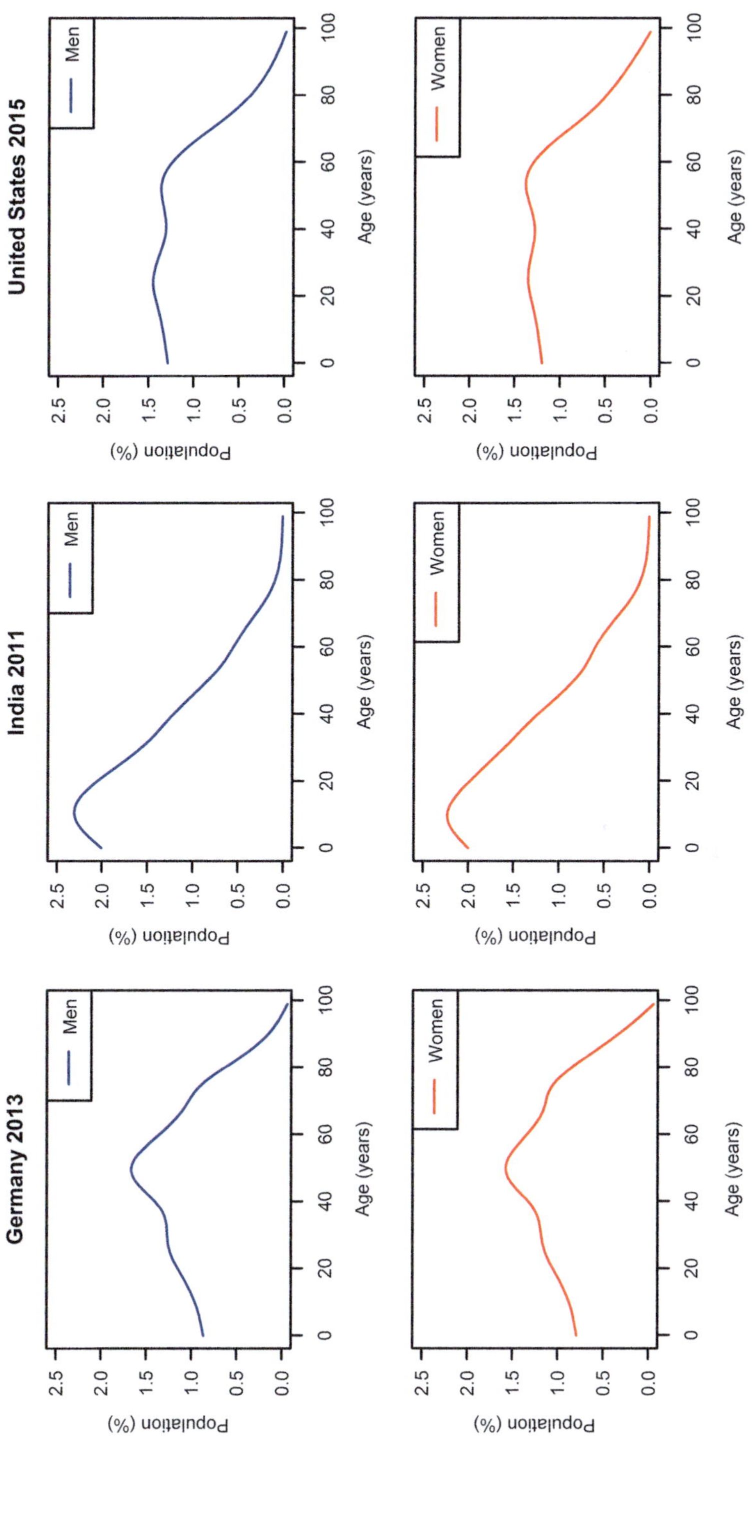

Fig. 13.4 Relative age distributions for men (top row) and women (bottom row) in Germany (left), India (middle) and the USA (right) in three years between 2011 and 2015

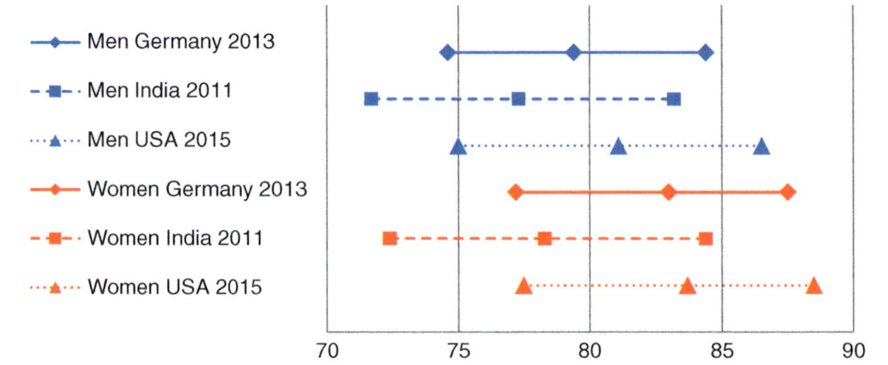

Fig. 13.5 First quartile, median and third quartile of the age of onset of dementia for men and women in Germany, India and the USA

Table 13.1 Quartiles of age of onset for men and women in Germany, India and the USA

		AOO (years)	
	Country, year	Median	First and third quartile
Men	Germany, 2013	79.4	74.6–84.4
	India, 2011	77.3	71.9–83.2
	USA, 2015	81.1	75.0–86.5
Women	Germany, 2013	83.0	77.2–87.5
	India, 2011	78.3	72.4–84.4
	USA, 2015	83.7	77.5–88.5

AAO age of onset

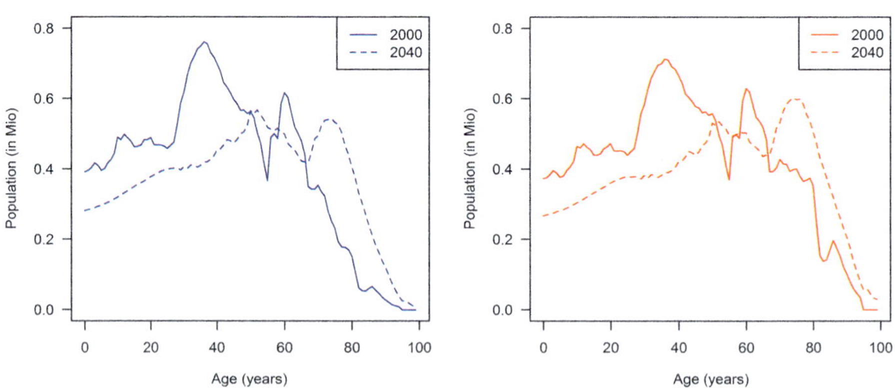

Fig. 13.6 Age distributions of men (left) and women (right) in Germany in the years 2000 (solid line) and 2040 (dashed line)

2040. Obviously, we can observe that there will be a substantial change in the age distribution over the considered period. To examine the question of how the change in age distribution over time affects the AOO of dementia, Fig. 13.7 shows the mean AOO over time for men and women according to Eq. (13.3) under the assumption that the age-specific prevalence and incidence do not alter with calendar time. While

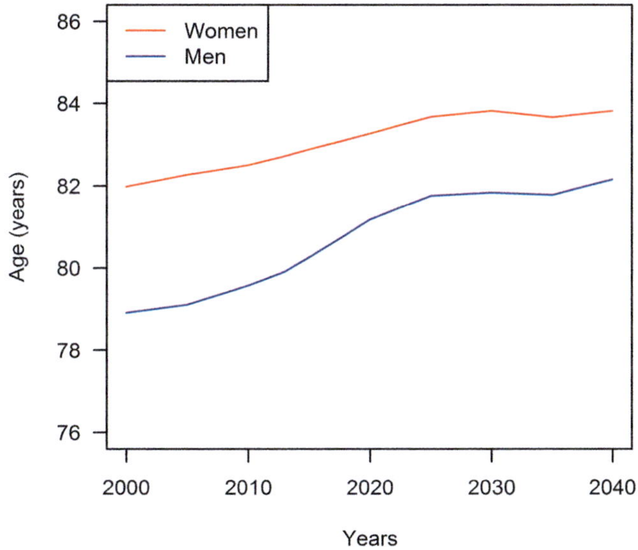

Fig. 13.7 Mean age of onset of dementia in Germany for men (blue) and women (red) over calendar time

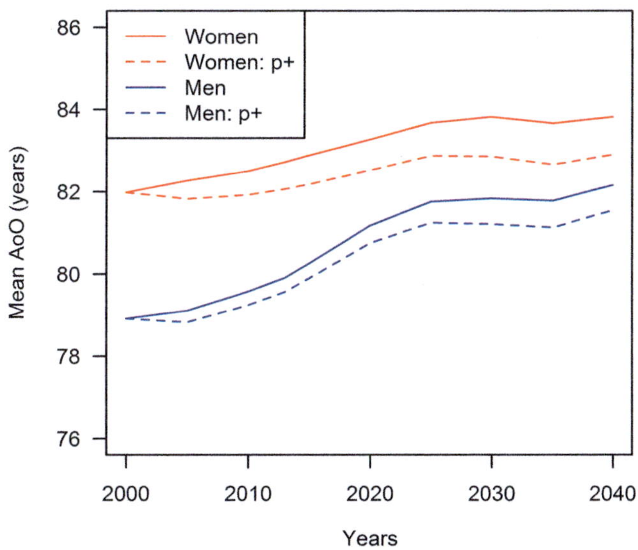

Fig. 13.8 Increasing mean age of onset of dementia over time. The solid lines show the age of onset under the assumption that there is no temporal change in the age-specific prevalence and incidence rate. The dashed lines show the more likely assumption of increasing prevalence (scenarios *p*+)

the mean AOO of dementia in the year 2000 is 78.9 and 82.2 years for men and women, respectively, in the year 2040 the mean AOO increases to 82.2 and 83.8 years in men and women, respectively.

So far, all of the results shown in this section are based on the assumption that for men and women the age-specific prevalence (p) and incidence rate (i) do not change with calendar time. It has been assumed that prevalence and incidence remain the same as shown in Fig. 13.1. However, this assumption is unlikely to be correct. In fact, it is more likely that the age-specific prevalence will increase over calendar time (Brinks and Landwehr 2014). If the prevalence is rising, the AOO of dementia will decrease according to Eq. (13.3). The effect on the AOO is shown as dashed lines in Fig. 13.8 in comparison to the scenarios without an increase of the prevalence (solid lines in Fig. 13.8). Instead of the mean AOO increasing to 82.2 and 83.8 years in 2040 in men and women, respectively, in the scenario with increasing prevalence the mean AOO increases only to 81.6 and 82.9 years in 2040, respectively.

13.4 Discussion

Based on the empirical observation that within the male and female sex the age-specific prevalence and incidence rate of dementia are approximately the same for all regions of the world (see Fig. 13.1), we have estimated the AOO of dementia in three countries from three different continents. For this, we have introduced the terminology of the illness–death model of a chronic disease. The illness–death model is a state model with the associated transition rates (incidence and mortality) between the states (see Fig. 13.2). The transition rates depend on several time scales (age a, calendar time t and duration d). The terminology of the illness–death model allows a straightforward derivation of the probability density of the AOO of a chronic disease [Eq. (13.3)]. Given the age-specific prevalence (p), the incidence rate (i) and the age distribution of the considered country (f_{POP}), the AOO can be calculated analytically. In this case, no epidemiological surveys of the AOO are necessary. Applied to dementia in the three countries, the distributions of the AOO are relatively stable. Men, on average, have a lower AOO of dementia than women (about 2–3 years). The median AOO ranges from about 77 to roughly 83 years of age in the three countries considered. The differences in the AOO between the countries stem from differences in the age distributions in these countries only.

If the age distribution of a country is changing over time, the AOO will change according to the analytical expression in Eq. (13.3). This effect has been demonstrated using data from Germany, where over a period of 40 years the AOO of dementia is increasing by approximately 3.2 and 1.8 years in men and women, respectively.

As mentioned in Sect. 13.1, the concept of the AOO of a chronic disease has been suggested as an alternative measure for disease frequency (Boshuizen and Greenland 1997). This measure was argued to be especially suitable and informative in chronic diseases with a high background risk where ratios of incidence rates cannot be interpreted as risk ratios. With a view to dementia and its high prevalence in older ages, there seems to be a high background risk in both men and women. However, it is not clear to us how much more informative the on average 2–3 years earlier onset of dementia in men than in women is than the age-specific incidence rate for men and women. The opposite seems to be the case: the lower AOO of dementia in men indicates a more frequent occurrence of dementia in men than in women. Regarding Fig. 13.1, this conflicts with the impression given by established epidemiological measures such as the prevalence and incidence. Thus, we would clearly advocate against the use of AOO as an alternative measure for the frequency of a chronic disease.

The cross-country comparisons and the effect of a temporal change of the age distribution on the AOO were based on the empirical observation that within the group of men and women the age-specific prevalence and incidence rate of dementia do not alter with time. Due to future medical progress, such as better care and treatment for the diseased, the future prevalence of dementia is likely to increase. We have shown in Fig. 13.8 that the AOO of dementia will decrease as a consequence of the increasing prevalence. Again, the mechanism of this somewhat paradoxical behaviour (higher prevalence leads to lower AOO) can be explained by Eq. (13.3). Apart from the age distribution f_{POP} of the underlying population, the quantities involved in Eq. (13.3) are related to the illness–death model (Fig. 13.2). Hence, we can say that the distribution of the AOO is tightly connected to the illness–death model and the associated transition rates.

Conclusion

In this chapter, we have demonstrated that the AOO depends on the age distribution in the sample population. Despite this, the AOO of the dementias is relatively stable across different regions. Generally, men are affected earlier than women. In addition, we have shown that AOO of a chronic disease is closely connected to the illness–death model of epidemiology. As the age-specific incidence rate of a chronic disease is more comprehensive and informative than a single epidemiological measure such as the AOO, this should, if possible, be subject to epidemiological surveys. The AOO can then be estimated using Eq. (13.3).

References

Bickel H. Demenzsyndrom und Alzheimer Krankheit. Eine Schätzung des Krankenbestandes und der jährlichen Neuerkrankungen in Deutschland [Dementia syndrome and Alzheimer disease: an assessment of morbidity and annual incidence in Germany]. Gesundheitswesen. 2000;62:211–8. https://doi.org/10.1055/s-2000-10858.

Bickel H. Stand der Epidemiologie. In: Hallauer J, Kurz A, editors. Weißbuch Demenz. Versorgungssituation relevanter Demenzerkrankungen in Deutschland. Stuttgart: Georg Thieme; 2002. p. 10–4.

Boshuizen HC, Greenland S. Average age at first occurrence as an alternative occurrence parameter in epidemiology. Int J Epidemiol. 1997;26:867–72.

Brinks R, Landwehr S. Age- and time-dependent model of the prevalence of non-communicable diseases and application to dementia in Germany. Theor Popul Biol. 2014;92:62–8. https://doi.org/10.1016/j.tpb.2013.11.006.

Brinks R, Landwehr S. A new relation between prevalence and incidence of a chronic disease. Math Med Biol. 2015;32:425–35. https://doi.org/10.1093/imammb/dqu024.

Brinks R, Landwehr S, Icks A, Koch M, Giani G. Deriving age-specific incidence from prevalence with an ordinary differential equation. Stat Med. 2013a;32:2070–8. https://doi.org/10.1002/sim.5651.

Brinks R, Landwehr S, Waldeyer R. Age of onset in chronic diseases: new method and application to dementia in Germany. Popul Health Metr. 2013b;11:6. https://doi.org/10.1186/1478-7954-11-6.

Brinks R, Hoyer A, Landwehr S. Surveillance of the incidence of non-communicable diseases (NCDs) with sparse resources: a simulation study using data from a National Diabetes Registry, Denmark, 1995–2004. PLoS One. 2016;11:e0152046. https://doi.org/10.1371/journal.pone.

Bruvik FK, Ulstein ID, Ranhoff AH, Engedal K. The quality of life of people with dementia and their family carers. Dement Geriatr Cogn Disord. 2012;34:7–14. https://doi.org/10.1159/000341584.
Campbell M, Machin D, Walters SJ. Medical statistics. 4th ed. Hoboken: Wiley; 2007.
Federal Statistical Office of Germany. Bevölkerung Deutschlands bis 2060. 13. koordinierte Bevölkerungsvorausberechnung [Population of Germany up to 2060]. 2015. https://www.destatis.de/DE/ZahlenFakten/GesellschaftStaat/Bevoelkerung/Bevoelkerungsvorausberechnung/Bevoelkerungsvorausberechnung.html. Accessed 23 June 2017.
Fratiglioni L, Rocca WA. Epidemiology of dementia. In: Boller CS, editor. Handbook of neuropsychology, vol. 2. Amsterdam: Elsevier; 2001. p. 193–215.
Fratiglioni L, Launer LJ, Andersen K, Breteler MM, Copeland JR, Dartigues JF, et al. Incidence of dementia and major subtypes in Europe: a collaborative study of population based cohorts. Neurologic Diseases in the Elderly Research Group. Neurology. 2000;54(Suppl 5):10–5.
Gao S, Hendrie HC, Hall KS, Hui S. The relationships between age, sex, and the incidence of dementia and Alzheimer disease: a meta-analysis. Arch Gen Psychiatry. 1998;55:809–15.
GBD 2015 DALYs, HALE Collaborators. Global, regional, and national disability-adjusted life-years (DALYs) for 315 diseases and injuries and healthy life expectancy (HALE), 1990–2015: a systematic analysis for the Global Burden of Disease Study 2015. Lancet. 2016;388:1603–58. https://doi.org/10.1016/S0140-6736(16)31460-X.
Green PJ, Silverman BW. Nonparametric regression and generalized linear models: a roughness penalty approach. London: Chapman & Hall; 1994.
Hendrie HC. Epidemiology of dementia and Alzheimer's disease. Am J Geriatr Psychiatry. 1998;6(Suppl 1):S3–S18.
Hofman A, Rocca WA, Brayne C, Breteler MM, Clarke M, Cooper B, et al. The prevalence of dementia in Europe: a collaborative study of 1980–1990 findings. Eurodem Prevalence Research Group. Int J Epidemiol. 1991;20:736–48.
Jorm AF, Jolley D. The incidence of dementia: a meta-analysis. Neurology. 1998;51:728–33.
Jorm AF, Korten AE, Henderson AS. The prevalence of dementia: a quantitative integration of the literature. Acta Psychiatr Scand. 1987;76:465–79.
Kapetanakis V, Matthews FE, van den Hout A. A semi-Markov model for stroke with piecewise-constant hazards in the presence of left, right and interval censoring. Stat Med. 2013;32:697–713.
Keiding N. Age-specific incidence and prevalence: a statistical perspective. J R Stat Soc A. 1991;154:371–412.
Keiding N, Holst C, Green A. Retrospective estimation of diabetes incidence from information in a prevalent population and historical mortality. Am J Epidemiol. 1989;130:588–600.
Keiding N, Hansen BE, Holst C. Non-parametric estimation of disease incidence from a cross-sectional sample of a stationary population. In: Gabriel JP, Lefèvre C, Picard P, editors. Stochastic processes in epidemic theory. Lecture notes in biomathematics, vol. 86. Heidelberg: Springer; 1990. p. 36–45.
Kukull WA, Higdon R, Bowen JD, McCormick WC, Teri L, Schellenberg GD, et al. Dementia and Alzheimer disease incidence: a prospective cohort study. Arch Neurol. 2002;59:1737–46.
Landwehr S, Brinks R. A comparative study of prevalence-based incidence estimation techniques with application to dementia data in Germany. Stat Med. 2016;35:768–81. https://doi.org/10.1002/sim.6736.
Launer LJ, Andersen K, Dewey ME, Letenneur L, Ott A, Amaducci LA, et al. Rates and risk factors for dementia and Alzheimer's disease: results from EURODEM pooled analyses. EURODEM Incidence Research Group and Work Groups European Studies of Dementia. Neurology. 1999;52:78–84.
Lobo A, Launer LJ, Fratiglioni L, Andersen K, Di Carlo A, Breteler MM, et al. Prevalence of dementia and major subtypes in Europe: a collaborative study of population-based cohorts. Neurology. 2000;54(Suppl 5):S4–9.
Lopes MA, Bottino CM. Prevaléncia de deméncia em diversas Regioes do mundo. Análise dos estudos epidemiolágicos de 1994 a 2000 [Prevalence of dementia in several regions of the world: analysis of epidemiologic studies from 1994 to 2000]. Arq Neuropsiquiatr. 2002;60:61–9.

Muench H. Derivation of rates from summation data by the catalytic curve. J Am Stat Assoc. 1934;29:25–38.
Murray CJL, Lopez AD. Quantifying disability: data, methods and results. Bull World Health Organ. 1994;72:481–94.
Office of the Registrar General and Census Commissioner, India. Series C, C-13 Single year age returns by residence and sex. 2011. http://www.censusindia.gov.in/2011census/C-series/c-13/DDW-0000C-13SC.xls. Accessed 23 June 2017.
Plassmann BL, Langa KM, Fisher GG, Heeringa SG, Weir DR, Ofstedal MB, et al. Prevalence of dementia in the United States: the aging, demographics, and memory study. Neuroepidemiology. 2007;29:125–32. https://doi.org/10.1159/000109998.
Qiu C, Kivipelto M, von Strauss E. Epidemiology of Alzheimer's disease: occurrence, determinants, and strategies toward intervention. Dialogues Clin Neurosci. 2009;11:111–28.
Ritchie K, Kildea D. Is senile dementia "age-related" or "ageing related"? Evidence from meta-analysis of dementia prevalence in the oldest old. Lancet. 1995;346:931–4.
Ritchie K, Kildea D, Robine JM. The relationship between age and the prevalence of senile dementia: a meta-analysis of recent data. Int J Epidemiol. 1992;21:763–9.
Rouanet A, Joly P, Dartigues JF, Proust-Lima C, Jacqmin-Gadda H. Joint latent class model for longitudinal data and interval-censored semi-competing events: application to dementia. Biometrics. 2016;72:1123–35.
Scazufca M, Menezes PR, Vallada HP, Crepaldi AL, Pastor-Valero M, Coutinho LM, et al. High prevalence of dementia among older adults from poor socioeconomic backgrounds in São Paulo, Brazil. Int Psychogeriatr. 2008;20:394–405.
The Canadian Study of Health and Aging Working Group. The incidence of dementia in Canada. Neurology. 2000;55:66–73.
Touraine C, Helmer C, Joly P. Predictions in an illness-death model. Stat Methods Med Res. 2016;25:1452–70.
U.S. Census Bureau, Population Division. National population projections - projected population by single year of age, sex, race, and Hispanic origin for the United States: 2014 to 2060. 2014. https://www.census.gov/programs-surveys/popproj.html. Accessed 23 June 2017.
Weyerer S. Altersdemenz. Bundesberichtserstattung des Bundes. Berlin: Robert Koch Institut; 2005. p. 28.
World Health Organization. World Health Report 2001. Mental health: new understanding, new hope. Geneva: World Health Organization; 2001.
World Health Organization and Alzheimer's Disease International. Dementia: a public health priority. 2012. http://www.who.int/mental_health/publications/dementia_report_2012/en/. Accessed 23 June 2017.
Zhang ZX, Zahner GE, Roman GC, Liu J, Hong Z, Qu QM, et al. Dementia subtypes in China: prevalence in Beijing, Xian, Shanghai, and Chengdu. Arch Neurol. 2005;62:447–53.
Ziegler U, Doblhammer G. Prävalenz und Inzidenz von Demenz in Deutschland [Prevalence and incidence of dementia in Germany]. Gesundheitswesen. 2009;71:281–90. https://doi.org/10.1055/s-0028-1119384.

14 Conclusions: From the Study of the Age of Onset to the Development of Age-Specific Interventions in Mental Health

Patrick D. McGorry, Norman Sartorius, and Giovanni de Girolamo

14.1 Overview and Implications of Age of Onset

Age of onset (AOO) provides the fundamental basis for understanding the epidemiology of mental disorders and developing targeted intervention and preventive strategies (Kessler et al. 2007). The compilation of chapters in this book provides a blueprint to guide such strategies through the comprehensive examination of AOO for the most relevant mental disorders. Despite the limitations of the evidence-base reviewed (e.g. various definition of AOO), commonalities in AOO were observed across most mental disorders. The majority of disorders emerged between childhood and young adulthood (e.g. schizophrenia, ADHD, bipolar, anxiety, alcohol use and eating disorders), although a broader AOO period extending well into adulthood was also observed, with the exception of the dementias, which are relatively contained within the later adult years and old age. It is also important to acknowledge other onset periods during adulthood that include the post-natal period (Munk-Olsen et al. 2006), menopause (Freeman et al. 2004) and midlife stages (Lang et al. 2011).

Although AOO is dispersed over the lifespan with early and late onset disorders possible, incidence rates for most mental disorders peak between adolescence and young adulthood, coinciding with the transition to adulthood when young people are

P. D. McGorry (✉)
Orygen The National Centre of Excellence in Youth Mental Health and Centre for Youth Mental Health, University of Melbourne, Parkville, VIC, Australia
e-mail: Pat.mcgorry@orygen.org.au

N. Sartorius
Association for the Improvement of Mental Health Programmes (AMH), Geneva, Switzerland
e-mail: sartorius@normansartorius.com

G. de Girolamo
Unit of Psychiatric Epidemiology and Evaluation, IRCCS St John of God Clinical Research Centre, Brescia, Italy
e-mail: gdegirolamo@fatebenefratelli.it

G. de Girolamo et al. (eds.), *Age of Onset of Mental Disorders*,
https://doi.org/10.1007/978-3-319-72619-9_14

on the verge of independence and about to embark upon their most fruitful years of productivity. It is also a time when mental disorders impose their greatest burden of impact (Gore et al. 2011), which can persist and accumulate through later adulthood, significantly impacting on employment and economic productivity (Gibb et al. 2010). While some features of mental disorders, such as self-harm, may resolve by the late 20s (Patton et al. 2014), a substantial proportion manifest chronicity or recurrence, and delayed treatment, undertreatment or lack of treatment can lead to poorer outcomes. Indeed delayed treatment is a risk factor for reduced response to treatment (Altamura et al. 2010; Perkins et al. 2005). Conversely, effective treatment during the early stages of illness can result in more favourable short- and long-term outcomes (Berk et al. 2011; Fusar-Poli et al. 2017; Hegelstad et al. 2012).

Ultimately, studying AOO aims to inform service development and clinical practice and guide research examining the epidemiology, treatment and prevention of mental disorders. A key value of the AOO approach is that it can identify critical windows for early intervention and preventive strategies, guiding the development and implementation of service models and evidence-based treatments that target individuals during high-risk developmental periods. Within this framework, age-specific and developmentally and culturally appropriate interventions and services, delivered in a timely manner, aim to prevent or delay the onset of mental disorders, reducing their significant burden at both an individual and societal level. In concluding this book, we discuss the implications of AOO on the management of mental disorders, particularly in regards to improving access and timing of interventions, and the prevention of mental disorders.

14.2 Access and Timing of Treatment

Despite most mental disorders emerging between adolescence and early adulthood, young people are the least likely age group to access treatment (Pottick et al. 2008). While stigma and individual beliefs can negatively influence young people's willingness to engage with mental health services (Rickwood et al. 2007), the design and scale of services available for this age group also form a barrier to accessing timely and appropriate care, which can be improved through better knowledge of AOO and its potential to select and organise appropriate sources of care. Firstly, primary health-care services typically focus on physical heath and especially cater for younger children and older adults, typically neglecting young people and their main health problem of mental ill health, and, secondly, stringent entry criteria into under-resourced and poorly designed specialist mental health services often disadvantage emerging adults with mental and substance use disorders. Traditional child and adolescent mental health service models with cut-offs at 16–18 years of age do not align with the epidemiological evidence demonstrating the tendency for mental disorders to develop or worsen during the transition from adolescence to adulthood. While only a minority gain entry to specialist care prior to the age of 18, failure to make the service transition between service cultures during this peak AOO period can result in the discontinuation of treatment during a critical period of development, with risky and often disastrous outcomes (McGorry 2007). Young people who require ongoing management and safe "scaffolding" are often faced with a lack of support in transitioning to adult services (Singh et al. 2010). Furthermore, those transitioning to an adult service culture, or attempting to make first contact as a young adult, can be locked out of services due to not meeting criteria for a serious (typically meaning "chronic") mental disorder (Lamb and Murphy 2013). Young people who are in the early stages of mental illness typically present with fluid, non-specific symptoms that do not meet diagnostic or severity criteria for entry into adult services, which are typically targeted towards a restricted subset of late-stage phenotypes or chronic mental disorders. Essentially, this means that young people with emerging distress, impairment, substance abuse, self-harm and/or suicidal behaviours are unable to access early, efficient and appropriate mental health care at a time most needed. This represents complete failure to grasp arguably the best preventive opportunity and best buy in the whole of health care.

To counter the misalignment between AOO of mental disorders and models of care, youth-friendly stigma-free services, including e-health, that span the most critical years of onset and the full spectrum of mental disorders have been established across a number of countries (Illback and Bates 2011; Oppetit et al. 2018; Iyer et al. 2015; McGorry et al. 2013, 2014b). This holistic youth service model is distinctly tailored to the unique developmental, psychosocial, biological and cultural needs of young people with emerging mental health needs. This enables appropriate and effective interventions to be delivered in a timely manner when the incidence and indeed prevalence of mental disorders are at its highest, increasing the treated incidence, eliminating the risk of discontinuing treatment during periods when care is most needed and effective and providing coordinated linkages with services for younger children and older adults, allowing optimal "soft" transitions in care across the lifespan as needed (McGorry et al. 2013). These services are also interwoven with community awareness campaigns (McGorry et al. 2014b), which have been shown to improve mental health literacy and reduce duration of untreated illness and barriers to help-seeking (Melle et al. 2004; Wright et al. 2006). To date, the evidence for early intervention and youth models of care has been compelling in demonstrating its cost-effectiveness, increased engagement and access and reduced rates of relapse and hospital admissions (Bird et al. 2010; Kessing et al. 2013; McGorry et al. 2009; Mihalopoulos et al. 2009; Stafford et al. 2013).

Although the distribution of AOO across the various age groups clearly indicates the need for increased investment in youth mental health services, this does not preclude similarly targeted early intervention services for younger children and older adults, which are also necessary for preventive efforts and ongoing management. This includes ADHD, anxiety and conduct disorder in younger children and in old age psychiatry, novel streams targeting early dementia and other mental health issues.

14.3 Prevention Strategies

AOO can also guide critical time points for pre-emptive measures that serve to prevent, or at least delay, the onset of mental disorders, reducing their impact and burden. In addition to targeting peak onset periods for mental disorders (i.e. childhood, adolescence and young adulthood) (McGorry 2011), prevention-based programmes targeting earlier developmental periods and key risk factors are required to prevent the emergence, or alter the trajectory, of mental illness (Ginsburg et al. 2015; Freedman et al. 2018). Although preventive measures for mental disorders spanning childhood and adolescence show promise, further research is needed to support their implementation (Lawrence et al. 2017; Le et al. 2017; Mendelson and Eaton 2018; Merry et al. 2011; Moreno-Peral et al. 2017). With regard to transition to first-episode psychosis, there are encouraging findings to suggest that conversion can be prevented or delayed following early intervention (Stafford et al. 2013; van der Gaag et al. 2013). While prevention of late onset disorders such as dementia and Alzheimer's remains elusive, modifiable risk factors and preclinical detection of Alzheimer's disease offer some hope in delaying or preventing their onset (Livingston et al. 2017).

Targeting modifiable risk factors that may have a cumulative effect is also critical for the prevention of other mental disorders where the onset is highest during the transition to adulthood. For example, seminal work from the Isle of Wight study revealed that the combination of two or more risk factors, rather than a single factor, increased the risk of a mental disorder (Rutter et al. 1975a, b). Thus, modifying any of these equivalent risk factors (e.g. marital discord, maternal mental illness, paternal criminality, bullying, overcrowding) may have a positive effect on altering risk for mental ill health and a range of outcomes. Risk factors typically connote risk for multiple syndromes and outcomes. For example, prevention and alleviation of childhood trauma, a common risk factor across various mental disorders, may further prevent the onset or lessen the severity of several mental disorders (de Graaf et al. 2002).

Further new opportunities for preventive and early intervention approaches, guided by the onset and trajectory of mental illness, are possible through the clinical staging approach (McGorry et al. 2006). Within this model, the various stages and potential progression of mental illness, ranging from asymptomatic to chronic illness, are described to guide diagnosis, management and prevention. The clinical staging model is particularly relevant to young people during high incidence periods for mental disorders due to its recognition of early-stage profiles often exhibited by this group (e.g. fluid, undifferentiated, non-specific microphenotypes). It also recognises that treatment approaches alter according to stage of illness, with asymptomatic and very early stages involving pre-emptive strategies that could be guided by neurobiological markers (McGorry et al. 2014a). Although clinical staging provides a useful heuristic framework to guide early intervention and prevention, further research is needed to determine its full potential in delivering timely, effective, safe and preventive strategies, particularly during high-risk onset periods.

Conclusions

The distribution of AOO across the lifespan, with its peak incidence and prevalence during the transition between adolescence and young adulthood, clearly indicates the need for prevention and early intervention programmes directed towards these and indeed later developmental life stages. Historical and current models of care for mental health have meant that young people with the greatest need of treatment are disadvantaged with services that are inaccessible, create discontinuity of care at critical periods and are inappropriate for their developmental, cultural, biological and psychosocial needs. While youth-specific stigma-free early intervention models have emerged, improving outcomes and reducing barriers to accessing care, additional efforts are needed to strengthen these services (McGorry et al. 2018) to promote equity of access and quality care for all young people across the full range of mental disorders and across the lifespan. Novel models of care such as these are underpinned, as in other areas of health care, by preventively oriented frameworks such as the clinical staging approach that strongly advocate the use of simple and safe interventions (e.g. mental health literacy, psychoeducation, exercise and problem solving) for at-risk groups and early-stage disorders. Widespread application of such interventions and youth-friendly early intervention models could significantly benefit those during at-risk periods and early-stage disorder. More sophisticated and dynamic approaches to health system design, guided by AOO, have the potential to further alleviate, and ultimately eliminate, much of the burden of mental disorders not only for young people but across all stages of the lifespan.

References

Altamura AC, Dell'Osso B, Berlin HA, et al. Duration of untreated illness and suicide in bipolar disorder: a naturalistic study. Eur Arch Psychiatry Clin Neurosci. 2010;260:385–91.

Berk M, Brnabic A, Dodd S, et al. Does stage of illness impact treatment response in bipolar disorder? Empirical treatment data and their implication for the staging model and early intervention. Bipolar Disord. 2011;13:87–98.

Bird V, Premkumar P, Kendall T, et al. Early intervention services, cognitive-behavioural therapy and family intervention in early psychosis: systematic review. Br J Psychiatry. 2010;197:350–6.

de Graaf R, Bijl RV, Smit F, et al. Risk factors for 12-month comorbidity of mood, anxiety, and substance use disorders: findings from the Netherlands Mental Health Survey and Incidence Study. Am J Psychiatry. 2002;159:620–9.

Freedman R, Hunter SK, Hoffman MC Prenatal primary prevention of mental illness by micronutrient supplements in pregnancy. Am J Psychiatry. (2018);21:appiajp201817070836. https://doi.org/10.1176/appi.ajp.2018.17070836. [Epub ahead of print] PubMed PMID: 29558816.

Freeman EW, Sammel MD, Liu L, et al. Hormones and menopausal status as predictors of depression in women in transition to menopause. Arch Gen Psychiatry. 2004;61:62–70.

Fusar-Poli P, McGorry PD, Kane JM. Improving outcomes of first-episode psychosis: an overview. World Psychiatry. 2017;16:251–65.

Gibb SJ, Fergusson DM, Horwood LJ. Burden of psychiatric disorder in young adulthood and life outcomes at age 30. Br J Psychiatry. 2010;197:122–7.

Ginsburg GS, Drake KL, Tein JY, et al. Preventing onset of anxiety disorders in offspring of anxious parents: a randomized controlled trial of a family-based intervention. Am J Psychiatry. 2015;172:1207–14.

Gore FM, Bloem PJ, Patton GC, et al. Global burden of disease in young people aged 10-24 years: a systematic analysis. Lancet. 2011;377(9783):2093–102.

Hegelstad WTV, Larsen TK, Auestad B, et al. Long-term follow-up of the TIPS early detection in psychosis study: effects on 10-year outcome. Am J Psychiatry. 2012;169:374–80.

Illback RJ, Bates T. Transforming youth mental health services and supports in Ireland. Early Interv Psychiatry. 2011;5(Suppl 1):S22–7.

Iyer SN, Boksa P, Lal S, et al. Transforming youth mental health: a Canadian perspective. Ir J Psychol Med. 2015;32:51–60.

Kessing LV, Hansen HV, Hvenegaard A, et al. Treatment in a specialised out-patient mood disorder clinic v. standard out-patient treatment in the early course of bipolar disorder: randomised clinical trial. Br J Psychiatry. 2013;202:212–9.

Kessler RC, Amminger GP, Aguilar-Gaxiola S, et al. Age of onset of mental disorders: a review of recent literature. Curr Opin Psychiatry. 2007;20:359–64.

Lamb C, Murphy M. The divide between child and adult mental health services: points for debate. Br J Psychiatry. 2013;202(Suppl 54):41–4.

Lang IA, Llewellyn DJ, Hubbard RE, et al. Income and the midlife peak in common mental disorder prevalence. Psychol Med. 2011;41:1365–72.

Lawrence PJ, Rooke SM, Creswell C. Prevention of anxiety among at-risk children and adolescents—a systematic review and meta-analysis. Child Adolesc Ment Health. 2017;22:118–30.

Le LKD, Barendregt JJ, Hay P, Mihalopoulos C. Prevention of eating disorders: a systematic review and meta-analysis. Clin Psychol Rev. 2017;53:46–58.

Livingston G, Sommerlad A, Orgeta V, et al. Dementia prevention, intervention, and care. Lancet. 2017;390(10113):2673–734.

McGorry PD. The specialist youth mental health model: strengthening the weakest link in the public mental health system. Med J Aust. 2007;187(Suppl 7):S53–6.

McGorry P. Transition to adulthood: the critical period for pre-emptive, disease-modifying care for schizophrenia and related disorders. Schizophr Bull. 2011;37:524–30.

McGorry PD, Hickie IB, Yung AR, et al. Clinical staging of psychiatric disorders: a heuristic framework for choosing earlier, safer and more effective interventions. Aust N Z J Psychiatry. 2006;40:616–22.

McGorry PD, Nelson B, Amminger GP, et al. Intervention in individuals at ultra-high risk for psychosis: a review and future directions. J Clin Psychiatry. 2009;70:1206–12.

McGorry P, Bates T, Birchwood M. Designing youth mental health services for the 21st century: examples from Australia, Ireland and the UK. Br J Psychiatry. 2013;202(Suppl 54):30–5.

McGorry P, Keshavan M, Goldstone S, et al. Biomarkers and clinical staging in psychiatry. World Psychiatry. 2014a;13:211–23.

McGorry PD, Goldstone SD, Parker AG, et al. Cultures for mental health care of young people: an Australian blueprint for reform. Lancet Psychiatry. 2014b;1:559–68.

McGorry PD, Ratheesh A, O'Donoghue B. Early intervention: an implementation challenge for 21st century mental health care. JAMA Psychiatry. 2018;75(6):545–6.

Melle I, Larsen TK, Haahr U, et al. Reducing the duration of untreated first-episode psychosis: effects on clinical presentation. Arch Gen Psychiatry. 2004;61:143–50.

Mendelson T, Eaton WW. Recent advances in the prevention of mental disorders. Soc Psychiatry Psychiatr Epidemiol. 2018;53:325–39.

Merry SN, Hetrick SE, Cox GR et al Psychological and educational interventions for preventing depression in children and adolescents. Cochrane Database Syst Rev. (2011); (12):CD003380.

Mihalopoulos C, Harris M, Henry L, et al. Is early intervention in psychosis cost-effective over the long term? Schizophr Bull. 2009;35:909–18.

Moreno-Peral P, Conejo-Cerón S, Rubio-Valera M, et al. Effectiveness of psychological and/or educational interventions in the prevention of anxiety: a systematic review, meta-analysis, and meta-regression. JAMA Psychiat. 2017;74:1021–9.

Munk-Olsen T, Laursen TM, Pedersen CB, et al. New parents and mental disorders: a population-based register study. JAMA. 2006;296:2582–9.
Oppetit A, Bourgin J, Martinez G, et al. The C'JAAD: a French team for early intervention in psychosis in Paris. Early Interv Psychiatry. 2018;12:243.
Patton GC, Coffey C, Romaniuk H, et al. The prognosis of common mental disorders in adolescents: a 14-year prospective cohort study. Lancet. 2014;383:1401–11.
Perkins DO, Gu H, Boteva K, Lieberman JA. Relationship between duration of untreated psychosis and outcome in first-episode schizophrenia: a critical review and meta-analysis. Am J Psychiatry. 2005;162:1785–804.
Pottick KJ, Bilder S, Vander Stoep A, et al. US patterns of mental health service utilization for transition-age youth and young adults. J Behav Health Serv Res. 2008;35:373–89.
Rickwood DJ, Deane FP, Wilson CJ. When and how do young people seek professional help for mental health problems? Med J Aust. 2007;187(Suppl 7):35–9.
Rutter M, Cox A, Tupling C, et al. Attainment and adjustment in two geographical areas. I. The prevalence of psychiatric disorder. Br J Psychiatry. 1975a;126:493–509.
Rutter M, Yule B, Quinton D, et al. Attainment and adjustment in two geographical areas. III. Some factors accounting for area differences. Br J Psychiatry. 1975b;126:520–33.
Singh SP, Paul M, Ford T, et al. Process, outcome and experience of transition from child to adult mental healthcare: multiperspective study. Br J Psychiatry. 2010;197:305–12.
Stafford MR, Jackson H, Mayo-Wilson E, et al. Early interventions to prevent psychosis: systematic review and meta-analysis. BMJ. 2013;346:f185.
van der Gaag M, Smit F, Bechdolf A, French P, Linszen DH, Yung AR, et al. Preventing a first episode of psychosis: meta-analysis of randomized controlled prevention trials of 12 month and longer-term follow-ups. Schizophr Res. 2013;149:56–62.
Wright A, McGorry PD, Harris MG, et al. Development and evaluation of a youth mental health community awareness campaign—The Compass Strategy. BMC Public Health. 2006;6:215. PubMed PMID: 16923195; PubMed Central PMCID: PMC1564138.

CPI Antony Rowe
Eastbourne, UK
September 20, 2019